Essential Readings in Case Management

Editor

Catherine M. Mullahy, RN, BS, CRRN, CCM
President
Options Unlimited
Huntington, New York

and

Aspen Reference Group

AN ASPEN PUBLICATION®
Aspen Publishers, Inc.
Gaithersburg, Maryland
1998

Library of Congress Cataloging-in-Publication Data

Essential readings in case management / editor Catherine Mullahy.—
2nd ed.
p.   cm.
A companion to: The case manager's handbook.
Includes bibliographical references and index.
ISBN 0-8342-1139-4 (pbk.)
1. Hospitals—Case management services—Handbooks, manuals, etc.
I. Mullahy, Catherine H.   II. Mullahy, Catherine H.   Case manager's
handbook.
RA975.5.C36E87
1998
362.1'1—dc21
98-14420
CIP

Orders: (800) 638-8437
Customer Service: (800) 234-1660

About Aspen Publishers • For more than 35 years, Aspen has been a leading professional publisher in a variety of disciplines. Aspen's vast information resources are available in both print and electronic formats. We are committed to providing the highest quality information available in the most appropriate format for our customers. Visit Aspen's Internet site for more information resources, directories, articles, and a searchable version of Aspen's full catalog, including the most recent publications: **http://www.aspenpub.com**
Aspen Publishers, Inc. • The hallmark of quality in publishing
Member of the worldwide Wolters Kluwer group.

Editorial Resources: Brian MacDonald
Library of Congress Catalog Card Number: 98-14420
ISBN: 0-8342-1139-4

Printed in the United States of America

1   2   3   4   5

Table of Contents

Contributors vii

Preface xiii

PART I   PROFILE OF A CASE MANAGER 1

    1—Nurse Case Manager Roles: Implications for Practice and
        Education 3
        Roberta M. Conti

    2—Redefining the Role of Clinical Nurse Specialists 15
        Julie N. Tackenberg and Anne M. Rausch

    3—Case Management as a Mindset 28
        Gloria G. Mayer

    4—Components of a Successful Case Management Program 39
        Sherry L. Aliotta

    5—Managed Care, Utilization Management, and Case Management
        in the Emergency Department 47
        Kelly S. Morgan

    6—The Johns Hopkins Hospital Launches Case Management Initiative 53
        Lawrence F. Strassner

    7—Case Management: Meeting the Needs of Chronically Ill Patients
        in an HMO 57
        Ronnie Grower, Bonnie Hillegass, and Fran Nelson

    8—A Look at the Newest Ethical Issues in Workers' Compensation 70
        Anne Llewellyn

PART II   THE CASE MANAGER'S UNIVERSE 73

    1—A Case Study of Nursing Case Management in a Rural Hospital 75
        Wanda Anderson-Loftin, Danette Wood, and Linda Whitfield

2—Population-Based Case Management 82
Faiga J. Qudah and Melissa Brannon

3—Telephonic Nursing: Empowering Patients at Risk for
Preterm Birth 95
Marianne E. Weiss and Annette K. Adams

4—In Case Management, Who's Watching the Store? Implementing
Practice Parameters and Outcomes 103
Kathleen Moreo

5—A Framework for Integrated Quality Improvement 106
Catherine Willoughby, Ginette Budreau, and Debra Livingston

6—The Integration of Primary Care and Case Management in
Chronic Disease 115
Cheryl Phillips-Harris

7—Managing and Redesigning the Continuum of Care: The Value
Chain Model 121
Kathy Fleschut, Chip Caldwell, and B. Eugene Beyt, Jr.

8—Managing Critical Pathway Variances 128
Janice Schriefer

9—Using Computer Systems To Enhance Case Management 142
Joy L. Luque, Michael J. Pereira, and James D. Brown

PART III CASE MANAGEMENT ADMINISTRATION AND FINANCIAL
CONSIDERATIONS 151

1—Activity-Based Costing for Hospitals 153
Suneel Udpa

2—Monitoring Case Management Cost Savings 168
Victoria Hekkers

3—Pricing Specialty Carve-Outs and Disease Management Programs
Under Managed Care 170
Kenneth T. LaPensee

4—Case Management and Home Health Care: An Integrated Model 180
Sherry L. Aliotta and Jo-Anne Andre

5—Tutorial: Causal Modeling and Patient Satisfaction 193
Dale N. Glaser and Barbara Riegel

6—Comprehensive Case Management: Implications for Program
Managers 203
L. Michele Issel

7—Effects of the Program-Management Model: A Case Study on
Professional Rehabilitation Nursing 213
Mary Ann Miller and Laban Darrel Miller

8—The Change Process and a Clinical Evaluation Unit at University of
    Massachusetts Medical Center 219
    Steven L. Strongwater

PART IV   CASE MANAGEMENT IN ACTION: CASES IN PROFILE 231

1—Trauma Critical Pathways: A Care Delivery System That Works 233
    Elizabeth E. Latini

2—Guidelines for Evaluation and Education of Adult Patients with Mild
    Traumatic Brain Injuries in an Acute Care Hospital Setting 237
    Kathy A. Lawler and Carol A. Terregino

3—The Challenges of Neurobehavioral Case Management 247
    Rick Aquado

4—Returning Brain-Injured Clients to Work: A Team Approach 250
    M. J. Schmidt and Mary Pat Murphy

5—Approaching Health and Wellness Issues for Those with
    High-Level Spinal Cord Injury 254
    Theresa M. Chase

6—The Effectiveness and Efficiency of an Early Intervention
    "Spinal Protocol" in Work-Related Low Back Injuries 258
    James M. Alday and Frank J. Fearon

7—HIV Continuum of Care: Challenges in Management 263
    *Robin I. Goldenberg, Stefanie H. Bell, Jacqueline Wright,
    Sharon E. Brodeur, Mary Ann Turjanica, Loretta Beckman, and
    Nancy Warker*

8—An Interdisciplinary Problem-Based Practicum in Case Management
    and Rural Border Health 274
    Marion K. Slack and Marylyn M. McEwen

9—Clinical Pathway Across Tertiary and Community Care After an
    Interventional Cardiology Procedure 284
    *Karen Doran, Barbara Sampson, Ruth Staus, Cathy Ahern,
    and Donna Schiro*

10—Creating a Practice Partnership: A Clinical Application of Case
    Management 296
    Colleen M. Lucas, Eric J. Dierks, and Nadine Parker

Index 309

Contributors

Annette K. Adams, RN, MSN
Coordinator for the Preterm Birth Prevention
    Program
Kaiser Permanente
Fontana, CA

Cathy Ahern, RN
Coordinator, Cardiac Rehabilitation
Immanuel-St. Joseph's Hospital
Mankato, MN

James M. Alday, MD
Medical Director
The Rehabilitation Institute
Northeast Georgia Medical Center
Gainesville, GA

Sherry L. Aliotta, RN, BSN, CCM
Regional Director of Case Management and
    Utilization Management
Prudential Health Care
Woodland Hills, CA

Wanda Anderson-Loftin, RN, MSN
Assistant Professor
Department of Nursing
Georgia Southern University
Statesboro, GA

Jo-Anne Andre, BSN, MN
Director of Continuing Care
Talbert Medical Management Corporation
Costa Mesa, CA

Rick Aquado, RN, CRRN
Neuro Behavioral Healthcare
Conroe, TX

Loretta Beckman, RN, MSN, CANP
Coordinator of Clinical Services
Office of HIV Services
Inova Health System
Fairfax, VA

Stephanie H. Bell, BSN, MBA
Director
Quality Leadership
Inova Home Health
Springfield, VA

B. Eugene Beyt, Jr., MD, MS
Chief Clinical Officer
General Health System
Baton Rouge, LA
Clinical Associate Professor
Health Systems Management
Tulane University
New Orleans, LA

Melissa Brannon, RN, PhD
Director ICM
Operations and Development
Integrated Care Management
Harris Methodist Health System
Arlington, TX

Sharon E. Brodeur, MPA
Director
Office of HIV Services
Inova Health System
Fairfax, VA

James D. Brown
Desktop Computer Specialist
PacifiCare of California
Cypress, CA

Ginette Budreau, MA, MBA, RN
Advanced Practice Nurse
Pediatric/Obstetrics and Gynecology Nursing
    Division
University of Iowa Hospitals and Clinics
Iowa City, IA

Chip Caldwell, FACHE
Vice President
Juran Institute
Wilton, CT

Theresa M. Chase, ND, RN
Patient Education Specialist
Craig Hospital
Englewood, CO

Roberta M. Conti, RN, PhD, CCM, FAAN
Assistant Professor
Coordinator
Graduate Program in Nursing Administration
George Mason University
Fairfax, VA

Eric J. Dierks, MD, DMD, FACS
Head and Neck Surgeon
Columbia Otolaryngology Group, Inc.
Portland, OR

Karen Doran, MSN, RN, CNSC
Cardiac Centers at Mercy and Unity Hospitals
Mercy Hospital
Coon Rapids, MN
Unity Hospital
Fridley, MN

Frank J. Fearon, DPT
Assistant Professor in the Graduate Physical
    Therapy Program
North Georgia College and State University
Dahlonega, GA

Kathy Fleschut
Quality Manager
CIGNA Healthcare of North Carolina
Charlotte, NC

Dale N. Glaser, PhD
Methods Analyst, Health Services Research
    and Development
Sharp Healthcare
Assistant Professor, Department of Psychology
    and Family Studies
United States International University
San Diego, CA

Robin I. Goldenberg, MD
Medical Director
Quality Management
Fairfax Hospital (Inova Health System)
Annandale, VA

Ronnie Grower, MA
Director of Quality Improvement and Research
Sierra Health Services, Inc.
Las Vegas, NV

Victoria Hekkers, RN, BSM, CCM
President
Intercare Network
Hartland, WI

Bonnie Hillegass
Assistant Vice President of Health Care
    Operations
Sierra Health Services, Inc.
Las Vegas, NV

L. Michele Issel, PhD, RN
Assistant Professor
School of Nursing
The University of Texas at Austin
Austin, TX

Kenneth T. LaPensee, PhD
Vice President
Health Economics Research
Physicians World Communications Group
Secaucus, NJ

Elizabeth E. Latini, MS, RN
Trauma Clinical Nurse Specialist
Regional Trauma Center
Robert Packer Hospital
Sayre, PA

Kathy A. Lawler, DPhil
Director, Neuropsychology Laboratory
Division of Neurology
Department of Medicine
Cooper Hospital/University Medical Center
Clinical Assistant Professor of Neurology
The University of Medicine and Dentistry
Robert Wood Johnson Medical School
Camden, NJ

Debra Livingston, MS, ARNP, CS
Administrative Associate
Medical/Psyciatric and Chemical Dependency
   Nursing Divisions
University of Iowa Hospitals and Clinics
Iowa City, IA

**Anne Llewellyn, RN, BPS-HSA, CCM,
   CCRN**
Co-owner
Professional Resources in Management
   Education
Fort Lauderdale, FL

Colleen M. Lucas, RN, MN, CS
Clinical Nurse Specialist/Case Manager
Patient Care Support Services
Legacy Portland Hospitals
Portland, OR

Joy L. Luque, RN, BSN
Chronic Long-term Case Manager
PacifiCare of California
Cypress, CA

Gloria G. Mayer, RN, EdD, FAAN
President
Friendly Hills HealthCare Network
La Habra, CA

Marylyn M. McEwen, MS
College of Nursing
University of Arizona
Tucson, AZ

Laban Darrel Miller, MA, PhD Candidate
Administrative Fellow
Cardinal Hill Rehabilitation Hospital
Lexington, KY

Mary Ann Miller, BSN
Assistant Program Manager
Cardinal Hill Rehabilitation Hospital
Lexington, KY

**Kathleen Moreo, RN, BSN, BPS-HSA,
   CDMS, ABDA**
Co-owner
Professional Resources in Management
   Education
Fort Lauderdale, FL

Kelly S. Morgan, MN, RN, CEN
Quality Review Manager
Vencor Hospital-Tucson
Tucson, AZ

Mary Pat Murphy, MSN, CRRN, CCM
Director of Clinical Services
ReMed Recovery Care Centers
Conshohocken, PA

Fran Nelson
Project Manager of Quality Improvement and
   Research
Sierra Health Services, Inc.
Las Vegas, NV

Nadine Parker, RN, MSN
Graduate Student
Department of Adult Health and Illness
Oregon Health Sciences University
Portland, OR

Michael J. Pereira
Clinical Data Systems Specialist
PacifiCare of California
Cypress, CA

Cheryl Phillips-Harris, MD
Director of Clinical Resources
Continuing Care Division
Sutter/CHS
Sacramento, CA

Faiga J. Qudah, RN, PhD
Senior Vice President of Integrated Care
    Management
Harris Methodist Health System
Arlington, TX

Anne M. Rausch, BSN, MPA
Director of Managed Care Programs
University Medical Center
Tucson, AZ

Barbara Riegel, DNSc, RN, CS, FAAN
Associate Professor, School of Nursing
San Diego State University
Clinical Researcher, Health Services Research
    and Development
Sharp HealthCare
San Diego, CA

Barbara Sampson, MS, RN
Assistant Clinical Nurse Manager,
    Telemetry
Abbott Northwestern Hospital
Minneapolis, MN

Donna Schiro, RN
Director of Nursing
Arlington Municipal Hospital
Arlington, MN

M. J. Schmidt, MA
Director of Operations
ReMed Recovery Care Centers
Conshohocken, PA

Janice Schriefer, MSN, MBA, RN, CCRN
Clinical Project Coordinator
Fletcher Allen Health Care
Burlington, VT

Marion K. Slack, PhD
Assistant Research Scientist/Teaching
    Associate
Department of Pharmacy Practice and Science
College of Pharmacy
University of Arizona
Tucson, AZ

Ruth Staus, BAN, RN
Staff Nurse, Telemetry
Abbott Northwestern Hospital
Minneapolis, MN

Lawrence F. Strassner, RN, MS, CNA
Director of Clinical Path Program
The Johns Hopkins Hospital
Baltimore, MD

Steven L. Strongwater, MD
Associate Chief Medical Officer
Clinical System
University of Massachusetts Medical Center
Worcester, MA

**Julie N. Tackenberg, RN, MA, MAOM,
    CNRN**
Clinical Nurse Specialist
Community Case Manager of Managed Care
    Programs
Arizona Health Sciences Center
Tucson, AZ

Carol A. Terregino, MD
Director of Clinical Research
Department of Emergency Medicine
Cooper Hospital/University Medical Center
Instructor of Clinical Surgery
The University of Medicine and Dentistry
Robert Wood Johnson Medical School
Camden, NJ

Mary Ann Turjanica, RN, MSN, CS, CRNP
Clinical Nurse Specialist
Medicine and HIV
Fairfax Hospital
Fairfax, VA

Suneel Udpa, PhD
Associate Professor of Accounting
School of Economics and Business
    Administration
Saint Mary's College of California
Moraga, CA

Nancy Warker, RN, CRNI
Program Manager, IV Therapy
Business Development
Inova Home Health
Springfield, VA

Marianne E. Weiss, RN, DNSc
Associate Professor
Marquette University College of Nursing
Milwaukee, WI

Linda Whitfield, RN, BSN
Director of Nursing
Candler County Hospital
Metter, GA

Catherine Willoughby, MA, RN
Nurse Manager
Child Psychiatry Unit
University of Iowa Hospitals and Clinics
Iowa City, IA

Danette Wood, RN, MSN, CNS
Nurse Case Manager
Candler County Hospital
Metter, GA

Jacqueline Wright, RN, MSN
Regional Vice President
Hospice of Northern Virginia
Fairfax, VA

Preface

Essential Readings in Case Management is a compilation of carefully selected readings intended to be utilized by instructors and students of case management as a supplement to *The Case Manager's Handbook, Second Edition.*

The selections have appeared in the following Aspen publications:

Inside Case Management
Nursing Administration Quarterly
Advanced Practice Nursing Quarterly
Quality Management in Health Care
Managed Care Quarterly
Journal of Rehabilitation Outcomes
Measurement
Journal of Head Trauma Rehabilitation
Home Health Care Management & Practice
Critical Care Nursing Quarterly
The Journal of Cardiovascular Nursing
Topics in Emergency Medicine
Journal of Nursing Care Quality
Health Care Management Review
The Health Care Supervisor
Family & Community Health

It is important to note that the field of case management continues to evolve and is represented by several professional disciplines. Found in virtually every sector of the private and public health care delivery system, case management has a wide range of models in a variety of practice settings. Payers and providers alike recognize the value of case management, and educators and students face many challenges as we prepare entry-level practitioners and advance the practice of the professionals.

The Case Manager's Handbook, Second Edition, provides the essential components, but because it is a single text, does not present in-depth discussion of the many variances, viewpoints, issues, and considerations represented in the field.

The selected articles for *Essential Readings in Case Management* are intended to promote discussion within educational settings, provide more in-depth information, stimulate the student as she comes to appreciate the differences and commonalities in case management practice, and enhance a greater understanding of this challenging professional role. Some of the readings offer analytical views, others portray controversial issues confronting hospitals, community-based programs and employer/payers, while still others focus on the technology and challenges in defining outcomes for the increasing number of case management programs. Understandably, the views expressed by the authors of these readings will vary and may even seem contradictory, but this, too, is a reflection of the ever-changing role and function of the case manager.

Articles have been designated in certain sections to correspond with similar sections in the textbook. These readings are not the only ones available, and continuous research by the student is encouraged. Within this compendium of articles, as well as the textbook, are listings of other recommended readings and references, and other authors are preparing manuscripts, books, newsletters, and articles as this is going to press.

To the authors of these articles, I express my appreciation for your valuable contributions. To the instructors and students who are utilizing *The Case Manager's Handbook, Second Edition,* and this companion publication, I encourage you to add to the growing body of case management writings. Your pilot programs, success stories, challenges, theories, and research will promote case management and empower future case managers.

PART I

Profile of a Case Manager

Nurse Case Manager Roles: Implications for Practice and Education

Roberta M. Conti

The high cost of health care has been and continues to be a national problem. Payer response has included a variety of initiatives, all of which focus on improved efficiency and increased accountability among those delivering health care services. Over the last decade, efforts to accomplish these two goals have resulted in a major paradigm shift from a patient-driven, fee-for-service system to a payer-driven, capitated managed care system.

To date, the new paradigm's fiscal success has been due primarily to the overlay of established utilization management techniques on providers. However, this approach suffers from the same limitations as its predecessor in that its focus is on the acute health care need and resource consumption dynamics. This focus is both inefficient and ineffective in dealing with clients with highly complex or extended term health care needs. Such clients represent a high risk of high cost. As such, they are best supported by a strategic approach to their health care resource consumption. Case management, a concept dominating health policy discussions and health care delivery, is proposed as the approach of choice for these clients.

Literature reviews demonstrate numerous case management practice models across the domains of social work, medicine, and nursing. As a result, significant diversity exists regarding the role behaviors, roles, and education of case managers. This article reports on a study designed to identify these components in nurses practicing in the Broker Model of Case Management.

The Broker Model of Case Management focuses on identifying client needs, matching appropriate health and community resources in a timely, cost-effective fashion, and monitoring the results of the match between the client's needs and the provided services. Case managers in this model frequently are employed by insurance companies or other payers. Recommendations and decisions consider both client needs and payer policy. The case manager in this model changes the service plan as needed, but provides no direct care or treatment personally.[1]

NURSES AND CASE MANAGEMENT

Nurses are a major group of health care professionals engaged in the Broker Model of Case Management. Historically, nurses have been sought by insurance companies to manage catastrophic cases because of their knowledge and understanding of medical and nursing practice. The health care industry's focus on case management to bring about coordination and cost-effectiveness of care has resulted in creation of a significant job market for nurses. Unfortunately, there is an absence of research on nurse case management, resulting in a lack of clear definition of the role, its role behaviors, and sources of learning.

Nurs Admin Q 1996; 21(1): 67–80

The concept of role has gained definitional clarity through creation of associated concepts such as role learning and role expectations. Hardy and Conway[2] define a role as a set of behaviors associated with a position in a social structure. This definition supports the premise that the role of the nurse case manager is demonstrated in the behaviors associated with the role. Identification and analysis of the role behaviors, roles, and education of nurse case managers will be beneficial not only to current and future nurse case managers practicing in the Broker Model, but also to policy makers, employers, and the nursing profession, the entity responsible to plan direction in education and promote enhanced practice patterns.

HISTORY OF CASE MANAGEMENT

The roots of case management can be traced to the early 18th century when the coordination of services for the sick and poor, and the conservation of public funds, was founded under the first Board of Charities in the State of Massachusetts. It has evolved out of the dual concern for efficient, quality service coordination and cost-effective service provision.[1]

Case management is rooted in a long history of social work efforts for service coordination, such as Chicago's Hull House, founded in 1889 to offer a variety of programs for immigrant populations. These programs contributed major value orientations to case management, such as worth of the individual and the provision of individualized treatment to assist clients toward self-support and self-sufficiency.[1] They also established the basis for today's case management standards that reflect the importance of trained staff and volunteers and the systematic collection of information.

Nursing's initial settlement house involvement was the Henry Street Settlement House, founded in New York in 1938 by Lillian Wald.[3] In the early 1900s, Wald suggested that Metropolitan Life Insurance Company organize a visiting nurse department to furnish case management nursing services to the company's industrial policyholders in the Manhattan section of New York. The company agreed and the result was cost-effective nursing services. By 1912, there were 589 Metropolitan Life nursing centers across the country.[3]

The case management services established by Metropolitan Life Insurance Company paved the way for creation of the Broker Model of Case Management. Today, companies such as Liberty Mutual Insurance employ rehabilitation nurses to manage services for injured policyholders. These Broker Model nurse case managers provide services by coordinating the services necessary to ensure recovery of the injured worker in a cost-effective environment.[4]

Client-level coordination, recognized in the 1970s as a distinct approach to case management, emerged as the result of the proliferation of categorical social programs in the 1960s.[5] The Allied Services Act of 1972 was the first congressional initiative to address case management. It required that social service programs be consolidated, offer a full range of services, and increase access to care. With passage of the Omnibus Budget Reconciliation Act of 1981, state Medicaid programs could implement case management systems that restricted the provider from or through whom a recipient could obtain primary care. These federal requirements prohibited case management from impairing access to services and required that a specific person or agency be responsible for locating, coordinating, or monitoring Medicaid services on behalf of the recipient. In addition, states had to demonstrate that case management was cost-effective.[6]

Nurses were not designated as case managers in federal case management programs or demonstration projects until the 1987 Medicare Nursing Practice and Patient Care Improvement Act and the 1989 Healthy Birth Act. Identification of role complexity and span of application resulted in the inclusion of case management in undergraduate and graduate curriculums in the early 1990s.

MODELS OF CASE MANAGEMENT

Numerous case management models are described in the social services, health care, and nursing literatures.[7–9] Articles began to appear in the social services literature in the late 1970s and early 1980s. Descriptive in nature, most focused on the expected functions of the case manager or the process of care delivery.[10–15] A review of the periodical literatures of social service, health care, and nursing from 1978 to 1992 identified two research studies in social services relative to models. Modrcin, Rapp, and Poertner[16] reported on an experimental design comparing two models of case management service to the chronically mentally ill, while Rothman[17] reported on a series of studies culminating in the development of an empirically based model for case management practice.

The health care and social services literatures have described case manager roles for more than 30 years. However, no research validating these descriptions has been forthcoming. Consequently, there is no general agreement in the human services field as to how the diversity and variability of these roles link to form a coherent model of practice.[17]

A search of the periodical literature from 1985 to 1992 identified three studies reporting on case manager roles.[17–19] Rothman[17] identified 14 functions of case management derived from a field survey of 48 case managers and an applied field study. Middleton[18] identified that the majority of case managers were involved in the tasks of service plan development, making agency contacts, recording and reporting, and evaluation of community services. Zimmerman[19] gathered data from case records, agency personnel, and the clients themselves in a program to provide integrated case management services for multiproblem children.

The nursing literature did not delineate practice behaviors unique to case managers. Instead, it focused on its convergence with other roles, such as with clinical nurse specialist,[20–22] nurse practitioner,[22] rehabilitation nurse,[23] and trauma nurse.[24] This literature posits that the practice of nurse case management is discipline specific and that nurse case manager role behaviors do not differ significantly from already existing nursing roles. Nurse authors demonstrated a lack of consensus regarding nurse case manager role behaviors, and no identified behaviors were ex-

amined within the context of a specific practice model or conceptual framework. Additionally, no formal professional nursing curriculum to teach the roles of nurse case managers and no studies that identified or described the role behaviors of nurse case managers in the Broker Model of Case Management were found.

CONCEPTUAL FRAMEWORK

The set of roles enacted by a case manager determines the degree of emphasis on service integration and coordination. Role theory provides the framework for identifying role behaviors. Roles are explained by the presumption that persons are members of social positions and hold expectations for their own behaviors and those of others.[25] A role is a composite of both the expected and the actual behaviors associated with a position.[2,26] Role behaviors are defined as anticipated behaviors to be performed by individuals who are engaged in that role in society. These anticipated behaviors can be influenced by learning and socialization and are known as role expectations.[2,27]

In this study, the conceptual framework of role theory called symbolic interactionism, as derived from the work of Mead,[28] Cooley,[29] and Blumer,[30] provided the basic definitions for identification and comprehension of communicated behaviors of nurse case managers. This framework posits that people create meaning from experiences via interactional responses to the situations in which they find themselves[31] and that they are constantly evaluating and acting upon events based on their interpretation of the meaning of these events.

METHODOLOGY

The qualitative fieldwork method and the survey method were used in this study, based on their consistency with the major tenets of symbolic interactionism. In the qualitative fieldwork method, the investigator performed ethnographic interviews, an approach intentionally unstructured to maximize discovery and description[32] and recognized as an established research method for studying social behavior. Since the roles of nurse case managers are reflected in social behaviors resulting from the multiple interactions characterizing their practice, ethnographic interviews provided an appropriate vehicle to identify and specify these behaviors.

The investigator conducted the interviews using a purposive sample of four practicing Broker Model nurse case managers selected at random from two offices of a national case management corporation located in the metropolitan Washington and Baltimore areas. Upon obtaining agreement from corporation management, the investigator contacted the identified nurses and provided them with an overview of the study. All agreed to participate.

The investigator interviewed each nurse case manager over two separate, one-hour sessions. The first interview, called the Grand Tour,[33] was guided by the opening question, "Tell me what it is you do as a nurse case manager." The investigator asked follow-up questions to maintain the interviewee's focus on a particular behavior, or to request expansion of interviewee comments. The investigator analyzed the transcripts from the first interview and compiled lists of the behaviors that described the nurse case manager's practice. The lists helped focus questions to guide the second interview.

For the second interview, called the mini interview,[33] the investigator provided each interviewee with a list of behaviors identified from their first interview and asked the following three questions: Do they accurately describe what you do as a case manager? Should any be grouped together because their meaning is the same? Can you define or describe in more detail what these behaviors mean to you? The investigator transcribed each of the eight audio-recorded interviews verbatim into a word processing software program and then into *The Ethnograph*, a software program that facilitates the management and reorganization of interview data.[34] Through use of a set of interactive, menu-driven computer programs, *The Ethnograph* performed the mechanical aspects of data analysis (i.e., coding, recoding, and sorting of data files

into analytic categories), as well as adding, deleting, or modifying the coding scheme. The investigator examined each line of verbatim text, searching for segments where the interviewee specified or alluded to a behavior associated with his or her practice. Each text segment was then "coded" with a label that specified a particular behavior.

The coding process resulted in identification of a total of 96 code words (nouns and verbs). Of these, only verbs were retained on the final word list to focus attention on the *action* component of the behaviors, and of these, only those verbs stated by two or more of the interviewees were retained on the final behavior code word list, resulting in a final total of 59 behavior code words. *The Ethnograph* sorted the behavior code words per transcribed interview for an alphabetical listing and a frequency list of the behavior code words. Finally, the investigator constructed a list of the behavior code words. From these data, the investigator constructed a list of all code words used across all eight ethnographic interviews and calculated their frequencies.

The next phase in data analysis involved clustering of code words. Code words were placed into clusters using *The Synonym Finder*[35] as the authoritative source for word meanings, with all code words displaying a similar meaning clustered together. For words not listed in this reference, *Roget's International Thesaurus*[36] was used as the authoritative source. Each cluster was labeled using the code word in it with the highest frequency of occurrence.

Clusters were rank-ordered according to the cumulative frequency counts of the words in each cluster. This resulted in a numerical value for each cluster. After identification of individual cluster scores, all cluster scores were totaled. Then each individual cluster score was divided by the total cluster score, resulting in a "weighted" cluster score. This value was multiplied by 40 to obtain the proportion share of instrument items for that cluster. All clusters with a proportion share of 0.5 or above were retained. Sixteen clusters with a proportion share of 0.5 or above were retained for further analysis.

The second data collection method used in this study involved construction of a survey instrument. Following the coding and clustering process applied to the interview texts, the investigator constructed a survey instrument consisting of statements of nurse case manager behaviors. The numerical values of the clusters guided the number of statements associated with each cluster. Using the retained clusters and the individual code words that made up each cluster, *The Ethnograph* extracted and printed all segments of text for each cluster.

Text segments for each cluster that resulted in clear, specific, and succinct first person declarative instrument items were selected for the instrument. Items were arranged so that no two like cluster items were next to each other. Respondents rated the behavior specified in each statement according to their own practice as a nurse case manager using a five-point Likert-type scale, which quantified the frequency with which each behavior was present in a nurse case manager's practice.

The final survey instrument consisted of a forced-choice demographic data section, a series of items developed from the coding results of the ethnographic interviews, and a selection choice for each identified case management behavior was learned. Content validity of the instrument was addressed by expert review of the instrument. Three doctorally prepared nursing faculty members with expertise in research, clinical nursing, and instrument development used an investigator-developed scale to rate the quality of each statement in terms of grammatical clarity and study-focused appropriateness. Grammatical clarity was defined as the degree to which the statement demonstrated declarative format (i.e., subject-verb-object), present tense of the verb, and focus on a specific behavior. Appropriateness was defined as the degree to which each statement was consistent with the focus of the study as reflected in the research questions. Scoring values of 3 (fully meets criteria), 2 (partially meets criteria), and 1 (does not meet criteria) were used.

Prior to fielding, the instrument was pilot tested using the four nurse case managers who participated in the ethnographic interviews. Upon their agreement to do so, each received a packet consisting of a cover letter and the survey instrument. Additionally, they were asked to make comments regarding the ease of completing the survey instrument, whether the frequency choices (definitions for A, B, C, etc.) were clearly stated and easily understood, and how long it took to complete the instrument. The investigator analyzed the responses and made minor editorial changes to the instrument. Reliability of the instrument was assessed by calculating a coefficient alpha for the 38 survey instrument items.

PERFORMANCE OF THE SURVEY

A nationally known nurse case manager employer agreed to participate by providing a sampling frame for the 100 nurses to be surveyed. The employer required a written letter of request and a copy of the research proposal for review. The agreement to participate stipulated that the investigator would agree to have the instrument reviewed by the appropriate corporate individuals prior to the mailing, and that anonymity of the participants be maintained by placing the responsibility for the actual mailing of the survey instrument with the corporate office. The organization approved the instrument for mailing without modifications.

SELECTION OF SURVEY PARTICIPANTS

The corporation identified a population of 283 nurse case managers located in 39 states. Names and addresses were identified by searching for specific job title codes and specific ZIP codes for each state. Based on investigator guidance, corporate staff obtained a systematic random sample from this population by selecting every third name, after an initial random point was established, until 100 nurse case managers were selected. Two sets of mailing labels were printed to support an initial mailing and follow-up mailing of the survey instrument.

The investigator delivered 100 postage-paid, sealed packets containing a cover letter, the survey instrument, and a postage-paid, self-addressed return envelope to the corporation for mailing. Two weeks following the initial mailing, the corporation sent the investigator's reminder postcard to the selected participants. Survey responses were analyzed using a computer program written in SPSSX.

FINDINGS—DEMOGRAPHIC CHARACTERISTICS

Table 1 depicts the characteristics of study participants. All 4 original interviewees and 57 of 58 survey respondents completed this portion of the instrument. Both groups were similar in terms of age, years in nursing, and years as case managers. Among survey respondents, nearly 45 percent had an associate degree or diploma as their highest level of nursing education, versus one in four.

VALIDITY AND RELIABILITY

The content validity of the text derived from the ethnographic interviews was evaluated by having each interviewee review her list of verbatim text and behavior words from the first interview. Collectively, the interviewees affirmed the accuracy of the behavior word lists, suggested a few word groupings, and provided enhanced descriptions of selected words.

The content validity of the survey instrument was evaluated via instrument review by two groups: doctorally prepared nurse faculty and the original interviewees.

IDENTIFICATION OF BEHAVIORS

Review of the final behavior code word list of 59 words determined numerous words to be synonyms, permitting their grouping into 27 clusters. Each cluster was labeled with the behavior code word in the cluster with the highest frequency of occurrence. Those clusters with a

Table 1. Demographic characteristics: Ethnographic interviewees and survey respondents

Characteristics	Ethnographic interviewees n = 4	Survey respondents n = 57
Mean age	48.5	40.3
Standard deviation	8.2	9.1
Range	41–57 (16)	29–57 (28)
Basic nursing education		
Diploma	2	25
BSN/BS	2	15
Associate degree	0	16
Highest nursing education		
Diploma	1	13
Associate	0	12
BSN/BS	2	23
MSN	1	3
Other	0	6
Mean years as a RN	26.3	16.6
Standard deviation	7.5	7.8
Range	20–35 (15)	5–35 (30)
Mean years as a case manager	3.3	3.2
Standard deviation	5.7 months	19.8 months
Range	3–4 yrs (1)	2 mo–9 yrs (8.8)

weighted cluster score of 0.5 or above were represented in the survey instrument. As a result, 16 clusters were retained for use in development of instrument items. These clusters represented 94 percent of the composite score of the original 27 clusters and generated a total of 38 survey instrument items.

FREQUENCY CHOICE SELECTIONS— SURVEY METHOD

The box presents the frequency choice options listed in the survey instrument. Initial review of frequency data revealed a strong selection pattern for choices "A" and "B" and a weak selection pattern for choices "C," "D," and "E." Based on these patterns of selection, analysis of frequency data was limited to choices "A" and "B." For the combined scores for choice A and choice B, all clusters demonstrated a frequency choice selection score of 80 percent or above. Table 2 summarizes the frequency choice selection cluster scores for choice A and choice B, and the combination of choices A and B.

Survey Instrument Frequency Choice Options

I include this behavior in my practice:

Choice A   with almost every client (80–99%) of the time)

Choice B   with most of my clients (60–79% of the time)

Choice C   with some of my clients (40–59% of the time)

Choice D   with a few of my clients (20–39% of the time)

Choice E   with an occasional client (0–19% of time)

SOURCES OF LEARNING

The survey instrument instructed respondents to indicate their primary source of learning for each behavior by placing a check in the appropriate box. However, some respondents selected both answers for one or more statements; thus the total number of responses exceeded the num-

---

Table 2. Percentage cluster scores for most frequent case manager behaviors

Cluster name	Choice "A" Almost every client	Choice "B" Most clients	Combined "A" and "B" choices cluster score
Monitoring	93	5	98
Problem solving	88	10	98
Expediting	65	33	98
Public relating	85	15	100
Communicating	82	13	95
Contacting	80	12	92
Planning	84	13	97
Explaining	78	20	98
Recommending	71	20	91
Coordinating	58	24	82
Documenting	61	21	82
Assessing	70	15	85
Negotiating	69	28	97
Educating	85	14	99
Brokering	62	26	88
Researching	52	36	88

ber of respondents. To account for this, the responses were totaled and a percentage score developed for each statement and cluster.

Analysis of responses demonstrated "on the job" to be the most common source of learning for respondents, with 70 percent or more selecting this choice for 32 of 38 statements. The remaining 6 statements involved an aspect of the nursing process and had a learning choice selection score of 30 percent or greater for "formal education" as the source of learning. Table 3 summarizes the percentage cluster scores for sources of learning. Ninety percent or more of survey respondents (n=58) indicated "on the job" as the source of learning for 3 of 16 clusters. For 10 of the remaining 13 clusters, 75 percent or more of the survey respondents selected "on the job" as the source of learning. Of the 3 remaining clusters, the percentages of respondents selecting "on the job" as the source of learning were 73, 69, and 68, respectively. Cumulatively, across all 16 clusters, 78 percent of respondents selected "on the job" as the source of learning, versus 22 percent who selected "formal education" as the source of learning.

Table 3. Percentage cluster scores: Sources of learning for nurse case managers

Cluster label	Formal education %	Source of learning on the job %
Monitoring	9	91
Problem solving	31	69
Expediting	9	91
Public relating	25	75
Communicating	22	78
Contacting	21	79
Planning	27	73
Explaining	20	80
Recommending	20	80
Coordinating	20	80
Documenting	22	78
Assessing	32	68
Negotiating	13	87
Educating	14	86
Brokering	4	96
Researching	18	82

ROLE EMERGENCE

Role theory is concerned with an important feature of social life, that of characteristic behavior patterns or roles. Consistent with the study's conceptual framework, survey respondents attached meaning to each of the behavior statements in the survey instrument and communicated this meaning through their frequency choice selections.

The pattern of frequency choices among the behaviors listed by the survey respondents supported the credibility of the designated cluster labels as appropriate identifiers of the roles of the nurse case manager in the Broker Model. Accordingly, the investigator transposed cluster labels into nouns and rank-ordered them according to their frequency of selection as indicated from survey statement frequency selections. Table 4 displays the results of this action.

DISCUSSION

Utility of conceptual framework

The findings from this study affirmed the tenets of symbolic interactionism and supported the validity of this framework as a means to understand and explain role behaviors and, ultimately, role enactment of nurses practicing under the Broker Model of Case Management.

Characteristics of study participants

The four nurse case manager interviewees and the 58 survey respondents were very similar in terms of age, gender, years in practice as an RN, and years in practice as a nurse case manager. Both groups demonstrated many years of experience in nursing practice, limited experience as nurse case managers, and equivalent patterns of basic and advanced education. Similarities also were evident in the percentage of nurses with BS or BSN and MS or MSN as their highest attained education level, with sizable percentages of survey respondents reporting the associate degree as both their basic and highest education level (28 percent and 21 percent, respectively).

Table 4. Cluster labels as representative of nurse case manager roles

Cluster label roles	Survey respondents' percent selection rate*
Public relator	100
Educator	99
Expeditor	98
Monitor	98
Problem solver	98
Explainer	98
Negotiator	97
Planner	97
Communicator	95
Contactor	92
Recommender	91
Broker	88
Researcher	88
Assessor	84
Documenter	82
Coordinator	82

* Selection rate = the frequency choice selection scores for the combination of choices "A" (almost all) and "B" (most).

Findings

The qualitative fieldwork method and the survey method proved to be appropriate research methods to identify and describe role behaviors and roles of nurse case managers practicing in the Broker Model. Both methods demonstrated consistency with key tenets of the study's conceptual framework in that both methods supported and affirmed their interconnectedness of meaning, interaction, and language.

Completion of the qualitative fieldwork method resulted in identification of a final set of 16 clusters of behavior code words, which generated 38 survey instrument statements. These statements reflected the meanings of the behaviors enacted by the nurse case managers interviewed. In the survey method, 58 nurse case managers from across the United States communicated the meanings of their role behaviors and roles as nurse case managers through completion of the survey instrument. Consistent with the tenets of symbolic interactionism, the meanings of these role behaviors were derived from social interactions (i.e., interactions between the nurse case managers and clients, colleagues, employees, vendors, and others). By reading and reflecting on the summary statements, respondents applied an interpretive process and modified their role and role behavior meanings. They then communicated these modified meanings via language (i.e., selection of a frequency choice for each statement).

Analysis revealed respondents indicated a frequency choice selection score for choices "A" (almost all clients) and "B" (most clients) that exceeded 80 percent for all clusters. These findings indicate these role behaviors were highly valued and well established.

As regards sources of learning, findings indicated most nurse case manager roles and attendant behaviors to be the product of employment and life experience and evolving outside the nursing education system. However, the behaviors of assessing, problem solving, and planning identified as learned via "formal education" mirror those associated with the nursing process. This finding suggests that the scope and depth of applicability of these nursing process behaviors extend to a diverse variety of roles, including those of the nurse case manager.

This study's most significant findings involve the number and types of roles identified from the nurse case manager behaviors. Of the 16 roles resulting from this process, 9 have received little or no mention in the nursing literature. As a result, the scope of practice of nurse case managers in general, and specifically in the Broker Model, has yet to be subjected to substantive examination and discussion by the profession. This situation must be reversed if dynamic role evolution is to occur.

CONCLUSIONS

Across the various models of case management, the largest number of nurses practice as case managers in the Broker Model, the model used by the health care insurance industry and self-insured corporations. Case management is a relatively new job market for nurses that requires assumption of multiple and complex roles not learned through formal education. This finding has significant implications for practicing nurse case managers, the nursing education system, the service network, employers, and the public served.

As more and more health care delivery systems turn to managed care, demand for case managers will increase. Identification and analysis of the role behaviors of nurse case managers will be beneficial not only to current and future Broker Model nurse case managers, but also to policy makers, employers, and the nursing profession as it plans direction in education and promotes enhanced practice patterns.

Nurse case managers in this study based their new role development on extensive clinical practice and life experience, indicating a willingness to step out of traditional nursing roles and into one with minimal role definition. An unexpected finding was that nearly 45 percent of study participants' highest level of education was less than a baccalaureate degree. This finding indicates that the complex roles of nurse case managers in this model are being performed in large part by technical nurses. Historically, technical nursing education has prepared nurses for practice in acute care settings where supervision of practice is consistently available. This study's findings indicate many technical nurses are breaking new ground as they practice independently in an arena in which the expectations of the role behaviors are distinctly different from the terminal teaching objectives of their nursing education programs.

Role identification resulting from this study revealed the majority of roles (13 of 16) are not espoused in the nursing literature as integral to nursing practice. The high selection of these behaviors reflects a need for nurse case managers to have knowledge of business practices, the integration of efficiency and effectiveness, and influential communications, in addition to their clinical knowledge. Additionally, findings regarding the sources of learning of role behaviors require addressing issues such as how an individual nurse case manager evaluates practice when the majority of learning of the practice takes place in the absence of standards of practice.

This study's findings indicate that nursing education must recognize that the traditional nursing curriculum, with its focus on therapeutic communication skills between nurse and patient, and the structured environment of organized nursing services will no longer prepare nurses for practice in the changing health care delivery system. The frequency choice selection by survey respondents indicate they are performing a complex level of communication skills within a role set that is beyond traditional organizational boundaries.

Nursing education must respond to the challenge of the movement of practice away from acute care and into more interdisciplinary, interdependent, and independent roles and must work with the corporate world to design new, innovative pathways that result in acquisition of complex communication skills. This action is consistent with a commitment to continuous improvement of curriculum content based on the realities of diverse roles and practice environments. Most important, employers of nurse case managers practicing under the Broker Model can use these findings to explain the position in job interviews, to develop accurate position descriptions, to organize orientation programs, to explain the relationship between these role behaviors and the roles they represent, and as a basis for evaluating performance.

These findings suggest several areas for future research on nurse case management:

- Is nurse educational level a criterion of importance in the practice of case management?
- What curriculum revisions are needed to ensure learning of key role behaviors via formal education?
- What impact does or can nurse case management have on attainment of patient-, payer-, nurse-, and employer-desired outcomes?

Academic-practice nurse case management collaborative ventures are the investment of choice for the 1990s, based on current Bureau of Labor Statistics analysis. Case management heads the list of the bureau's projections of growth in the health care professions, with a greater than 250 percent increase in case manager positions by the year 2003. Given the present diversity in the conceptualization of case management, attempts to delineate the roles of the nurse case manager will have significant application to health care reform policy and to the paradigm of managed care. This study has demonstrated that nurse case manager roles can be clearly explicated through identification and analysis of the behaviors associated with these roles.

REFERENCES

1. Weil, M., and Karls, J. *Case Management in Human Service Practice*. San Francisco, Calif.: Jossey-Bass, 1985.

2. Hardy, M., and Conway, M. *Role Theory: Perspectives for Health Professionals*. Norwalk, Conn.: Appleton-Century-Crofts, 1978.

3. Kalisch, P., and Kalisch, B. *The Advance of American Nursing*. Boston, Mass.: Little, Brown, 1986.

4. McBride, S.M. "Rehabilitation Case Managers: Ahead of Their Time." *Holistic Nursing Practice* 6, no. 2 (1992): 67–75.

5. Blazyk, S., Crawford, C., and Wimberley, E. "The Ombudsman and the Case Manager." *Social Work* 46 (1987): 451–53.

6. Spitz, B., and Abramson, J. "Competition, Capitation, and Case Management: Barriers to Strategic Reform." *The Millbank Quarterly* 65, no. 3 (1987): 348–69.

7. Desimone, B.S. "The Case for Case Management." *Continuing Care* 7, no. 7 (1988): 22–23.

8. Papenhausen, J. "Case Management: A Model of Advanced Practice?" *Clinical Nurse Specialist* 4, no. 4 (1990): 169–70.

9. Brault, G.L., and Kissinger, L.D. "Case Management: Ambiguous at Best." *Journal of Pediatric Health* 5, no. 4 (1991): 179–82.

10. Roberts-DeGennaro, "Developing Case Management as a Practice Model." *Social Casework: The Journal of Contemporary Social Work* 68, no. 8 (1987): 466–70.

11. Zawadski, R.T., and Eng, C. "Case Management in Capitated Long-term Care." *Health Care Financing Review Annual Supplement* (1988): 75–81.

12. Austin, C. "Case Management in Long-Term Care: Options and Opportunities." *Health and Social Work* 2 (1983): 16–30.

13. Kemp, B. "The Case Management Model of Human Service Delivery." *Annual Review of Rehabilitation* 2 (1981): 212–37.

14. Netting, F.E. "Case Management: Service or Symptom?" *Social Work* 37, no. 2 (1992): 160–63.

15. O'Connor, G.G. "Case Management: System and Practice." *Social Casework: The Journal of Contemporary Social Work* 69, no. 2 (1988): 97–106.

16. Modrcin, M., Rapp, C., and Poertner, J. "The Evaluation of Case Management Services with the Chronically Mentally Ill." *Evaluation and Program Planning* 11, no. 89 (1988): 307–14.

17. Rothman, J. "A Model of Case Management: Toward Empirically Based Practice." *Social Work* 36, no. 6 (1991): 522–27.

18. Middleton, J. "Case Management in Mental Retardation Service Delivery Systems: A View from the Field." Ph.D. diss., University of Pennsylvania, 1985.

19. Zimmerman, J.H. "Negotiating the System: Clients Make a Case for Case Management." *Public Welfare* 45, no. 2 (1987): 23–27.

20. Nugent, K. "The Clinical Nurse Specialist as Case Manager in a Collaborative Practice Model: Bridging the Gap Between Quality and Cost of Care." *Clinical Nurse Specialist* 6, no. 2 (1992): 106–11.

21. Norris, M., and Hill, C. "The Clinical Specialist: Developing the Case Manager Role." *Dimensions of Critical Care Nursing* 10, no. 6 (1991): 346–53.

22. Schroer, K. "Case Management: Clinical Nurse Specialist and Nurse Practitioner, Converging Roles." *Clinical Nurse Specialist* 3, no. 4 (1991): 189–94.

23. Mound, B., et al. "The Expanded Role of Nurse Case Managers." *Journal of Psychosocial Nursing* 29, no. 6 (1991): 18–22.

24. Simmons, F. "Developing the Trauma Nurse Case Manager Role." *Dimensions of Critical Care Nursing* 11, no. 3 (1992): 164–70.

25. Biddle, B.J. "Recent Developments in Role Theory." *Annual Review Sociology* 12, no. 2 (1986): 57–68.

26. Biddle, B.J. *Role Theory: Expectations, Identities, and Behaviors*. New York, N.Y.: Academic Press, 1979.

27. Biddle, B.J. *Role Theory: Expectations, Identities, and Behaviors*. 2nd ed. New York, N.Y.: Academic Press, 1985.

28. Mead, G.H. *Mind, Self and Society*. Chicago, Ill.: University of Chicago Press, 1934.

29. Cooley, C.H. *Human Nature and the Social Order*. New Brunswick, N.J.: Transaction Publishers, 1991.

30. Blumer, H. *Symbolic Interactionism: Perspective and Method*. Englewood Cliffs, N.J.: Prentice Hall, 1969.

31. Williams, B. "The Utility of Nursing Theory in Nursing Case Management Practice." *Nursing Administration Quarterly* 15, no. 3 (1991): 60–65.

32. McCall, G.J. and Simmons, J.L. *Issues in Participant Observation*. Reading, Mass.: Addison-Wesley, 1969.

33. Spradley, J.P. *The Ethnographic Interview*. Chicago, Ill.: Holt, Rinehart & Winston, 1979.

34. Tesch, R. "Computer Programs That Assist in the Analysis of Qualitative Data: An Overview." *Qualitative Health Research* 1, no. 3 (1991): 309–25.

35. Rodale, J. *The Synonym Finder*. Emmaus, Pa.: Rodale Press, 1978.

36. Roget, P. *Roget's International Thesaurus*. New York, N.Y.: Thomas Y. Crowell, 1962.

Redefining the Role of Clinical Nurse Specialists

Julie N. Tackenberg and Anne M. Rausch

Over the last two decades, health care has seen a major shift in its focus of service and methods of care delivery. These changes have created opportunities and challenges for clinical nurse specialists (CNSs) to redefine and reconfigure their role activities of expert practice, consultation, education, research, and administration/management to better meet societal health care needs. The community case manager is an example of how a CNS role can be reconfigured. Fiscal constraints, restructuring of the care delivery system, and public demand for increased services are moving the industry to innovative and challenging collaborations. Although tumultuous and unpredictable, it is an environment in which the CNS as a community case manager can promote holistic interaction with the client while attempting to explore fiscally responsible health care choices.

THE ENVIRONMENT

In order to appreciate the role of the CNS as a case manager within the community, it is important to understand the environmental changes that have influenced the present status of the health care industry. Three forces that have moved the health care system to its present position include technological advancements, societal pressures, and the corresponding response

Adv Prac Nurs Q 1995; 1(1): 37–48

of the internal health service environment. The major external pressures have developed on two different fronts. The first wave of change came in the late 1950s. Because of increased availability of media coverage for marketing of products and the protective services of consumer advocate groups, the public became educated and litigious consumers. This self-advocacy heightened awareness of consumer rights not only in the purchase of manufactured products, but also in the procurement of expendable services. Repeated clamor for improved quality and accountability have influenced the business world to incorporate its customer into the identification and description of quality services. Those corporations that have failed to respond to this trend have experienced a significant decline in their profits. Because the emphasis was on manufactured goods rather than service, the health care industry was not on the forefront of this first wave of change.

The burgeoning customer expertise that resulted, developed against a background of costly technological advancement as space age developments, were applied to the public sector. Indeed, this advancement was part of the clamor for quality. Lighter, better, faster, and stronger became the comparative marketing tools of the era. As technological advancements were applied to health care, quality of care came to mean utilization of the latest diagnostic and treatment technology. The new consumer was vocal in establishing and obtaining this standard of care, necessitating delivery of nursing care to occur in the hospital rather than the home. This combination increased both hospitalization and technology and continued to drive health care costs upward, eventually leading to the regulation of costs within federally supported institutions.

In an attempt to control monetary expenditures, the federal government implemented a system of reimbursement based on diagnosis-related groups (DRGs) of medical disease. This new system, implemented in 1984, required a review of medical management in light of appropriate services delivered in a timely fashion with the measurable patient outcomes of recovery/response to treatment. One of the concepts to gain momentum in response to this new method of business was the need to maintain the health care dollars within the provider system of care. Verticalization of services soon followed, as well as the development of health maintenance organizations (HMOs), insurance/provider systems, and managed care with capitated dollars. A new health care delivery environment now exists that is starkly different than that of the early post-World War II era.

A vertically integrated health system according to Conrad (1990, p. 10) is "an arrangement whereby a health care organization (or closely related group of organizations) offers, either directly or through others, a broad range of patient care and support services operated in a functionally unified manner." Vertical organization requires both administrative and clinical collaboration among the interested parties. Geographic proximity and overlap of service boundaries are both important factors in defining vertical services. These boundaries, generally local or regional, define the service market. Secondary and tertiary health care services for the chronic or terminal client need to be augmented by home health, skilled nursing facilities, rehabilitation services, and long-term care. Given the perspectives of geography and process, it is easy to understand vertical integration of services as the "linkage of services that exist at different stages in the production process of health care" (Conrad, 1990, p. 10).

Another dimension, that of linking health insurance with delivery of health care services, exists in the integration of current health care. With this linkage/integration, the insurer/delivery system manages the care process rather than just pays the bills "because it dictates by whom and where services will be provided, effectively channeling the population" (Conrad, 1990, p. 12). Both financial and delivery systems become responsible for the economic health of the organization. This is the current environment as physician groups and hospital corporations assume the challenge of providing adequate health care with contracted dollar amounts. These contracted organizations are then at risk for assuming the burden of mismanaged health care dollars.

During the past decade, the aging population has also moved the health care industry toward vertical integration. Older individuals experience more chronic disabilities that require more frequent pre- and post-acute treatment, as well as rehabilitation and long-term care. Older persons are a population at risk that requires extensive use of health care resources. This growing population has forced many institutions to review their organizational structure to provide the necessary services along the entire continuum of health care delivery.

Services such as health promotion and disease prevention, offered by an acute care firm, demonstrate the organizations' commitment to serve a population base in the health maintenance aspect of the health care continuum. Today, surviving corporations are those that offer the depth and breadth of services necessary to manage the health care dollars within their market area (Figure 1). Without complete vertical integration within an organization, it is necessary to subcontract for services to manage contractual obligations. It is essential to refocus the goals from marginal overutilization of services to maximize profitability by delivery of appropriate, clinically sound utilization of services. This approach is critical under capitation and other contracts as well.

THE DEVELOPMENT OF MANAGED CARE SYSTEMS AT ARIZONA HEALTH SCIENCES CENTER

Managed care is "a comprehensive system which includes helping people know when they need care, what kind of care they need, and how

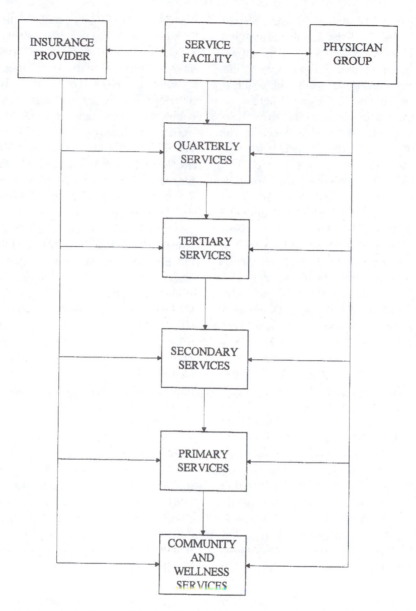

Figure 1. A model of vertical delivery of health care. Verticalization of health care services requires a broad spectrum of services that can be provided either directly or indirectly to the consumer. Definition and control of service market is enhanced by geographic boundaries, breadth of services, and clinical and administrative support.

to obtain that care in the most efficient, cost-effective way possible" (Holt, 1990, p. 27). As developed at the Arizona Health Sciences Center (AHSC), managed care is seen as an opportunity to streamline our systems to provide quality patient-centered care while continuing to focus on our teaching and research mission. Approxi-

mately 30% of client lives are covered under capitated contracts at AHSC. The expectation is that within 5 years all programs will be capitated. It became imperative to develop a system in anticipation of the future environment.

A review of all available services pointed to the need to streamline services through a continuum of care. The continuum focuses on activity levels from wellness through quaternary services, each in a variety of settings. The settings incorporate the community programs with inpatient, outpatient, and home health. The goal is to provide an ideal continuum of care where a system of case managers orchestrate patient care services. The continuum of care, overlaid with the system of case managers, was developed to manage capitated contracts.

Under capitation economics, profitability is directly related to controlling costs through the appropriate utilization of services. Capitation economics demands that there are appropriate utilization of services and that program membership continues to grow. Community case management facilitates these goals by managing avoidable hospital admissions and by increasing member satisfaction with the plan. Community case management also allows for control over a population that inherently demands high-technology services from a university setting.

A vital component to the managed care system is the role of the case manager. As a practice modality, case management has its roots in North American social casework. During the 1970s and 1980s, this method of intervention was used to address problems of service fragmentation and cost containment issue of long-term care (Beardshaw & Towell, 1990; Thornicroft, 1991) with varying degrees of success (Worley, 1991). Since that era, however, the increasing number of dependent people in the community, and the Care in the Community Project that increases accessibility of health services (Cambridge, 1990) and other projects have indicated case management is an integral component of quality care outcomes (Department of Health, 1989).

Conceptually, the goals of case management are to achieve normalization, choice, and dignity for the individual (Department of Health, 1989). To accomplish this requires the institution to be "innovative and flexible." The professional in this framework must be accessible and advocacy oriented (Thornicroft, 1991). Recently, Challis, Chessum, Chesterman, Luckett, and Traske

(1985) reported that studies at Gateshead and Darlinton supported that case management be expanded to include health as well as social provisions, taking it out of the social casework format.

When the managed care programs were under development, it seemed reasonable that one community case manager would act as a team leader to facilitate care for a predetermined number of clients through the entire continuum. The Medicare Risk program was selected as a pilot for the concept due to the rapid outcomes measures related to high utilization of the population. As a practical matter, however, a system of case managers was developed. In this model, a clinical case manager facilitates care provided in the hospital setting. Upon discharge, client health care concerns are communicated to the community case manager. The home health staff also performs a case management role when care is required in the home. The physician office coordinators (RNs) play a significant role in the case management system as educators and in identifying appropriate referrals. Social services implements hospital discharge plans and the utilization managers authorize services and ensure that subcontracts are honored.

Concerns of the primary care physician were also considered in the development of the AHSC case management model. The system supports the primary care physician to enable him or her to focus on quality patient care, relying on strong communication links and clear role definition.

The community case manager is most closely linked to the program goals of monitoring costs and intervening when there is a potential avoidable admission. As a pivot point for the system of case managers, it is clear that a high-level performer is indicated in this role. The community case manager must have good problem solving skills, clinical expertise, a grasp of available resources, and the ability to communicate well. The community case manager must also be motivated and have the flexibility to act independently in nontraditional settings. The community case manager must fully understand and communicate the plan limitations and liabilities related to managed care.

THE EVOLVING ROLE OF THE CNS

Throughout the developments in the 20th century, the role of the CNS has responded to the changing needs and values of society. Cited by Boone and Kikuchi (1977) as a response to the demands of post-World War II health care, the first post-graduate programs for the advanced CNS were developed in 1954 (Sills, 1983). The role of these first psychiatric CNSs was to provide clinical decision making based on scientific theory and to close the gap between theory and practice (Montemuro, 1987).

In the literature, between 1965 and 1980 the CNS was described by nursing leaders as having the following four major role functions: practitioner, consultant, educator, and researcher. The bedside practitioner component of the role allowed the CNS to directly impact client outcome and improve nursing standards by acting as a role model for the staff nurse. The consultant role was envisioned as providing expert clinical information to caregivers outside the immediate site of the specialist's practice. In the consultant role, the CNS could provide expert services either within the institution of practice or externally within the community as a representative of the institution. As an educator, the CNS was responsible for the education of both the client and family. Modalities for fulfilling this role include either individual teaching or group instruction, with the specialist in charge of material development and evaluation. Although it is acknowledged that the CNS practices in an optimal position to encounter nursing problems that lend themselves to systematic study (Girouard, 1983), the research aspect of the role has not traditionally been rewarded in the service setting (Montemuro, 1987). As master's-prepared practitioners, Hodgman (1983, p. 81) suggests that the "research practice of the clinical specialist needs to be on the evaluation, communication, and utilization of the new knowledge to improve practice rather than the discovery of new knowledge."

Implementation of the DRG system resulted in many new strategies as health care institutions attempted to remove the inefficiencies from the health care process. Reimbursement, according to DRG, was tied into length of stay for each admission along with a window of readmission. Within the nursing arena, this change brought both a renewed interest in standards of care and nursing care plans to identify appropriate nursing interventions and provide measurable outcome criteria as well as early development of appropriate discharge plans. To guide the general nursing staff in provision of effective and efficient care, a new emphasis was placed on the nursing clinical expert. The emphasis on shortened length of stay has encouraged movement of the CNS from the traditional academic hospital into both smaller community hospitals and into the community itself.

As a profession, nursing is linked to the needs and values of the social system in which it exists (Larson, 1977). Advanced practice roles, such as the CNS, are defined as anticipated behaviors to be performed by individuals who are engaged in a certain role within society (Biddle & Thomas, 1979). Role behaviors are anticipated by both the individual and by society and can evolve based on personal experience of the individual and changing needs of society (Biddle & Thomas, 1979). The role of the CNS is therefore influenced not only by the larger societal changes, but also by the organizational culture and needs. Between 1960 and 1980, emphasis was placed on the educator role of the CNS (Yokes, 1966) and recommendations were for the CNS to be positioned within the staff development/continuing education department (Pinkerton, 1978). A 1986 survey by Robichaud and Hamric found that patient care (40%) rather than education (27%) consumed the majority of the role responsibilities of the CNS. However, the responsibilities of practice continues to be practitioner, educator, consultant, researcher, and change agent/executive, although the degree of involvement in each role varies with the individual and the institutional needs. Despite the setting, the focus of the CNS practice continues to be client-based. According to the American Nurses' Association (ANA) Council of CNSs, "To fulfill the clinical nurse specialist's role, the nurse must have a client-based practice" (ANA, 1986, p. 2). Hamric (1989, p. 10) reiterates this, stating that "essential to the definition of the CNS is the focus of practice on the patient/client/family. Regardless of the setting, the CNS's practice is directed toward improving patient care and nursing practice."

By definition, the CNS has a major role in the delivery of innovative, cost-effective, quality care. Encompassed in this responsibility is the need to be current with innovations of the health care delivery systems as well. Providing leadership in the area of managed care and implementation of new nursing roles is the current challenge that faces not only the provider institutions but also the CNS (Holt, 1990).

CASE MANAGEMENT AT AHSC

At the AHSC, case management is in the final stages of implementation. Development of the continuum of care philosophy placed case management at a critical point within the institution and externally within the community (Figure 2). The clinical specialist, positioned as a case manager, has a more active role in promoting cost containment and utilization of services than previously defined. Efficacy of placement of the clinical specialist in this role has recently been documented by Schull (1992). The innovative component of this framework is the placement of the clinical specialist in the community and homes of the clients to facilitate the core health tasks of the individual.

Nationally, older persons have been recognized as a group at risk for excessive consumption of health care resources. Few HMO corporations are willing to incorporate this population because of a high dollar utilization pattern. As the market for members begins to tighten, however, the older sector of the population is coming under the auspices of managed care. At AHSC, this is the first population to be addressed by the case management model, with a CNS in the case manager position.

Providing services within a vertical framework necessitated development of the concep-

tual case management model by all members of the health care team. This was a lengthy process as territories and operations were defined and redefined with the new goal in mind. As presented in Figure 3, the team focused on utilization of all existing services within the organization as well as those of the community. The role of the case manager remained that of a clinical expert and client advocate. To provide the best clinical decision for the patient, this role was free of utilization and authorization responsibilities. This task was the responsibility of the utilization review (UR) nurse who represented the concerns and interests of the parties at risk: primarily the institution and the HMO. Obviously, a collaborative relationship was necessary in order to provide the best service to all customers.

Within this framework, the clinical specialist as case manager uses the indirect intervention approach as defined by Moxley (1994). Using this orientation, the case manager at AHSC focuses on "systems intervention, community gatekeepers, and social support for the clients" (p. 66). This linkage and support mission in the AHSC model promotes self-help rather than absolute control of service delivery.

Occasionally the client may not be eligible for services, if only temporarily. In these situations the case manager may assume a direct intervention approach characterized by working "directly with the client to improve skills of self-care, service acquisition, and self-monitoring" (Moxley, 1994, p. 66). These interventions may take the form of direct nursing skills, counseling, or behavioral management or caregiver support. Direct intervention is the exception within the AHSC model.

COMMUNITY PARTNERSHIP

Underlying implementation of case management is the concept of partnering with the health care consumer. Partnership is a form of communicating and relating that allows mutual respect (Newman, Lamb, & Michaels, 1990). Partnership is the opposite of domination that is seen in present society as the models of patriarchy or

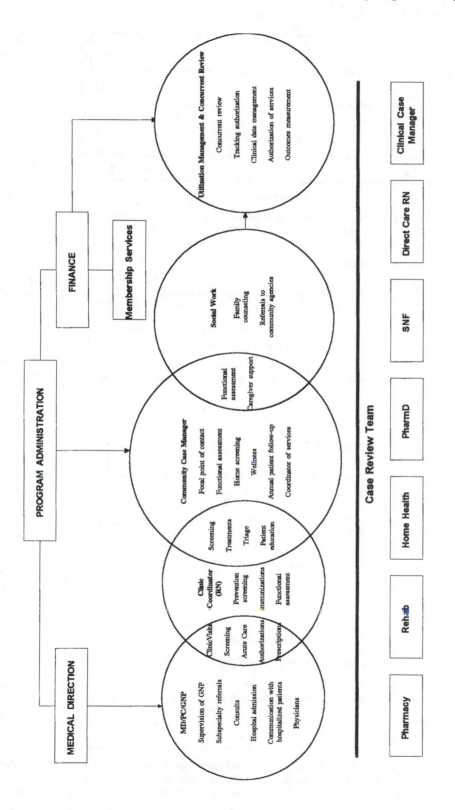

Figure 2. Community case management roles and communication. A graphic representation of the team concept related to community case management at AHSC. Courtesy of Arizona Health Sciences Center, Tucson, Arizona.

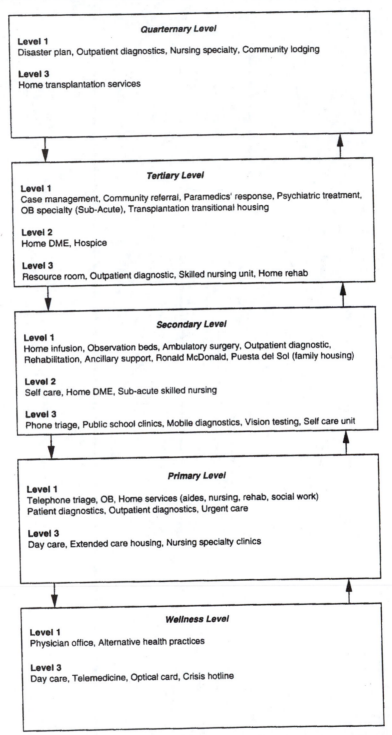

Figure 3. AHSC continuum of care model. Within the AHSC continuum of care, the individual may move through all levels of service. Health care and wellness activities can be obtained in the community, the home, the physician's office, skilled nursing facilities, or supervised homes. Courtesy of Arizona Health Sciences Center, Tucson, Arizona.

matriarchy. These dominator models that "rank" individuals are the most prevalent patterns of societal relationships. Partnership is not paternalistic but rather open to change and growth. It is a concept that links people and avoids equating diversity with either inferiority or superiority (Eisler, 1987, p. xvii). The language of each model is reflective of its relational philosophy (see box). Partnership is a process built on trust (Eisler, 1990). Applied to case management practice, this concept allows the client to determine the parameters of "normalization" to be achieved by the relationship with the health care system. This approach promotes a client choice of interaction with the environment and respect for that choice. As a professional, the case manager must advocate for these choices. The consequences of the decision may be relational, financial, or related to quality of life and must be supported nonjudgmentally by the case manager. It is this aspect of community case management that offers the foundation of all the role behaviors that define the clinical specialist.

Unique to case management is the opportunity not only to select clients, but also the decision to terminate care. Unlike Medicare guidelines that dictate the conditions in which home health nursing services can be rendered, case management is without such concrete guidelines (Newman et al., 1990). Based on the partnering concept, termination is a mutual decision, but it is based in a relationship that may be renewed as needed.

Case finding, which is a task identified by the Department of Health (DOH), occurs through the cooperative efforts of nurses along the continuum. The in-house case manager identifies high-risk patients at the time of discharge. Monitoring of the discharge plan and follow-up care becomes the responsibility of the community case manager. If brokerage for further services is needed, this again requires collaboration with the patient's community physician, as well as the utilization and service personnel. Additional services may include the following:

1. home health skilled nursing;
2. home health aides;

Key Words Comparison of the Dominator and Partnership Models

The language of the partnership and dominator models reflects the principles supporting each philosophy:

Dominator model	Partnership model
fear	trust
win/lose orientation	win/win orientation
power over	power to/with
male dominance	gender partnership
control	nurture
ranking	linking
one-sided benefit	mutual benefit
manipulation	open communication
destruction	actualization
hoarding	sharing
codependency	interdependency
left-brain thinking	whole-brain thinking
negative condition-	positive conditioning
ing	empathy with others
violence against	working in teams
others	integration
taking orders	international
alienation	partnership
nuclear arms race	peace
war	openness/
secrecy	accountability
coercion	participation
indoctrination	education
conquest of nature	respect of nature
conformity	creativity

Source: Copyright © 1990, R. Eisler and D. Loye.

---

3. adjunct therapies such as physical therapy, occupational therapy, and psychiatric counseling; or
4. social services to assist with housing, financial, and home situations.

A knowledge of the available services within the vertical corporation and the earliest entry level into the health care system is one of the most effective cost-containment tools of the case manager.

Determination of risk level is made by using the criteria of the Carondolet case management program: ". . . people who are cognitively and emotionally challenged, lacking in sufficient family support, and have a high probability for sudden physiologic imbalance" (Michaels, 1992, p. 79). Referrals are made from the community and hospital setting using these criteria of case selection.

CASE STUDY

M.J. is an example of an individual in which a change placed her at risk for sudden decline of cognitive abilities. M.J. is a 73-year-old woman with a medical history of diabetes, celiac sprew syndrome, uncontrolled hypertension, and ulcerative colitis. She has an ostomy that needs daily care. She has a psychiatric history of possible schizophrenia and anxious depression.

According to friends, M.J. was independent in her living until a recent move into the Tucson area. At that time her housing situation became acute as she realized her income would not allow her the flexibility she had enjoyed in a small, rural Arizona community. Her psychiatric disorders put her at risk, and the worry over financial matters dissolved her coping abilities. She began to obsess on these issues and was unable to move forward in her life.

M.J. was also at risk due to poor relations with her children. Although she had two daughters, she was estranged from the older one, and would not impose on the younger daughter who had children and financial worries of her own. The latter daughter had power of attorney over M.J.'s bank accounts from an out-of-state position.

At the time of referral from the clinic where M.J. had her first introductory visit with the physician, M.J. was anxious, demonstrated excessive motor activity, and was unable to focus or make decisions. Goal setting with M.J. was difficult. Given her income, her solutions were unrealistic. She was introspective enough to realize she needed supervised housing, if only temporarily, and was willing to initiate the process for state support and a locally situated fiduciary.

Since M.J. had only one contact in the community, a support system was negotiated with her. Using her religious affiliation and community resources, plus the social service staff of the institution, M.J. was linked with individuals who would be available when needed to direct her anxiety. This partnering of concerned and compassionate individuals aborted the pattern of trips to the emergency department and urgent care that had begun to emerge prior to the establishment of this support system. It also placed M.J. in control of her situation. The case manager made daily trips or phone calls to M.J., established a medication box, an event calendar for orientation, and designed a progress report, as well as coordinated physicians' visits and financial proceedings.

Although the situation has not totally been resolved at the time of this writing, M.J. has reviewed her housing options and finds them satisfactory to her life needs. Assistance will be provided in these homes until she is able to assume more responsibility for herself. Financial review is now provided locally. Family relations remain unchanged. It was a difficult process for everyone, but M.J. was given the opportunity for informed choices throughout the process and helped build her self-reliance for "right" decisions without an exaggerated dependency on her physician or other support personnel over time. The case management team, over time, developed a sensitivity to M.J.'s life patterns, which will be the basis for a more effective relationship in the future.

DETERMINING "RISK"

Another mechanism for identification of individuals at risk for decreased health maintenance (other than referral) is use of a functional/home assessment. Developed in conjunction with geriatricians and preventative health physicians, this five-page questionnaire covers support systems, finances, physical abilities, health behaviors, medications, recent health resource use, and self-health determination.

Risk determination was made using medical diagnosis, findings of the functional assessment, use of urgent care/emergency department services, and complexity of medication regimen. A home visit and further assessment by the clinical specialist was made for those identified as high-risk individuals. Questionnaires that were not returned required a follow-up phone call to determine if the person was too frail to complete the survey or without adequate resources. The home visit usually includes a physical assessment to determine the current status of the client. This baseline is essential to develop further options for early interventions and wellness behaviors. A preventative focus can also be provided by the case manager as the physical environment is reviewed, and the need for appropriate improvements (air conditioners, roof repair, or placement of safety aids) are presented and negotiated.

The functional assessment is used in conjunction with the results from the HCFA SF36 Health Status Survey to determine the total population characteristics. A clear understanding of the potential risk of the entire population enables program management to project client needs, program response, and establish productivity measures.

Experience has shown that the home visit, as conceptualized at this institution, is a critical piece of community case management. In most instances, the term *case manager* indicates an emphasis on cost-effectiveness as well as quality (Newman, Lamb, & Michaels, 1990). In either the community or in the home of the client, the focus shifts from control by the expert to building of client self-reliance and self-determination. This shift provides the client an opportunity for fiscal responsibility rather than just being viewed as a passive recipient of health care and its cost.

PULLING THE CONCEPT TOGETHER

Operationalizing the team concept at University Medical Center (UMC) is the weekly case review. This team meeting encourages exchange of information regarding clients/patients in various stages of management. Interdisciplinary representatives, including physicians, participate in this collaborative effort. Brainstorming at this time results in both innovative plans of care and identification of team responsibilities. Interventions may either be intense for crisis management or long-term and future-oriented.

Communication with the hospital staff and clinic nurses is vital to the success of case management. As the client moves along the continuum, these resources provide the case manager with an opportunity to reconnect with the client during a new phase of health service. Open communication between all points of client contact allows for continuity of care for any high-utilization population.

THE WELLNESS PERSPECTIVE

Although managed care strives for early intervention of health problems, it also is designed to encourage health maintenance behaviors. Within the AHSC model, two programs of wellness opportunities are under design. The first approach consists of the traditional combination of didactic education related to medical diagnosis. Following this presentation is group discussion and support. This component of the program is intended to focus on problem solving and sharing as it relates to the problem at hand. Practical nutrition and cooking classes are another option, as are the exercise and activity modalities that are offered. Typically, this includes mall walking, water aerobics, and other low-impact activities.

For those who are interested in alternative modalities of self-help, other options are available. This will include stress management programs, massage, therapeutic touch, Tai Chi, herbal remedies, and music therapy. This variety of self-care modalities encourages the individual to find a means by which to maintain health that is effective, pleasurable, and consistent and more integrative of the holistic mind-body-spirit healing connection.

INITIAL PROGRAM EVALUATION AND FUTURE GOALS

The initial phases of the program have met with great success for the Medicare population. The community case manager bridges the gaps in the system providing continuous quality care for the client. There has been a decline in unnecessary admissions as clients are directed to alternative services at an earlier place in their process along the health continuum. In order to evaluate ongoing success, admissions, emergency department presentations, use of pharmacy, and customer satisfaction will be monitored. These indicators will be quantified in terms of cost savings to the program and wellness behaviors of the client. Future goals include expanding the program to all populations taking into account the individual population characteristics.

•   •   •

Community case management is a new arena of practice for the CNS. In the present health care environment, the challenges of working with complex medical conditions and cost containment have been extended to the community environment. Within this setting, the CNS is able to use advanced theoretical knowledge and decision-making skills to allow client self determination within the chosen health care system. Providing that care either directly or through coordination of services requires collaborative expertise. Working with the community member to implement those services as a partner requires communication skills and implementation of the educator role of the clinical specialist. Efficient resource management when orchestrating client care uses the management and administrative skills of the CNS. Meaningful evaluation of individual client and aggregate population's utilization of service, functional status, and clinical outcomes required the CNS to use evaluation and research skills.

As a professional responding to the needs of society, there is a commitment by the CNS in community case management to fiscal responsibility combined with quality outcomes. Appropriate matching of services to the client's needs and choices is a major component of this fiscal responsibility as health care moves into the 21st century.

REFERENCES

American Nurses' Association. (1986). *Council of clinical nurse specialists: The role of the clinical nurse specialist.* Washington, DC: ANA.

Beardshaw V., & Towell, D. (1990). Assessment and case management: Implications for implementation of "caring for people." *King's Fund briefing paper, 10.* King's Fund London.

Beecroft, P., & Papenhausen, J. (1989). Who is the clinical nurse specialist? *Clinical Nurse Specialist, 3*(3). 103–104.

Bergen, A. (1992). Case management in community care: Concepts, practices, and implications for nursing. *Journal of Advanced Nursing, 17,* 106–113.

Biddle, B. J., & Thomas, E. J. (1979). *Role theory: Concepts and research.* Melbourne, FL: Krieger Publishing.

Bigbee, J.L. (1984). Territoriality and prescriptive authority for nurse practitioners. *Nursing and Healthcare, 5,* 106–110.

Boone, M., & Kikuchi, J. (1977). The clinical nurse specialist. In B. LaSor & R. Elliott (Eds.), *Issues in Canadian nursing.* Scarborough: Prentice-Hall.

Cambridge, P. (1990). Ways forward. *Community Care, 37,* 25–28.

Challis, D., Chessum, J., Chesterman, J., Luckett, R., & Traske, K. (1985). *Case management in social and healthcare: The Gateshead community care scheme.* PSSRU. University of Kent, Canterbury.

Department of Health. (1989). *Caring for people.* London, England: Author.

Eisler, R. (1987). *The chalice and the blade: Our history, our future.* San Francisco, CA: HarperCollins.

Eisler, R., & Loye, D. (1990). *The partnership way: New tools for living and learning, healing our families, our communities, and our world.* San Francisco, CA: HarperCollins.

Girouard, S. (1983). Implementing the research role. In A.B. Hamric & J.A. Spross (Eds.), *The clinical nurse specialist in theory and practice.* Philadelphia, PA: W.B. Saunders.

Hamric, A.B. (1989). History and overview of the clinical nurse specialist. In A.B. Hamric & J.A. Spross (Eds.), *The clinical nurse specialist in theory and practice.* Philadelphia, PA: W.B. Saunders.

Heine, C.A. (1988). The gerontologist nurse specialist. *Clinical Nurse Specialist, 2*(1), 6–11.

Higgins, J. M., Ponte, P., James, J., Fay, M., & Madden, M. J. (1994). Restructuring the CNS role for a managed care environment. *Clinical Specialist, 8*(3), 163–166.

Hodgman, E. C. (1983). The CNS as researcher. In A. Hamric & J. Spross (Eds.), *The clinical nurse specialist in theory and practice.* New York, NY: Grune & Stratton.

Holt, F. M. (1990). Managed care and the clinical nurse specialist. *Clinical Nurse Specialist, 4*(1), 27–32.

Larson, M. S. (1977). *The rise of professionalism: A sociological analysis.* Berkeley, CA: University of California Press.

Lyon, J. C. (1993). Models of nursing care delivery and case management: Clarification of terms. *Nursing Economics, 11*(3), 163–169.

Mahn, V. (1993). Clinical nurse case management: A service line approach. *Nursing Management, 24*(9), 48–50.

Mason, D. J., et al. (1992). Promoting the community health clinical specialist. *Clinical Specialist, 6*(1), 6–13.

Meisler, N., & Midyette, P. (1994). CNS to case manager: Broadening the scope. *Nursing Management, 25*(11), 44–46.

Michaels, C. (1992). Carondelet St. Mary's nursing enterprise. *Nursing Clinics of North America, 27*(1), 77–85.

Montemuro, M. A. (1987). The evolution of the clinical nurse specialist: Response to the challenge of professional nursing practice. *Clinical Nurse Specialist, 1*(3), 106–110.

Moxley, D. P. (1994). Outpatient program development. In M. R. Donovan, & T. A. Matson (Eds.), *Outpatient case management: Strategies for a new reality.* Chicago, IL: American Hospital Publishing.

Newman, M., Lamb, G., & Michaels, C. (1990). Nurse case management: The coming together of theory and practice. *Nursing and Healthcare, 12*(8), 404–408.

O'Rouke, M. W. (1989). Generic professional behaviors for the clinical nurse specialist. *Clinical Nurse Specialist, 3*(3), 128–132.

Pinkerton, S. (1978). Administrative support for the clinical specialist organizationally placed in the C.E. department. *Nursing Administration Quarterly, 2,* 53–58.

Robichaud, A., & Hamric, A. B. (1986). Time documentation of clinical nurse specialist activities. *The Journal of Nursing Administration, 16,* 31–36.

Rogers, M., Riordan, J., & Swindle, D. (1991). Community-based nursing case management pays off. *Nursing Management, 22*(3), 30–34.

Schaffer, C. (1994). A new era for case management. *Continuing Care* (June), 20–23.

Schull, D. E., Tosch, P., & Wood, M. (1992). Clinical nurse specialists as collaborative case managers. *Nursing Management, 23*(3), 30–33.

Sills, G. (1983). The role and function of the clinical nurse specialist. In N. L. Chaske (Ed.), *The nursing profession: A time to speak.* New York, NY: McGraw-Hill.

Thornicroft, G. (1991). The concept of case management for long term mental illness. *International Review of Psychiatry, 3,* 125–132.

Worley, N. (1991). Advisor to the team. *Nursing Times, 87*(33), 38–40.

Yokes, J. A. (1966). The clinical nurse specialist in cardiovascular nursing. *American Journal of Nursing, 66,* 2,667–2,670.

Case Management as a Mindset

Gloria G. Mayer

The term *case management* has traditionally been associated with the insurance industry, in particular, with the rehabilitation model used in dealing with long-term workers' compensation cases. More recently, case management and managed care have been linked together. In the hospital, case management and critical paths are complementary, and on the ambulatory care side, the case management process has been associated with the care of the frail elderly and the chronically disabled. However, there has been very little written about case management practiced on all patients, in all environments, and as a philosophic mindset of patient care delivery.

Case management, perhaps partly because it has been used to respond to a whole range of problems, including poor provider coordination, inflexible benefits, lack of use of alternative care models, fragmentation of services, costly service duplication, and disorganization of complicated health care problems, has been given many definitions. White, for example, defined case management as "a service function directed at coordinating existing resources to assure appropriate and continuous care for individuals on a case-by-case basis."[1] According to her, case management

- is individualized,
- is holistic,
- enhances self-care and self-determination,
- provides continuity of appropriate care,

- maximizes independence through enhancing functional capacity,
- utilizes a wide range of services, and
- coordinates existing resources.

The focus of case management is the organization and sequencing of services and resources to respond to an individual's health care problem.[2]

The goals of the case management process are based on the individual needs of the patient. In general, however, case management should

- ensure continuity of care between all continuum points of care;
- provide early detection and intervention;
- improve and facilitate interdisciplinary communication and care planning;
- organize, delineate, and plan for complex multiple problems;
- utilize and cooperate with existing services to best meet the needs of patients;
- help strengthen the alliance between families and professional health providers;
- maximize the health of patients by increasing social support and health education;
- identify problems and needs and seek solutions through appropriate high-quality care;
- improve patient and caregiver satisfaction with the care provided and the care delivery system;
- coordinate the delivery of care;
- deliver cost-effective, high-quality care; and
- enhance independent living capability and maximize the quality of life of patients.

Quality Management in Health Care 1996; 5(1): 7–16
© 1996 Aspen Publishers, Inc.

Knollmeuller has reviewed the literature on case management and has identified seven models of case management[3]:

1. single-entry model (used in delivering institutional, ambulatory, and in-home services to elderly clients),
2. nursing center model,
3. health maintenance organization model,
4. public health model,
5. acute care model,
6. hospital-based model, and
7. preadmission certification model

Although these models are motivated by different objectives, in all of them the case manager is the coordinator of care and is responsible for patient outcomes. In the Friendly Hills HealthCare Network model, all providers and caregivers are responsible for coordination of care and the movement of patients through the various levels of care. The levels of care are called continuum points, and there are specific tools that assist the caregiver at each point. The continuum points and tools used are described in the following sections.

THE FRIENDLY HILLS HEALTHCARE NETWORK MODEL

The Friendly Hills HealthCare Network is a physician organization that services over 400,000 capitated lives in southern California. It is a fully integrated delivery system and has

- a 274-bed acute care hospital (Friendly Hills Regional Medical Center),
- 45 regional medical officers,
- 483 providers,
- 383 physicians (63 percent are primary care physicians),
- 100 allied health professionals,
- 4,000 employees,
- multiple outpatient pharmacy and vision service centers,
- an ambulatory surgery center,
- a hemodialysis center, and
- an imaging center (including magnetic resonance imaging [MRI]).

It contracts with 25 health maintenance organizations (HMOs), has 43 capitated contracts, and 95 percent of its gross revenues come from global capitation. It has 410,000 capitated members, including

- 280,000 commercial members,
- 100,000 Medi-Cal (Medicaid) members,
- 23,000 senior members, and
- 7,000 point-of-service (POS) members.

It is an affiliate of Caremark-Physician Resources Division, which was recently purchased by MedPartners IPA Networks.

Since Friendly Hills HealthCare Network receives global capitation for most of its patients and is responsible for all services provided, including all the health care venues, a philosophy of case management was adopted for all patients. Seven patient care continuum points (Figure 1) are the basis of the network's model, and no one is ever discharged from the system (every patient just accesses care along the continuum). The role of the caregiver is to identify which continuum point the patient has come from and which continuum point is currently most appropriate and to facilitate movement to that point. The seven continuum points are these:

1. primary preventive care,
2. ambulatory care,
3. acute care,
4. tertiary care,
5. home care,
6. long-term care, and
7. hospice care.

Patients access health care based on their individual needs and on the level of care required. There are clinical tools available at each continuum point that facilitate and coordinate care, and each continuum point has linkages to the other points of care. Examples of the types of care and tools are as follows.

Primary preventive care

This continuum point stresses prevention and includes

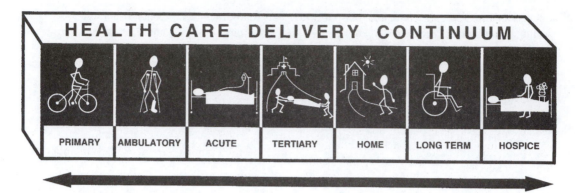

Figure 1. Friendly Hills Healthcare Network's seven continuum points.

- opportunities for education,
- screening for risk, and
- prevention of disease.

Patients at this point may have occasional contacts with a health care provider and routine follow-up care. Tools that are available at this point include

- general health education classes,
- prenatal care,
- smoking cessation classes,
- a cancer follow-up clinic,
- a cholesterol clinic,
- nutrition counseling,
- a flu shot clinic,
- health fairs,
- pharmacy reviews of current drugs,
- well-baby examinations,
- mammography,
- routine physicals,
- a caring for the caregiver class, and
- a telephone advice system.

Ambulatory care

This continuum point focuses on diagnosis and treatment in the ambulatory setting and includes the typical visit to the doctor for a specific health problem. Included in this point of care may be initial treatment and regular visits and management to control a chronic problem. Tools and resources for this access point include

- a posthospitalization follow-up clinic,
- a Coumadin clinic,
- a wound management clinic,
- community resource referrals,
- a cast clinic,
- a diabetic clinic,
- cardiac rehabilitation, and
- an asthma clinic for kids.

Acute care

This point of care is represented by a medical crisis that requires hospitalization, such as an acute myocardial infarction. Patients are managed through a multidisciplinary team approach. The main goal here is to manage care through very active case management and move the patient to the next point on the continuum. Tools used to move the patient along include

- active discharge planning,
- team meetings,
- critical paths (MAPS),
- social services,
- ethical case reviews,
- a chaplain program,
- patient and family education, and
- nutrition counseling.

Tertiary care

At the fourth continuum point, patients experience a complex, life-threatening condition that requires specialized care given at a tertiary care facility or a regional "center of excellence." Patients who may require this type of service include newborns who need a Level III neonatal intensive care unit and patients undergoing cardiovascular bypass surgery, neurosurgery, or complicated cancer surgery. A clinical nurse specialist follows each patient and coordinates all care. It may be this nurse who, in collaboration with the physician, moves the patient to the next most appropriate continuum point. Tools needed at this point include

- a condition-based provider network,
- patient care tracking systems,
- follow-up clinics,
- coordination of posthospitalization care,
- systems for communicating between centers,
- outreach education programs, and
- transportation systems.

Home care

This point of care encompasses the independent or semi-independent phase of an episode of illness. Care at home can be managed by the patient or family with or without supervision. The patients at this point may have a chronic illness such as diabetes or hypertension or continuing disabilities such as blindness. Tools needed here include

- community resources and referrals,
- health education,
- telephone follow-up,
- home health providers, and
- periodic provider home visits.

Long-term care

Long-term care is characterized by increasing disability or fluctuation of condition needing observation and care but not hospitalization. Nursing homes or rehabilitation centers are used for continued rehabilitation postacute phase, for prolonged recovery of more common conditions, or for any deficit in self-care requiring assistance. Tools needed here include

- a network of long-term institutions,
- community resource referrals,
- geriatric nurse practitioners,
- a transportation system,
- ethical case reviews,
- advanced directives,
- physical and occupational therapy and other special therapy, and
- a caregiver support group.

Hospice

The seventh continuum point is the period of time consisting of the weeks or days immediately preceding death. This level of care is created specifically for patients who are terminally ill and need palliative care. The hospice care planning is individualized for each patient and family as death approaches. Tools needed include

- social services,
- pain management programs,
- chaplain programs,
- a caregiver support program, and
- advanced directives.

All of the professional staff at Friendly Hills HealthCare Network understand the seven continuum points of care and understand the patient care management issues that arise in moving patients from point to point. Since the network never discharges any patient from the system, it needs to case manage each patient and attempt to place the patient at the most appropriate point of care.

SPECIALTY CASE MANAGEMENT

Complicated patients who require services across two or more continuum points frequently get lost in the system or find navigation of the many points of care difficult. For this type of patient, case managers with advanced degrees in a particular area are utilized to intensively case manage the patient and family. The goals of specialty case management are to

- optimize patients' self-care abilities,
- enhance quality of life or adjustment to an altered health status,

- prevent unnecessary rehospitalization and duplication of efforts,
- provide high-quality health care and decrease fragmentation across settings, and
- promote cost containment.

The specialty case manager's interventions include

- advanced physical, psychosocial, and cultural assessments;
- assessments of care being received and analyses of alternatives;
- goal setting performed in conjunction with patients, families, and other members of the health care team; and
- the provision of private as well as community resources.

The specialty case managers have master's degrees in cardiopulmonary, oncology, maternal and child health, or nephrology. We have five clinical nurse specialists, and they each have two to three RN assistants. These assistants are trained in utilization management, HMO benefit design, case management, and patient relations. They are also very knowledgeable about community resources and assist the clinical nurse specialists in a variety of ways, including follow-up of a care plan. The case management team's (clinical nurse specialist and assistants) caseloads average 5–40 patients, depending on the intensity of case coordination and the patients' individual needs. For example, a neonate may require long-term case management whereas a patient who undergoes bypass surgery may need intensive case management for only a short period of time. Therefore, it is difficult to dictate a specific caseload. Factors that affect the productivity of the case managers include the

- complexity of the patient assessment,
- complexity of care,
- duration of intensive case management,
- potential for telephonic case management,
- geographic location of patients,
- type of facilities where patients reside if outside of home (e.g., board and care, long-term care center, rehabilitation center),

- family participation in care,
- support services needed by patients,
- management information systems available to case managers,
- clerical support available, and
- technical support available.

CASE IDENTIFICATION

Patients may be selected for specialty case management by several methods. In the ambulatory setting, the following utilization-based criteria may be used:

- frequent and inappropriate office visits,
- numerous no-shows and cancellations,
- complicated chronic medical conditions requiring complex treatment arrangements,
- noncompliance with treatment,
- use and abuse of multiple medications,
- chronic use of the emergency department or urgent care,
- high risk of ambulance use, 911 calls, or hospitalization,
- misunderstanding of the managed care system, and
- chemical misuse.

Possible demographic or social criteria include these:

- old age–related frailty,
- disability,
- difficult living arrangements or limited financial resources,
- limited or lack of informal support system,
- limited cognitive capacity, and
- sensory impairment.

Any new patient who has been hospitalized in the past three months is a candidate for intensive case management. Figure 2 lists questions that may be useful in identifying high-risk patients that could benefit from case management.

There are other specific criteria for each type of patient (e.g., see the box entitled "Case Management Criteria for Maternal and Child Health"). However, each medical group or hospital has to define its own criteria for case man-

Does the patient live alone?	Yes	No
Does the patient take five or more medications?	Yes	No
Is there anyone capable and/or available to care for the patient if he/she becomes sick/injured?	Yes	No
Does the patient have difficulty controlling bladder and/or bowel functions on a daily basis?	Yes	No
Does the patient have episodes of any of the following: disorientation, confusion, wandering, impaired decision making?	Yes	No
Does the patient walk only with assistance or is he/she unable to walk?	Yes	No
Does the patient have multiple illnesses or disabilities that require regular medical care?	Yes	No
Does the patient have difficulty accomplishing activities of daily living, such as meal preparation, housework, bathing, etc.?	Yes	No
Has the patient been hospitalized in the past three months?	Yes	No

Figure 2. Questionnaire used to identify high-risk elderly patients. Reprinted with permission from the Center for Research in Ambulatory Health Care Administration, 104 Inverness Terrace East, Englewood, Colorado 80112-5306; 303-799-1111. Copyright 1990.

---

agement. For example, if a hospital is only responsible for care in the hospital, ambulatory identification of potential patients for case management would be of little concern. On the other hand, case rates or diagnosis-related group (DRG) reimbursement motivate institutions to perform aggressive case management. Again, if a group is responsible for pharmacy manage-

ment, use of multiple medications becomes a criteria for case management.

Identification of a patient needing case management can come from any caregiver in the system, but typically patients in high-risk groups are considered the prime candidates (see box entitled "Hospital Criteria for Identifying Patients in High-Risk Groups").

Case Management Criteria for Maternal and Child Health

- Patients with three or more acute and/or tertiary care admissions in one year for the same diagnosis.
- All tertiary care center high-risk obstetrics and neonatal intensive care unit admissions or transfers.
- Infants and children sent home with more than one home health nursing visit, oxygen, complex infusion therapy, or ventilator.
- Any child referred for or a recipient of an organ transplant or cardiovascular surgery.
- A chronically ill child with involvement of multiple systems and/or a need for multiple services.

- Pediatric patients seen in the emergency department or urgent care once per month or more frequently with the same symptoms or diagnosis.
- Pregnant patients seen in the emergency department, urgent care, or labor and delivery once per month or more frequently with the same symptoms or diagnosis.
- Pregnant patients receiving home uterine monitoring.
- Patients readmitted to acute care within one month of previous discharge.
- Patients with two or more specialty referrals to tertiary center ambulatory care services.

Hospital Criteria for Identifying Patients in High-Risk Groups[1]

1. Age
   - Seventy years of age or older, living alone or with a non-capable caregiver
   - Under age 18—suspected abuse, neglect
   - Mentally retarded, regardless of age
   - Individuals of all ages who are admitted from or anticipate being transferred to nursing homes, residential care homes, or specialty hospitals
   - Pregnant minors (under 16 or as defined by local government)
2. Residence
   - Any person admitted who does not reside in the area normally served by the hospital and who may need follow-up treatment and care
   - Transfers from other facilities
   - Unclear or no known place of residence ("street people," indigent, abandoned)
3. Behavioral factors
   - History of noncompliance with health care plan
   - Re-admissions (within 15 days, 30 days, 60 days)
   - Attempted suicide/suicidal tendencies
   - Possible or active substance abuse (alcohol, chemical)
   - Manipulative, aggressive, or other behavioral problems
4. Social/family
   - No identification—John/Jane Doe
   - No next of kin and/or guardianship need
   - Interfamily problems
   - No known social support system
   - Domestic violence
   - Spiritual distress
5. Medical
   - Multiple trauma
   - Head and spinal cord injury
   - Handicapped—visual, hearing, paralysis, and other progressive degenerative or debilitating conditions
   - Chronic conditions—COPD, CHF, CVA, or any condition that may impair body function and growth
   - Abuse—physical, psychological, failure to thrive
   - All psychiatric patients
   - History of multiple hospitalizations within a short period of time
   - Joint replacement
   - Terminal illness
   - AIDS
   - Patients taking multiple medications (OTC and prescription)
   - Obstetrics—high-risk or complicated pregnancy, single parent, minor, adoption
   - Nutritional problems—TPN, anorexia
   - High technology—ventilators, apnea monitors
   - Transplants—immunosuppressant therapy
6. Nursing care/social service
   - Patients in need of follow-up treatment, teaching, and/or referral to other agencies (home care, day care)
   - Patients with inadequate financial resources
   - Patients being currently serviced by other agencies
   - Patients who may require special equipment in the home (durable medical equipment)
   - Patients with changes in body image (stoma, plastic repair, burn)
   - Patients with cognitive deficiencies
   - Patients requiring supportive care—transportation, housekeeping, shopping, laundry

Source: Reprinted with permission from E.G. Hartigan, Discharge Planning: Identification of High-Risk Groups, *Nursing Management,* Vol. 18, No. 12, pp. 30–32, © 1987, Springhouse Corporation.

In collaboration with other team members, the specialty case manager coordinates the plan of care, monitors patient outcomes, and communicates changes in the patient's condition. Although all providers at Friendly Hills Health-Care Network are considered case managers, the advanced skill of the specialty case managers allows them to handle the complex needs of complex patients. The network must support this type of case management by empowering the case managers to expedite treatment using the most appropriate treatment options available. It is at this level that additional health care benefits may be needed to reduce the total cost of caring for the patient. The decision flowchart (Figure 3) provides the specialty case manager with the control needed to truly case manage. For example, suppose a patient is at high risk for falling but does not have durable medical equipment as a benefit. In this case, it may be more cost-effective to give the patient a $35 walker rather than wait for a fall, a broken hip, and an emergency department visit. Of course, if the specialty case manager can get the walker paid for or donated, that would be preferable. However, it is important to view the patient as our patient for life, and preventive measures today pay for themselves in the future.

To understand the case management process more fully, consider a patient who has had a coronary artery bypass graft (CABG) and experienced many of the continuum points. Goals

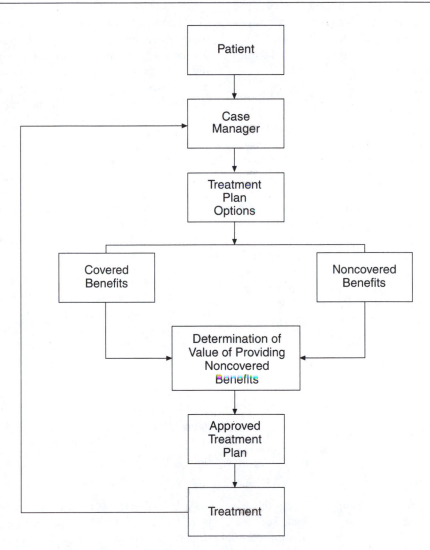

Figure 3. Case management decision flowchart.

and outcomes are defined, and specific tools are available to assist the patient at each continuum point. (The case manager who has a master's in cardiopulmonary disease designed this process and is ultimately responsible for ensuring the patient achieves the desired outcome with the help of the case management assistants.)

The case manager is called to help the patient in the primary and ambulatory setting when the patient is identified as needing a CABG. The patient and family are thoroughly prepared for the bypass surgery and are encouraged to attend several educational programs prior to surgery. The administrative procedures are completed and exact details are reviewed with the patient.

Goals and outcomes for the patient and family at this point include these:

- The patient and family are oriented to the plan of care.
- The authorization process is completed in a timely manner.
- Cost-effectiveness is optimized by reducing duplication of services by different institutions.
- Quality of care is enhanced by accurately assessing patient and family needs and providing required resources.
- The patient and family are educated regarding surgical and postoperative expectations.
- A plan of care is instituted to optimize the patient's movement through preoperative, operative, and postoperative processes.

In the tertiary care setting, the patient's goals are

- a six-day length of stay,
- discharge to home without delays or difficulty,
- no postoperative complications,
- patient and family satisfaction with care, and
- no duplication of services.

At this point, the case manager may visit the patient at the tertiary care center to make sure the plan of care is being followed, to continue to prepare for discharge if needed, and to coordinate communication with all the caregivers across the continuum.

After discharge, the patient should be able to

- optimize self-care at home,
- attain an adequate understanding of the medication regimen and follow-up instructions,
- return to work or to the level of functioning that existed prior to the acute illness, and
- utilize appropriate resources as needs arise.

The case manager coordinates ambulatory care visits, assists in communication between the surgical team and the cardiologist, visits the patient as needed, keeps in contact with the patient telephonically on an ongoing basis, and assists in the timely transition from home health services to outpatient visits. The case manager is a general problem-solver and assists the patient and family throughout the transition period.

Follow-up goals include

- a reduction of cardiac risk factors,
- an increase in confidence in managing the condition,
- an increase in the patient's coping skills, and
- a successful transition back to the primary continuum point of care.

Again, the case manager assists the patient and the family by general counseling, meeting the patient at the ambulatory visits to assess progress, reviewing lab and X-ray data, and encouraging the patient to attend the "Coping with Cardiac Disease" classes. A summary of the patient flow through the continuum is contained in Figure 4.

This program, like others that follow the same patient throughout the continuum, appears to result in more favorable patient outcomes and higher patient satisfaction at a reduced cost.

•   •   •

At Friendly Hills HealthCare Network, each provider is considered a case manager utilizing its seven continuum points as a model of patient care and patient flow. The object is to consider

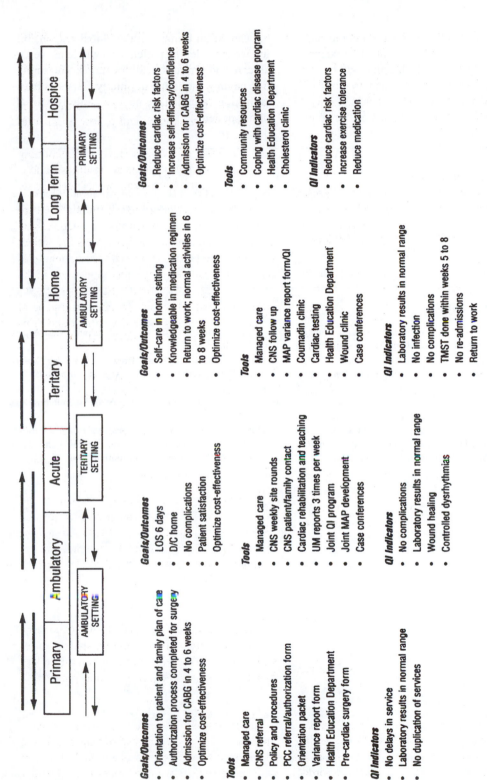

Primary	Ambulatory	Acute	Teritary	Home	Long Term	Hospice

AMBULATORY SETTING	TERTIARY SETTING	AMBULATORY SETTING	PRIMARY SETTING

Goals/Outcomes
- Orientation to patient and family plan of care
- Authorization process completed for surgery
- Admission for CABG in 4 to 6 weeks
- Optimize cost-effectiveness

Tools
- Managed care
- CNS referral
- Policy and procedures
- PCC referral/authorization form
- Orientation packet
- Variance report form
- Health Education Department
- Pre-cardiac surgery form

QI Indicators
- No delays in service
- Laboratory results in normal range
- No duplication of services

Goals/Outcomes
- LOS 6 days
- D/C home
- No complications
- Patient satisfaction
- Optimize cost-effectiveness

Tools
- Managed care
- CNS weekly site rounds
- CNS patient/family contact
- Cardiac rehabilitation and teaching
- UM reports 3 times per week
- Joint QI program
- Joint MAP development
- Case conferences

QI Indicators
- No complications
- Laboratory results in normal range
- Wound healing
- Controlled dysrhythmias

Goals/Outcomes
- Self-care in home setting
- Knowledgeable in medication regimen
- Return to work; normal activities in 6 to 8 weeks
- Optimize cost-effectiveness

Tools
- Managed care
- CNS follow up
- MAP variance report form/QI
- Coumadin clinic
- Cardiac testing
- Health Education Department
- Wound clinic
- Case conferences

QI Indicators
- Laboratory results in normal range
- No infection
- No complications
- TMST done within weeks 5 to 8
- No re-admissions
- Return to work

Goals/Outcomes
- Reduce cardiac risk factors
- Increase self-efficacy/confidence
- Admission for CABG in 4 to 6 weeks
- Optimize cost-effectiveness

Tools
- Community resources
- Coping with cardiac disease program
- Health Education Department
- Cholesterol clinic

QI Indicators
- Reduce cardiac risk factors
- Increase exercise tolerance
- Reduce medication

Figure 4. Case management goals and outcomes, tools, and quality improvement indicators for elective coronary artery bypass surgery. Note: CABG = coronary artery bypass graft, LOS = length of stay, D/C = discharge, CNS = clinical nurse specialist, PCC = patient care committee, UM = utilization management, QI = quality improvement, TMST = treadmill stress test. *Source:* Reprinted from A. Jacoby et al., Patient Management Systems: Use of Clinical Nurse Specialists as Advanced Case Managers in an Integrated Health Care Delivery System, in *Making Capitation Work*, G.G. Mayer, A.E. Barnett, and N.P. Brown, eds., © 1995, Aspen Publishers, Inc.

the total episode of care as the outcome rather than one or two continuum points. For example, if another day or two in the hospital will result in a discharge to home rather than to a nursing home, we would advocate the added stay to avoid the additional patient transfer. Since global capitation brings with it global responsibility, we consider the patient as a whole as well as all care and services in all locations. The capitation payment structure definitely assists us in establishing case management as a mindset for all of our patients.

REFERENCES

1. White, M. "Case Management." In *The Encyclopedia of Aging,* edited by G.L. Maddox. New York, N.Y.: Springer, 1986.

2. Merrill, J. "Defining Case Management." *Business and Health,* July-August 1985, pp. 5–9.

3. Knollmeuller, R.N. "Case Management: What's in a Name?" *Nursing Management* 20, no. 10 (1989): 38–42.

SUGGESTED READINGS

Barnett, A.E., and Mayer, G.G. *Ambulatory Care Management and Practice.* Gaithersburg, Md.: Aspen Publishers, 1992.

Hartigan, E.G. "Discharge Planning: Identification of High-Risk Groups." *Nursing Management* 18, no. 12 (1987): 30–32.

Jacoby, A., et al. "Patient Management Systems: Use of Clinical Nurse Specialists as Advanced Case Managers in an Integrated Health Care Delivery System." In *Making Capitation Work,* edited by G.G. Mayer, A.E. Barnett, and N.P. Brown. Gaithersburg, Md.: Aspen Publishers, 1995.

Mayer, G.G., Barnett, A.E., and Brown, N.P. *Making Capitation Work.* Gaithersburg, Md.: Aspen Publishers, 1995.

Mayer, G.G., Madden, M.J., and Lawrenz, E. *Patient Care Delivery Models.* Gaithersburg, Md.: Aspen Publishers, 1990.

Schraeder, C., et al. *Case Management in Primary Care: A Manual.* Englewood, Colo.: Center for Research in Ambulatory Health Care Administration, 1990.

Components of a Successful Case Management Program

Sherry L. Aliotta

Case management is one of the most touted interventions in the health care industry, with many managed care organizations scrambling to implement such programs within their systems.

A recent study indicates that, of those HMOs surveyed, 86 percent are planning to implement or expand their case management programs.[1] However, the study also indicates that these decisions have been reached without the benefit of meaningful information to validate the financial and outcomes impacts of such programs.

FHP, Inc., is a large staff, IPA, and mixed model HMO. FHP/Quality Continuum was the subsidiary that housed the organization's case management operations. Using experience gained from being director of case management operations in FHP/Quality Continuum, and as a consultant in evaluating and assisting HMOs in implementing case management programs, the author has found that health care organizations can implement a successful program by following these basic steps:

- Define case management and organizational goals.
- Assess organizational strengths and capacities.
- Identify, assess, and select patient cases.
- Create, monitor, and evaluate outcome measures.

Managed Care Quarterly 1996; 4(2): 38–45

DEFINING CASE MANAGEMENT AND ORGANIZATIONAL GOALS

Case management is defined as "a collaborative process which assesses, plans, implements, coordinates, monitors, and evaluates options and services to meet an individual's health needs through communication and available resources to promote quality, cost-effective outcomes."[2]

Through case management, an organization can ensure that health care services are available to meet the needs of its population. The primary focus is a coordinated dialogue between providers and patients to help guide patients through a continuum of services, rather than to "compartmentalize" their care.

Many people erroneously classify programs that are primarily utilization review/management programs as case management programs. However, there are many inherent differences between the two (Table 1).

Unlike case management, traditional utilization management models are designed primarily to control costs, ensure medical necessity, and identify trends. Moreover, traditional utilization management places an undue emphasis on acute care episodes where reducing length of stay and effective discharge planning are remaining options.

Using the case management, or more active approach, an organization stands the greatest chance of improving quality and reducing overall costs because of its focus on early intervention and emphasis on a continuum of care. The goal of this

Table 1 Case Management and Utilization Management Comparison

Case management (Proactive)	Utilization management (Reactive)
Meant to be actively identifying patients at risk for exacerbation of chronic illness and intervening in a manner that has a positive effect on the outcome.	The patient presents for service. At this point there is already an illness or perception of illness. The only decision is how to treat the illness.
Focuses on the continuum of care (ideally from enrollment).	Focuses on the episode of illness.
Focuses on a small number of patients at a high level of intensity.	Focuses on a large number of patients at a low level of intensity.
Focuses on medically appropriate care.	Use of prior authorization and concurrent review to evaluate medical necessity.

approach is to maintain the patient at the most appropriate level of care—preferably as far left on the continuum as possible (Figure 1).

The first step in implementing a case management program involves creating a case management definition such as that noted above and establishing program goals that fit the health plan's philosophy of care and expected outcomes. For instance, a health plan may decide its goals for a particular program or group of patients are lowering admission rates, improving clinical outcomes, reducing cost of care, or improving satisfaction. Whatever an organization's goals, they should reflect that plan's culture and philosophy of care. Moreover, senior management should be apprised of these efforts and its support sought.

In a well-structured case management program, case managers oversee this continuum, and seek to intervene early to prevent a patient's condition from progressing in severity by placing the patient in alternative settings, where appropriate. They also follow a low volume of patients at a high level of intensity. They often have contact with these patients several times per day, gaining familiarity with the patient's medical, social, and overall course of care. This approach shifts the emphasis from site of care to the patient's health care needs. Some advances, including those in home care, have increased the amount and type of services that can be safely provided in the home.

ASSESSING ORGANIZATIONAL STRENGTHS AND CAPACITIES

Many organizations have the proper resources already in place to launch a case management program, but need assistance in properly allocating them. A health plan should examine its existing utilization and case management capacities to uncover strong and weak areas. Depending on the plan's internal capacity to conduct such a review, having an independent consultant conduct an analysis is another option that could save the plan dollars and time.

The organizational assessment should focus on several key capacities: a health plan's relations with its providers; its staff, and staff training and recruitment efforts; data availability; and plan incentives. All these areas will play a role in how a plan designs its case management program.

Provider relations

A major part of the success of this effort is the relationship between the health plan and its providers. Because different providers have different relationships, models and focus vary with organizations. The case management model is most effective when it addresses the organization's quality and cost issues. For example, a medical group usually has complete control of ambulatory cost and quality, which has an impact on overall care.

Many case management programs are planned to operate independently of the physi-

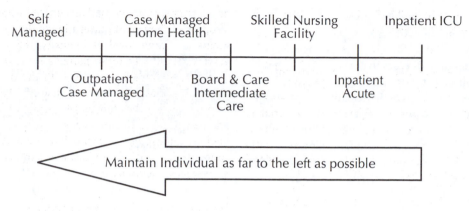

Figure 1. Continuum of care.

cian team, which in many cases ends up alienating the very physician group and clinicians needed to achieve the case management program's goals. At FHP/Quality Continuum, managers avoided this scenario by enhancing the newly launched Primary Care Delivery System (PCDS). The PCDS is a system of care that allows patients to select their own primary care physician, and the patient and physician work together as a team to meet the patient's health care needs.

Each case management approach is designed to maximize the relationship between patient and physician, and support the physician in managing a complex panel of patients. This commitment to partnership with the physician has been successful. In a recent survey, 93 percent of FHP physicians responded that case management was of value to them in their practice. The physicians also gave high marks to the collaborative role of the case manager and the long-term health maintenance approach of case managers.

Staffing and training

Sufficient resources are necessary to implement a case management program. This may sound obvious; however, many organizations expect to achieve monumental results without investing resources, such as staff, staff training, time, and equipment. A defined plan for such investments and criteria aid this effort—and this investment does not always need to cost money. Sometimes it just means using some creativity to make the most out of current resources, including human resources. For instance, rather than insisting that all of the registered nurses (RNs) hired have previous case management experience, FHP/Quality Continuum made a decision to accept RNs who may require training in case management. Since case management was a new concept within the organization, this allowed FHP to retain RNs that were employed by FHP, but lacked case management experience.

This decision also allowed the plan to use the strong pool of internal talent within the organization and maximize the knowledge of FHP systems this group possessed. Furthermore, these characteristics were identified as those that contributed to success as a case manager: creativity; flexibility; knowledge of community and company resources; prior nursing experience; and organizational, interpersonal, and problem-solving skills.

Once a part of the organization, the case manager must be supported with adequate training and job orientation. Even an experienced case manager benefits from an educational program that outlines the company's approach to case management. A comprehensive presentation of the company's case management philosophy and practice provides the new case managers with a common frame of reference. At FHP/ Quality Continuum, an eight-hour course was created that all new case managers are required to take, regardless of prior experience.

One of the most common questions concerns the proper ratio of cases to case manager, yet this ratio will vary according to each organization's needs. At the FHP/Quality Continuum program, the ratio is 45 cases to one case manager in the ambulatory care program, and 25–30:1 for the catastrophic program. Human resources will typically be an organization's largest investment as qualified staff are essential to the success of the program.

Data availability

The availability of data will drive the design of a successful case management model; thus, data systems must be established at the onset of the program. The data collected must be consistent with the goals and objectives of the program. Currently available data are a logical starting point. There are several essential data elements an organization must have available (see box). The extent to which each item is significant will depend on the organization's goals for case management. For example, if a health plan's goal is to reduce readmissions for the same or related diagnosis, then a plan will want detailed data on the frequency for the same or related diagnosis. However, if a plan aims to reduce admission rates for a particular group of patients, plan managers should be able to readily access data on current admission rates.

Many companies undertake massive vendor searches to meet their data needs without a real understanding of those needs. FHP/Quality Continuum's initial case management data capture system was a modified Paradox database. The system modifications continued as the program evolved and requirements were defined. Finally, an internally developed system was necessary to meet the expanded data needs. Many vendors were invited to submit proposals and stage demonstrations; however, none of the systems was adequate to meet the program needs. Because of FHP's initial approach to data management, staff were aware of their requirements, which enabled the plan to make the appropriate decisions.

Essential Data Elements

Demographics (e.g., age, sex)

	Diagnostic data
Utilization data (e.g., acute care days, skilled care days, office visits, home health visits)	Cost data (e.g., services unit or per diem costs of care)
Program data (e.g., referral source and reason, number of patients followed by CM)	Outcome data (e.g., clinical and financial)
Activity data (e.g., types, frequency, duration of case management activities)	Cost data (e.g., program cost, unit and aggregate)
Pharmacy data (e.g., medication usage)	Narrative data (e.g., patient level documentation)

Defining report requirements can be a complicated process. The program definition and goals will provide assistance in developing reporting guidelines. Traditional report questions must first be answered. What information is needed and who needs it? When is it needed? Where is the information available? How should it be transmitted? Who will interpret the reports and how can staff be trained to do so? In FHP's case, reporting has helped the organization identify and correct various problems and document its successes. Reporting must be a focus of continuous quality improvement.

Depending on the health plan's data availability, some organizations may need to purchase or design additional, more sophisticated data systems. Basic data systems can be developed with minimal investment to support early case management efforts while the organization more fully assesses its needs.

Financial incentives

While the case management model presented in this article (and the experiences of FHP/Quality Continuum, which uses this model) can be applied in virtually every setting, the degree to which it is effective and the way it is carried out may vary. The model is most effective when the organization's desired outcome is to reduce the number of hospital admissions and length of stay by use of outpatient and ancillary services. Despite financial incentives, the quality of care improvements make a case management program a worthwhile investment.

IDENTIFYING, ASSESSING, AND SELECTING PATIENT CASES

In order to be effective, case management must be proactive in its approach to patient care by defining the populations it will serve using statistics gleaned in the early planning phase. Once the population has been defined, individual members of that population must be selected and assessed for the appropriateness of case management intervention.

One of FHP/Quality Continuum's target populations was a group defined as "frail elderly." Characteristics of the population were developed such as age, numbers of chronic illnesses, and numbers of medications. FHP created systems that would assist in identifying members consistent with this profile for further review. One method used is the Health Assessment Questionnaire (HAQ), which is sent to new senior enrollees for FHP coverage. The returned HAQ is reviewed by a case manager to screen for high-risk indicators, and the appropriate follow-up is conducted. This procedure is being revised to incorporate a computer scored algorithm that will enhance FHP's case finding capabilities.

Assessment determines which of the patients identified through case finding are appropriate for case management. The terms screening and assessment are often used interchangeably, but are distinct. Screening is defined as the processes by which a system of managed care uses targeting criteria to select potential recipients of case management.[1] This is often accomplished by referrals from health care professionals. Assessment is the process by which the staff gathers information required to accept targeted enrollees for case management and to manage their care.[1] Methods of assessment vary, but should include a systematic approach. FHP/Quality Continuum case managers used internally developed behavioral indicators as well as standard geriatric assessment tools to complete the assessment process.

Plan managers should also accurately define the major diagnostic groups and evaluate the incidence and prevalence of disease states. In many cases, health plan managers may believe that all individuals with "high risk" diseases should be "case managed." However, approaches that manage high-risk persons on an individual or population basis, such as asthma care, enable an organization to address the typical drivers of chronic illness (see box) while managing the individual outliers.

The age of the health plan's members will guide an organization's care program and resource allocation in terms of human resource investment and costs. At FHP/Quality Continuum, the management of the senior population—those patients over age 65 or disabled Medicare-eligible patients under age 65—accounts for 83 percent of program costs. Simply stated, the Medicare population requires more case management services than the commercial (under 65) population. The data also indicate that at any point in time 1.25 percent of the FHP Medicare risk population, and 0.25 percent of the commercial population, are being followed by case managers. Over the course of a year, approximately 10 percent of the population receives some case management intervention. Certain aged populations will require increased intensity.

Drivers of Disease Cost[5]

Patient Compliance
Prevention
Rapid Resolution
Acute Flare Ups
80-20 Rule (80 percent of resources go to 20 percent of problems)

Once screening and assessment are completed, case managers must identify the areas for intervention. FHP/Quality Continuum developed a problem classification system to perform this function. The system is based on behaviors that can be identified and affected by case management intervention. Each problem behavior is tied to a corresponding expected outcome. For example, if a diabetic is not taking insulin properly, the expected outcome is that the patient takes the insulin as prescribed to manage the individual's illness. Behavioral areas include: health access; safety; medications; treatment and outcomes; diagnosis; and financial. The system has helped position FHP/Quality Continuum to evaluate the impact in resolving problems, and focused the attention of case managers on goals and outcomes.

The patient care plan is the vehicle for resolving identified problems. The care planning process should be multidisciplinary, meaning that the case manager, the primary care physician, and the patient must establish the plan collaboratively. Excluding any one of those individuals is a critical error that will likely result in failure of the plan.

Once the decision to proceed with the case management program is made, and the work of analyzing systems, defining data needs, developing procedures, and hiring qualified staff is complete, the case management functions must be clearly defined. A resource for health plans is the Case Management Society of America (CMSA), which has established standards of care for case management that serve as a sound platform on which to build a program.

The CMSA standards are a guide for achieving excellence in case management. Although nonbinding, the CMSA hopes the guidelines will serve as a framework for public policy, education, practice, and research. The standards of care covered in the CMSA document include: assessment/case identification and selection; problem identification; planning; monitoring; evaluating; and outcomes.[3]

To aid a continuum of care focus, an organization can develop case management criteria as a means to create a set of quality standards and show organizational support and commitment. FHP introduced such standards to its outpatient clinic program. Part of the outpatient clinic administrator's management incentive is based on successfully meeting these standards. One of the FHP standards is that the clinic must have a case manager with an identified caseload of patients.

Written policies and procedures also help ensure consistency, and consistency allows for measurements. The benefits of procedure manuals are well known, and case management is no exception. Policies and procedures are important in conveying the program's essence to new staff, review organizations, and regulators. Many of the procedures were field tested before being included in the procedure manual. One common pitfall of the procedure manual is demonstrated by a situation in which the author was reviewing a case management program and was presented with a very well-written procedure manual. There was only one problem. The program existed only in the pages of the manual. Obviously, there are programs that illustrate the opposite. The clear solution is somewhere in the middle, but to the extent possible existing practice should be documented to meet the requirements of licensure and demonstrate compliance with the standards of various accrediting organizations such as the National Committee for Quality Assurance (NCQA).

CREATING, MONITORING, AND EVALUATING OUTCOME MEASURES

Once the plan is crafted, the case manager is responsible for initiating the interventions and monitoring the program's effectiveness. The case manager must judge the plan's capability to meet the program's outcome goals for the patient using both objective and subjective data. It is not uncommon to modify a plan based on patient progress, or the lack of progress. A key case management responsibility involves monitoring this information with progress reports to the health care team.

Documented outcomes measurements based on objective criteria are essential to evaluating a plan's success. The establishment of expected outcomes at the onset of care planning assists the case manager in evaluating the effectiveness of case management in achieving those outcomes. At FHP the various outcomes to be measured are a part of the data system. The case managers input the data as they work with the patient; the data are then used to generate reports on individual and overall outcomes.

Case management outcomes are numerous, and measurement of the outcomes is usually an evolutionary process. In the early design phase, FHP attempted to identify not only areas of concern, but areas staff would be interested in as the program evolved. With the FHP/Quality Continuum program, the initial outcome measurement was financial savings. As the program matured, measurements became more sophisticated. In this evolution, the measurements proceeded from financial and utilization based to measurement of process outcomes. Clinical outcomes and patient satisfaction outcomes are now in the forefront of the plan's developmental activities.

Financial savings is one of the most universal measures of case management effectiveness, and frequently is the indicator that gains and sustains management support. Case management saves money even though very few companies have undertaken any accurate analysis.[4] The FHP/Quality Continuum program has consistently yielded savings. In the first year of operation the program saved nearly four million dollars.

The methodology for the calculation of savings should be presented and agreed upon in advance. The FHP savings methodology yields extremely conservative results. However, they are universally accepted within the organization. Financial results and utilization improvements are readily obtained measures of effectiveness.

The next step in FHP's evolution toward comprehensive outcomes measurement was process measurement. The organization approached process measurement by implementing "clinical trax," guidelines developed by FHP for specific high-risk diagnostic findings, such as a breast mass, to reduce fragmentation, improve continuity, and decrease the time from first discovery of the finding to treatment. These "clinical trax" improved the process times and practice variation in several areas.

In all of FHP's outcomes measurement initiatives, the ability of the case manager to achieve the identified expected outcome is documented. The next step in FHP outcomes evolution is to evaluate the effectiveness of achieving the desired process outcome in improving the clinical status of the patient. The newly implemented data system will assist us in taking the next step. Establishing the data requirements to reach this step may seem like a formidable task, but it starts with documenting the expected outcomes of the program. It is also wise for the organization to look at long-term, in addition to short-term, outcomes.

Finally, patient and physician satisfaction is another measurement of case management effectiveness. Standard tools are available to assist with this task, but consideration should be given to the development of individualized instruments, which are invaluable in measuring the specific objectives of an organization's program.

ANTICIPATING THE PITFALLS

Three basic pitfalls can reduce the effectiveness of a case management program. First is a concept referred to as *layering.* Layering occurs when an organization "layers" job duties and responsibilities on its case manager. The most common example of this pitfall is combining the concurrent review nurse duties with the case management duties. The concurrent review nurses have immediate demands on their time with inpatient activities. Active case management activities are the first casualty, and the model quickly returns to traditional utilization management.

A second pitfall is dilution. In this situation, the case manager has only case management duties but has an overwhelming number of patients to manage. The most common cause of this pitfall is poor patient identification. The most frequent targeting problem involves poor assessment. Patients that are "screened out" are not properly assessed and are accepted into case management when not appropriate. Often, novice case managers will continue to manage patients beyond a point where intervention is effective. Both poor assessment and inappropriate retention prevent case managers from focusing on the truly high-risk patients.

Finally, "narrowing" may occur, which involves limiting the scope of case management activities in a manner that prevents the high-risk patient from getting early intervention. This pitfall most commonly occurs in disease-specific programs. For example, one program reviewed only patients with congestive heart failure (CHF). Because CHF was the diagnosis that re-

sulted in numerous hospital admissions, clinic managers felt it essential to case manage these patients. The result was that case managers literally declined patients with obvious problems in order to case manage less needy CHF patients. Disease management is a worthwhile initiative but requires a separate strategic integration plan.

Clearly, case management is an effective strategy in improving health care quality and enhancing cost effectiveness. In order to achieve the maximum results, great care is required from inception to implementation. A careful analysis of a health care organization's current situation and implementation of systems based on its strengths and organizational goals will place it ahead on the success curve.

REFERENCES

1. Pacala, J.T. et al. *Case Management in Health Maintenance Organizations: Final Report*. Washington, D.C.: Group Health Foundation, 1994.

2. Case Management Association of America. *Standard of Practice for Case Management*. Little Rock: CMSA, 1995.

3. Ibid.

4. Pacala et al., *Case Management*.

5. Zitter, M. *Special Report: Disease Management*. The Zitter Group, November, 1995.

Managed Care, Utilization Management, and Case Management in the Emergency Department

Kelly S. Morgan

The essence of delivering patient care in a managed care environment is the efficient organization of patient care delivery. Efficient organization supports specific patient outcomes that are realized within fiscally responsible and efficient time frames. Positive outcomes are achieved through the appropriate utilization of resources, with both the sequence and the amount of resources applied being noted.

Hospitals, in response to the need to improve efficiency, have implemented internal efforts to control costs.[1] The methods used include the implementation of utilization review (UR) processes, staff restructuring, personnel reductions, and case management. UR is used to assess the intensity of care the patient is receiving. Specifically, UR seeks to ensure that the care is both necessary and appropriate. The goals of unit staff restructuring are to change the mix of caregiver skill levels and lower the overall cost of providing a unit of service. Decreasing the number of personnel in an organization focuses on health care professionals and administrative staff and aims at improving efficiency while decreasing wage expenses. Case management closely monitors each individual patient's progress with the goal of ensuring efficient use of resources in the shortest possible period of time.

This article discusses changes that support the delivery of managed care in the emergency department (ED) setting. It begins by examining some basic tenets of managed care and their effect on the hospital environment. UR and case management are then examined as adjuncts to the delivery of patient care in the ED. Although improved personnel efficiencies and staff restructuring assist in cutting the wage costs associated with patient care delivery, UR and case management work to improve the efficiencies of patient care. Efficient patient care management must be established to deal with the economic restraints imposed by a managed care environment.

GROWTH OF MANAGED CARE

Managed care systems have become a major form of health care delivery and financing in the United States. Initially, managed care consisted of health maintenance organizations (HMOs). The definition of a managed care system then expanded to include almost any form of health care insurance coverage that limits the enrollee's choice of health care providers and the enrollee's ability to self-refer to specialty physicians.[2]

The growth of the HMO market in recent years reflects the tremendous growth in managed care systems. According to the Group Health Association of America, by 1992 approximately 550 HMOs existed in America, covering the health care needs of more than 38.6 million individuals. HMO members represented 15% of the overall US population and 18% of the population younger than 65 years. This

Top Emerg Med 1996; 18(4): 50–57

membership volume has more than doubled since the beginning of 1986. In addition, more than half of all active physicians have HMO patients in their patient population. Finally, the American Hospital Association found that, in 1990, 48% of hospitals had HMO contracts.[2] With the current focus on cutting Medicare costs through contracting with HMOs, even more of our population will receive its health care in a managed care environment.

RESOURCE MANAGEMENT

The evaluation of health care interventions and the resources necessary to provide them is carried out by managed care organizations (MCOs). These MCOs focus on the efficiency and cost effectiveness of interventions across the system. With managed care systems, decisions related to the allocation of resources are often not made by direct health care providers. Resource allocation decisions are mandated prospectively by the administrators of the health care system and are communicated during the contracting process.

Cost-effectiveness analysis is used by managed care systems to evaluate health care interventions. Cost-effectiveness analysis enables managed care policymakers or administrators to set priorities and make decisions regarding the amount of resources allocated to a given program. The objective is to maximize the net health benefit to a target population while taking fixed resources into account. In this analysis, gains and losses are valued equally across the population.[3]

As the infiltration of managed care expands and government payers and private insurers continue their attempts at limiting the patient's length of stay, hospitals are finding that only the most acutely ill patients are being admitted for inpatient care and that the allowed number of patient days is decreasing. The decreased census and increased acuity result in a double impact on the hospital coffers. Because the intensity of service delivery to the patient is highest during the first hours after admission, these are the highest-cost days for the hospital. The lower-cost, higher-profit patient days near the end of the patient's stay have been eliminated from the time authorized by the payer.

GROWTH THROUGH EFFICIENCY

The growth of the managed care market demonstrates the ability to maximize the health care dollar through efficient resource utilization. The methods used to achieve efficiency include both financial management and patient care management. Financial management is accomplished through consolidation of purchasing power and services, use of disincentives to discourage waste and duplication of resources, and enhancement of the primary care physician role. Patient care management includes the limitation of inappropriate and unnecessary care, promotion of outcomes measurement, and promotion of wellness and prevention. A key goal of managed care is the development of a patient care delivery system fully supportive of managed care's objectives. Accomplishment of this goal may be achieved by adapting current patient care delivery systems or through the development of new models involving consolidation and integration.

HOSPITALS

As managed care systems grow, the hospital model is being redefined. No longer can a hospital afford to offer all services to all people for a set price. Hospitals now must consider themselves in the business of health care delivery and financing. Hospitals offering managed care services, such as enrollment, billing, claims processing, data analysis, member services, and provider relations, are in the greatest demand. Many hospitals now offer these services to specific groups by forming partnerships with MCOs.[2]

CONSOLIDATION

Consolidation is another adaptation to patient care delivery used by hospitals and managed care systems to increase efficiency and control costs. Consolidation refers to the joining together of services through ownership. Consolidation may refer to one hospital buying another facility in the area, evaluating the services of both facilities, and discontinuing duplicated services. It may also refer to the purchase of smaller systems, the purchase of physician groups, or the purchase of a hospital or extended care facility. [2] In the ED environment, an example of consolidation may involve a health care organization buying two or more hospitals with trauma programs and then consolidating the trauma services to provide a single level I trauma facility.

INTEGRATED PARTNERSHIPS

Integrated partnerships represent a model in which the hospital and physicians form one organizational entity. Although integration requires strong contractual agreements, there exists no ownership relationship between the hospital and physician group. The hospital and physician group join together to provide total patient care service packages. One example of integration may involve joint contracting agreements between a university medical center and the medical school–based physician group. Through their integrated partnership, the hospital and physician group then contract as one with an HMO to provide care for a given population.

The increased efficiency through combination of services theoretically enhances the partnership position in contracting for managed care system members. Through integration, the hospital works closely with the physicians, thereby allowing an enrolled member to receive health care in a nearly seamless environment. Although benefiting the managed care systems and their members, integrated partnerships limit the number of managed care systems with which hospitals contract as a result of the high level of commitment required by the managed care system.[2]

UTILIZATION MANAGEMENT

Utilization management (UM) is a critical process used by hospitals and managed care systems to assess and evaluate the resources that are devoted to patient care. UR, a concept that came into vogue during the 1980s, is the process by which the utilization of hospital resources is monitored. UM takes UR past the stage at which resource allocation is monitored and reviewed. It reflects the management of the utilization of health care resources.[4]

UR is primarily a cost containment activity. Utilization activities utilize established criteria to measure resource allocation and appropriateness of patient care. UM staff use the criteria chosen by the health care system to ensure the necessity and appropriateness of the care provided. The selection of the criteria for use in the UM process will reflect the goal and primary mission of the organization. Regardless of the criteria used for benchmarking, utilization modalities encourage fiscally responsible use of patient care resources.[4]

Any member of the health care team can perform data collection for UR. The development and implementation of the UM tools and the analysis of the data are most appropriately performed by professional staff. UM is achieved through prospective, concurrent, and retrospective techniques.[5]

Prospective review

Prospective reviews are performed on several types of patient groups. Preadmission certification determines the actual need for a patient's admission or treatment in a hospital. This preadmission screening can even be applied to an admission for an ED for treatment. Patients may be approved for the entire admission or for stabilization, or payment for treatment may be denied and arrangements made for the enrollee to be transferred to another facility. Surgical procedures are also reviewed on a prospective basis. For many nonemergency surgical procedures, a second opinion is required.

Prospective review is most often experienced in the ED setting during the triage process. When the patient presents for treatment, an acuity level is assigned based on the patient's complaint, history, and physical status. For example, the facility's three-level triage acuity system allows for emergent, acute, and urgent care assignments. Rather than treatment in the high-cost ED being authorized, those managed care patients presenting to the ED for urgent care with appropriate complaints may be referred to the managed care–run urgent care center by the physician gatekeeper.

Concurrent review

Concurrent reviews of patient care are performed during a patient's hospitalization. Concurrent review of specific treatments focuses on the necessity for and the quality of those treatments. Ongoing review of the patient's progress toward the designated outcomes is achieved through discharge planning. During discharge planning, quality analysts seek to transition the patient as quickly as possible from the expensive acute care setting to an alternative system of care. Alternatives include home health providers, long-term acute care facilities, and rehabilitation centers.

It may seem difficult to imagine performing concurrent review on ED patients because of the short length of stay for these patients. If applied as an aspect of patient education and discharge planning, however, concurrent review can be appropriate. Data related to the efficacy of medications or treatments can be collected as the interventions are performed and evaluated. With data collection and analysis, ED treatment processes can potentially be streamlined and made less costly.

Retrospective review

Retrospective reviews are used for the evaluation of care already delivered. Retrospective reviews often focus on care delivery in short-stay units, such as the ED. These reviews are helpful in measuring the efficacy of a program, determining whether a specific examination has been ordered as well as its appropriateness, and documenting regulatory compliance.

Retrospective reviews are of great benefit in that the records can be reviewed using an interdisciplinary approach. The retrospective review of urgent care utilization is one example of an interdisciplinary retrospective review. During the review, the nurse manager may evaluate the appropriateness of triage, the medical director may focus on the utilization of specific tests, and the financial manager may focus on the appropriateness of the billing level. Data from the review can then be used to improve the utilization of any of the services evaluated.

Data collected from retrospective reviews may also be used for contracting between the hospital and the managed care system. Nosocomial infection rates, patient outcome data, and a system's continuous improvement information are examples of information that is useful in the contracting process.

ASSOCIATED SAVINGS

UR is thought to save managed care systems 10% to 15% on hospital expenditures. One study performed in 1988 evaluated the total impact that UR had on one managed care system covering more than 200 employers.[5] The investigators determined that the UR program, which included preadmission, on-site, and concurrent review, lowered hospital expenditures by 11.9%. An 8.3% savings in total expenditures was also noted.

CASE MANAGEMENT

A significant trend in health care and professional nursing during the past several years has been the incorporation of nursing case management into the health care delivery model of an institution. Hospital administrators have realized that they must change their model of health care delivery to survive the impact of the uncertain health care reimbursement initiatives of managed care, Medicare, and other payers. A case management model has been viewed as a critical component in promoting strong management practices, quality care, and a sound financial position.[6]

Roles and responsibilities

Nursing case management has been defined as a system of patient care delivery that focuses on the achievement of outcomes within effective time frames and with appropriate use of resources. It encompasses the entire episode of illness and crosses all settings in which the patient receives care.[7] The focus of such a system of patient care delivery is the well-coordinated continuity of care. Coordinated care is established through collaboration of the health care team and embraces the opportunity to reduce wasted time, energy, and materials to achieve a greater financial return. Improvements in the efficacy of the delivered care occur while professional development and job satisfaction are provided for the health care providers.

The role and definition of the case manager vary in different types of health care organizations. Case manager roles often involve responsibilities associated with patient education, insurance, UM, risk management, organizational performance, and discharge planning. The case management process primarily involves six stages[4]:

1. case screening of the patient
2. assessment of the treatment plan
3. coordination and development of the treatment and discharge plans
4. ongoing evaluation
5. implementation of the final plan
6. final evaluation and postdischarge follow-up

Nursing case management in this delivery model assumes responsibility and accountability for establishing, with the other health care team members, plans and processes called critical paths.[8] Critical paths explain what should happen to a patient on an ongoing basis for each diagnosis and episode, along with the proper interventions needed to achieve a specific outcome within the allotted acceptable treatment period for the illness.

Case management works to identify variances and to intervene whenever a variance from the critical path occurs, thus ensuring that the planned processes are being carried out and adaptations to the plan are made as appropriate. In keeping variances to a minimum, case managment, through the use of the critical path, helps decrease hospital, health care, and payer costs. Patient complications are also minimized as a result of timely intervention for any variances. This interdisciplinary approach begins with patient admission to the hospital system and ends at discharge.

It is the registered nurse who, as a skilled clinician, can best meet the requirements of the case manager role. The nurse, trained as a direct care provider, develops an ongoing relationship with the patient and family. Nurse case managers are responsible for assessing, coordinating, and collaborating with physicians and others to plan the patient's care and achieve the standard outcome. Nurses are the principal members of the health care team who are in a functional and organizational position to provide the detailed and regular assessment required for effective operation of the case management model. Nurses are also able to maintain contact with all the other health care team members on a continuous basis.

Case management in the ED can be achieved in several ways. Ideally, a full-time ED case manager can be assigned to coordinate the case management activities within the department. In addition to providing continuity in the service, the designated case manager can interact with other case managers within the system. The case manager can coordinate case management activities using the shift's charge nurse or patient care coordinator to provide referrals, intervene on an emergent basis, and communicate perceived trends and issues.

Outcomes and case management

The nursing case management model provides a significant foundation to support the standardization, collection, and analysis of information directly related to specific processes and patient outcomes. Through benchmarking, or the comparison of similar data, different hospitals can determine how they rank in providing high-quality, cost-effective care. Insurers and employers can utilize these comparisons to determine whom to reward with additional business, and individual providers can feel secure in the knowledge that their patients are receiving consistent and proven care. Internally, hospitals can use the information to augment and strengthen their continuous performance improvement programs, thus fostering the concept that cost control and quality standards are a fundamental part of everyday hospital activity.[9]

Additional organizational benefits to the hospital result from adopting the nursing case management model. One benefit is the potential for decreases in the length of patient hospitalizations. Decreased lengths of stay result from the use of critical paths and allow the hospital to decrease its direct patient care costs because the plan of treatment is defined earlier in the episode. Variations from the critical path will be more easily identified and corrected on a more timely basis. In addition, the tests and procedures appropriate to the diagnosis will be identified and appropriately limited.[10]

A benefit that the hospital can also expect is improved professional staff retention. The recognition of nursing staff and the importance of their role as case managers to the patient, the hospital, and other members of the health care team supports an increased level of job satisfaction. Increased staff retention saves hospital costs in terms of staff recruitment and replacement. Increased retention also supports the continuity of care for the hospital and managed care populations.

CONCLUSION

As managed care infiltrates our health care environment, steps must be taken to ensure the quality of care rendered in the ED environment. UM and case management can provide the tools necessary to ensure that the delivery of patient care occurs in a cost-efficient manner while also improving the quality of that care. By extending beyond the walls of the ED, both these processes also have the potential for improving the continuity of care throughout the managed care environment.

Our health care environment is influenced by strong financial limitations, decreased resources, and outside controls. The ED environment can no longer support being all things to all persons. We must demonstrate the delivery of patient-focused care while being willing to pursue and advocate all effective health care delivery options. In this new environment, multiple paradigms are truly becoming the norm.

REFERENCES

1. Scott CD, Jaffe DT. From crisis to culture change. *Healthcare Forum J.* 1991;34:32–38, 40–41.

2. Friedman E. Managed care: Where will your hospital fit in. *Hospitals.* April 5–18,1993:18–23.

3. Detsky AS, Naglie IG. A clinician's guide to cost-effectiveness analysis. *Ann Intern Med.* 1990;113: 147–154.

4. Powell SK. *Nursing Case Management: A Practical Guide to Success in Managed Care.* Philadelphia, Pa: Lippincott; 1996.

5. Wallack SS. Managed care: Practice, pitfalls, and potential. *Health Care Financ Rev.* 1991(annual supplement):27–33.

6. Sovie MD. Redesigning our future: Whose responsibility is it? *Nurs Econ.* 1990;8:406–411.

7. Etheredge ML. *Collaborative Care: Nursing Case Management.* Chicago, Ill: American Hospital Association; 1989.

8. Guiliano KK, Poirier CE. Nursing case management: Critical pathways to desirable outcomes. *Nurs Manage.* 1991;22:52–55.

9. Bergman R. The measuring stick. *Hosp Health Netw.* 1993;67:36–42.

10. Firman J. Case management: Quality care today. *Hosp Mater Manage Q.* 1991;12:22–25.

The Johns Hopkins Hospital Launches Case Management Initiative

Lawrence F. Strassner

As health care reform and components of managed competition begin to infiltrate the health care system, changes in financial risk, increasing accountability, performance documentation, and outcome measurements are shifting the health care provider's focus from planned care to managed care. Managed care—once only applied to high cost, chronically ill, and disabled patients—is now being expanded to include all patients.

Consumers are demanding an integrated interdisciplinary health care system that provides comprehensive care from birth to death, not just events or episodes of care during hospitalization. They are becoming more emphatic about the need to maintain and sometimes improve the quality of care that is provided while simultaneously guaranteeing access and affordability of care.

To respond to these challenges, many hospitals across the country have established formal initiatives for monitoring, measuring, and managing clinical processes. The initiatives are often found in the form of hospital case management programs and implementation of critical pathways.

THE CASE MANAGEMENT INITIATIVE

The Johns Hopkins Hospital, a quaternary/tertiary academic medical center located in downtown Baltimore, is responding to this new era by developing an integrated case management system that measures and improves processes of care and patient outcomes.

The case management initiative was led by the vice presidents of nursing, medical affairs and performance Improvement under a re-engineering effort of the care delivery and processes with support from APM, Inc., a leading health care consulting firm. A re-engineering task force consisting of physicians, nurses, social workers, an admitting office administrator, home health nurse, and performance improvement/utilization management nurses, and their supervisors was created to establish the case management program at Hopkins.

Guiding principles identified from the organization re-engineering efforts were used to set the direction for establishing case management. These principles are as follows:

- to optimize patient outcomes respecting the unique needs and wishes of each patient;
- to support the missions of research, education, and the advancement of knowledge and community service;
- to provide access to comprehensive services for all individuals;
- to maximize efficiency and eliminate redundancy through interdisciplinary integrated communication, information systems, and documentation;
- to make clinical decisions that are data driven where care is provided;

Inside Case Management 1996; 3(8): 5–7

- to maximize patient outcomes through partnership and professional collaboration within a multidisciplinary context; and
- to coordinate care to achieve quality patient outcomes through affordable cost-effective care delivery.

CASE MANAGEMENT MODEL

At Hopkins, case management is defined as a multidisciplinary clinical system that coordinates patient care services for specific patient populations in order to ensure high quality, affordable, and efficient care. The model for the acute care inpatient setting case management includes a triad team of the registered nurse case manager, social worker and performance improvement/utilization management nurse (PI/UM nurse). (See Exhibit 1.) Together these individuals form a team and are aligned according to a particular patient service.

The task force identified the importance of maintaining the current decentralized approach to patient care and the importance of establishing a model that was flexible enough to accommodate variations in patient populations and settings. A "cookie cutter" approach would not meet the needs of the institution. Discipline specific core functions were identified that are applicable regardless of patient population or setting. These core functions are the foundation of the case management program (see Exhibit 2). Depending on the patient population and setting, the model may be implemented with variations around these core functions.

For example, in pediatrics, the case managers and social workers spend a significant amount of their time coordinating complex discharges. For the general pediatric infant service, 75 percent of this population require case management. In cardiac surgery, case managers spend more time coordinating the acute care episode. They perform clinical interventions such as discontinuing pacer wires, managing cardiac arrhythmias through approved protocols, monitoring resource utilization by house staff and attending physician, and facilitating the discharge process according to the critical pathway.

CASE MANAGEMENT PILOT

The general pediatrics and adult interventional cardiology services were chosen as the pilot services. Case managers were already in place and functioning in these services. Many of the case managers were previously clinical specialists within those departments and already had established working relationships with the physicians, nurses, social workers, and performance improvement nurses. Social workers and PI/UM nurses were also in place. Some were assigned by geographical unit, others assigned by service. One of the goals of the pilot was to realign the case manager, social worker, and PI/UM nurse by service, and establish a more formalized relationship and structure to facilitate case management functions.

Using the core functions established by the reengineering task force, the case manager, social worker, and PI/UM, identified as the case management triad team, worked with a clinical support/facilitator. This individual was appointed by the vice presidents of nursing, medical affairs, and performance improvement, to assist the triad team to further define each member's role as they related to pediatrics and cardiology.

Exhibit 1. The Johns Hopkins Hospital Case Management Triad Team

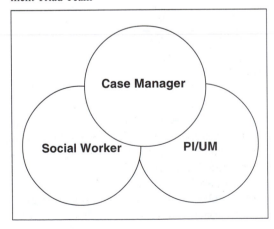

Exhibit 2. Core Functions of the Case Management Triad

Case Manager
- Assess patients' clinical and discharge planning needs for the episode of care.
  - Preadmission clinical screening
  - Assess appropriateness for clinical path
  - Identify risk factors for complex patients
- Using the skills and knowledge of an advanced practice nurse, coordinate/communicate multidisciplinary care plan, facilitate implementation of patients' progress toward outcomes and act as a clinical resource for the multidisciplinary team.
- Monitor resource utilization according to the plan of care or critical path.
- Coordinate services among multidisciplinary care team and ensure appropriate hand-offs to other providers (e.g., home care, managed care case manager).
- Coordinate complex discharge planning interventions.
- Facilitate achievement of quality, cost, and service outcomes, including input into development and revision of critical paths.

Social Worker
- Based on admission screen/referral begin preplanning for complex psychosocial discharge needs.

- Collaborate with case manager/PI /UM nurse to develop and execute complex discharge plans.
- Form psychosocial assessment development, implement and document patient goals and care plans.
- Perform counseling and other interventions as needed to address patient/family psychosocial.

PI/UM
- Access insurance information and present in daily rounds.
- Communicate with payers to obtain recertification of acute patient days.
- Accessibility to and discussion with on-site reviewers.
- Collect and track population specific performance improvement measures and clinical outcomes data.
- Identify documentation needs in the medical record and communicate finding to the case manager and/or physician.
- Concurrently optimize coding into the medical record.
- Review all readmissions.
- Review all insurance payment denial with case management team.

Another goal of the pilot was to test the applicability of the core functions identified for the triad team and identify redundancies and barriers to coordinating care.

During the pilot, the triad team met daily and discussed each patient on the service. The case manager led the daily discussions, which included topics such as patient insurance coverage, expected length of stay, discharge planning needs, acute inpatient plan of care, and psychosocial needs. The case manager screened all new admissions with input from the social worker and the PI/UM nurse using a screening tool developed for the pilot. This tool assisted the triad team in identifying patient needs, establishing a plan of care, and assigning responsibility for the execution of the plan.

PILOT FINDINGS

The triad model was successful in coordinating high quality, cost-effective patient care. Each discipline made a significant and unique contribution to the overall care of the patient. There was minimal overlap in the functions of each role.

The PI/UM nurses role changed the most. Some of the new functions included attending daily rounds and providing insurance information, such who is the insurance provider, what are the covered benefits, and what is the expected length of stay (certified days) as defined by the payer for each patient being case managed.

The PI/UM nurse also was to have accessibility to the payer's on-site reviewer and discuss findings or concerns with this reviewer as needed. They also optimized coding by providing information to the case manager and/or physician regarding clinical documentation requirements as it relates to reimbursement and regulatory requirements.

Case managers and social workers expressed minimal changes in their roles as a result of this pilot. There was more of a clarification of roles vs. a major restructuring. They did indicate there was a higher level of coordination and integration of the plan of care due partly to structured daily communication rounds and alignment of the team by service.

The daily communication meeting was essential in coordinating the care with physicians, nurses, other members of the multidisciplinary care team, and the payers. Through daily review of the patient's plan of care, clinical condition, and early identification of documentation issues, coding of diagnosis, procedures, and complications was also optimized.

The screening tool also assisted the triad in early identification and assignment of responsibilities of patient care needs.

Prior to implementing the model across the organization, several issues need to be addressed. These include system issues such as physicians' rotating schedules and daily rounds; number of services per triad; integration and accessibility of clinical and administrative information systems and data; role of the managed care office nurse; and organizational education about the case management model.

QUALIFICATIONS AND EDUCATION OF THE CASE MANAGER

The case manager is a master's-prepared registered nurse with expertise as a clinical practitioner and a skilled manager of clinical systems and health care finances that impact patient care. She/he has five years of acute care experience and a minimum of three years experience in the specialty area, and may be formally educated in the nursing role of clinical specialist and/or nurse practitioner.

The case manager possesses advanced interpersonal skills, demonstrates general computer skills, and has an ability to analyze complex data sets. She/he must be able to function effectively in a fluid, dynamic, and rapidly changing environment.

Early in establishing the model it was identified that the case manager, though an expert clinician, did not have the experience and education to integrate finance, quality, and clinical care. In an effort to prepare the case manager for these roles, a core group of clinicians, administrators, and faculty of The Johns Hopkins Hospital and Johns Hopkins University School of Nursing developed the Case Management Academy.

This week-long intensive in residence course instructs case managers in: a) financing systems such as capitation, global billing contracts, and the realities of managed care penetration, b) genesis and evolution of case management and case management models, c) roles and requirements of case managers practicing in various settings, d) clinical quality improvement and patient outcomes, e) critical paths and variance analysis, f) insurer/payer partnership, and g) legal and ethical responsibilities. The case managers also participate in a self-assessment and critique of videotaped case managers in action using actual cases.

NEXT STEPS

Currently small task forces are working on identified system issues and planning is underway to implement the model with the revised system supports in early September 1996, for the entire Pediatric, Cardiology, and Cardiac Surgical Adult Services. Qualitative and quantitative measures are also currently being reviewed and defined to evaluate the model.

Case Management: Meeting the Needs of Chronically Ill Patients in an HMO

Ronnie Grower, Bonnie Hillegass, and Fran Nelson

Individuals who need to access numerous health care services are often faced with negotiating a complex health care delivery system. In fee-for-service models, health care services can be fragmented and disorganized, having a negative impact on the quality of care and increasing costs. HMOs may eliminate some barriers to care by providing a continuum of services. By integrating case management into health care delivery, high-risk cases can be managed to ensure that the patient receives the appropriate level of care in the least restrictive and most cost-effective setting.

By offering a spectrum of services as alternatives to hospitalization and an extensive case management system, Health Plan of Nevada (HPN) has been able to manage high risk cases effectively. On a case-by-case basis, staff propose care plans based on desired outcomes, the least amount of invasion and restriction, and the most appropriate care setting.

The following article describes the Health Plan of Nevada's case management program, how it has evolved within the corporation, how it functions today, gaps that have been identified within the system, and a proposed model to better meet the needs of the chronically ill.

Managed Care Quarterly 1996; 4(2): 46–57

ORGANIZATIONAL OVERVIEW

Sierra Health Services, a managed care holding company, operates several subsidiaries that compose a vertically integrated health care delivery system. Health Plan of Nevada (HPN), one of SHS's wholly owned subsidiaries, is a federally qualified and state-licensed health maintenance organization. HPN currently serves over 115,000 commercial group members. Since 1985, HPN has offered a Medicare-risk product, Senior Dimensions, which currently provides coverage to approximately 25,000 senior citizens in Nevada.

HPN provides care through a mixed group/network model HMO, with most of the primary physician health care, specialty services, and extensive alternative care services provided by SHS's other wholly owned subsidiaries. This integration of medical care, case management, home health, hospice, mental health, and volunteer services enables access to comprehensive services, enhances quality, and controls costs. An extensive case management system, alternative care network, and computerized information system offer a health care delivery system that supports members through a continuum of care and ensures that members are cared for in the least restrictive, most cost efficient, safe environment.

HPN provides a full range of services including ambulatory care, subacute care, inpatient acute care, rehabilitation services, nursing home care, extensive home health services, mental health and substance abuse services, and a hospice program. To enhance services to the frail and chronically ill, several innovative programs have been developed. Highlights of these programs are presented below.

SENIOR DIMENSIONS SERVICE CENTER

One unique aspect of HPN is its Senior Dimensions Service Center, a walk-in resource center for its Medicare-risk contract members. Senior Dimensions Service Center staff recognize and assist members with their special needs, specifically supporting multiproblem patients by assisting them with accessing medical care and social services (e.g., arranging medical appointments, referrals for durable medical equipment, financial aid, and transportation), providing member service support (e.g., explaining benefits, providing health education information), and offering supportive volunteer programs. The concept of the "one-stop shop" has proven to be very successful.

With a staff of fourteen, including a social worker, a nurse, member services representatives, and administrative and clerical staff, the Senior Dimensions Service Center assists more than 1,000 walk-ins and more than 3,000 phone call requests per month. The staff is also responsible for administering the new member orientation program.

All new Senior Dimensions members are invited to attend a monthly new member orientation session. The primary focus of the orientation is to highlight member benefits, offer preventive services, and conduct risk assessments. Prior to new member orientation, members receive a packet of information that includes the following risk assessment questionnaires: Personal Health and Social History (PHSH), Drug History and Screen, and Pulmonary Screen. Approximately 85 percent of new members return these risk assessment forms, and approximately 56 percent attend new member orientation.

RISK ASSESSMENT

The PHSH form assesses activities of daily living (ADLs), instrumental activities of daily living (IADLs), comorbidity, and the need for immediate medical services, durable medical equipment, patient education, or case management. If a PHSH is not received after the initial mailing, the new member is contacted by the Senior Dimensions Service Center staff, and another PHSH form is mailed. If it is not completed and returned within 60 days, a closure letter is sent to the member, and a copy of the letter is included in the medical record. This update to the medical record serves as a notification to the physician provider that, when the member accesses service for the first time, the PHSH is still outstanding and needs to be completed. It also serves as notification to the provider of a member with potential compliance issues.

Upon receipt, the PHSH forms are reviewed by Senior Dimensions Service Center staff to identify those members responding positively to questions identifying medical and psychosocial risk factors. These members are followed up with a phone call, and if they meet predefined criteria, are referred directly to home health, durable medical equipment (DME), or complex case management. The PHSH form is then placed in the medical record for reference by the provider.

This process has proven effective in identifying high-risk patients at the time of enrollment; however, it does not "discover" those members who have experienced a change of health status. HPN has begun to develop methods to enhance its ability to identify these members.

VOLUNTEERS

HPN began its first volunteer program in 1989 to give individuals an opportunity to use their skills, contribute to their community, and assist HPN members. The volunteer program was designed to enhance the services offered to patients and customers by providing services the staff would not otherwise be able to provide. Through participation in the HPN Volunteer Program, many individuals receive needed socialization and enhanced self-esteem. HPN benefits from the involvement of volunteers who act as ambassadors within the community. More than 40,500 hours of service have been volunteered since 1989. Presently there are 55 active volunteers who have volunteered over 3,800 hours of service in the first five months of 1995.

Volunteers hold a variety of positions throughout the SHS subsidiaries. The following are examples of volunteer functions:

Friendly companion

Assists homebound members with letter writing, paper work, reading, and other duties as agreed upon by the volunteer and the client. The volunteer may also provide limited errand running for the client within five miles of the client's home. The volunteer, however, can not transport the clients at any time while volunteering. Friendly companion visits usually last one to three hours per week. Documentation of the visit is completed following each visit and submitted to the volunteer coordinator monthly, with contact available daily.

Friendly caller volunteer

Calls homebound members once every couple of weeks to check on them and to provide socialization and a friendly discussion. The volunteer may also direct clients to appropriate community resources for further assistance.

"Thinking of you" cards

Cards mailed by volunteers once a month to provide a nice pick-me-up for the client. Cards generally contain a nice greeting and friendly poem.

Health fair volunteer

Conducts blood pressure checks, inputs risk assessment data into health risk appraisal machine (computer program), distributes information, and conducts height and weight measurement.

Senior dimensions service center volunteer

Assists at blood pressure clinics and special projects and collates and sorts items for new member orientation and health promotion clinic.

SMA clinic volunteer

Assists in the medical records department, the laboratory, and/or the surgery waiting area, making patient reminder phone calls and administering patient callback surveys, organizing the physician's library, filing and collating papers, and greeting and directing patients.

Wheelchair repair

Wheelchairs are repaired by volunteers for low-income members upon request.

HOME HEALTH

HPN extensively utilizes its home health benefits to support the multiproblem patient to remain in or return to his or her home. Family Healthcare Services (FHS), a wholly owned subsidiary of SHS, is the primary provider of home health services to HPN members. FHS is a full service home health care agency licensed by the state of Nevada and certified by Medicare and Medicaid.

HPN has taken a liberal approach to interpreting the Medicare-risk contract in its provision of home health services. The following are some examples of how HPN utilizes the home health benefit:

1. Skilled nursing for IV therapy. When patients are unable to learn procedures and do not have a caregiver, skilled nursing visits can be made at a frequency necessary to administer IV medications. These medications are a covered benefit paid for under a capitated arrangement FHS has with HPN.
2. As an alternative to hospitalization, skilled nursing visits may be provided for round-the-clock care.
3. Respiratory therapy services to evaluate patients' pulmonary needs and to make recommendations, as needed, to physicians.

4. Home health aide services for limited respite care (for patients requiring assistance with two or more ADLs).
5. Home health aide services for extended hours (8 to 12 hours) for a short period of time until the patient improves, or until other arrangements are made (i.e., placement or private hire).
6. Home health services can be provided to members residing in group homes. In these instances, HPN monitors the patient's environment, health status, and services provided by the group home.

SUBACUTE AND REHABILITATIVE CARE

HPN has been an innovator in the management of patients in the subacute setting. HPN uses subacute and skilled nursing facilities for medical or rehabilitative treatment as an alternative to acute facility stays. Therapy services are offered that are over and above the standard Medicare-risk program to avoid extended hospitalizations and institutionalization. HPN case managers determine whether rehabilitation is appropriate, regardless of the Medicare three-day hospital stay requirement. In addition, rehabilitation services may be authorized when strengthening is required to recover from acute functional loss following hospital admission; however, the patient may not have a "typical" rehabilitation diagnosis.

In 1990, HPN was the driving force in the development of a subacute facility in the Las Vegas area. HPN determined that *medical* as well as rehabilitative care could be delivered safely in a less restrictive, lower-cost setting than the acute hospitals. What makes HPN's subacute unit unique is that other programs admit primarily rehabilitative patients, while HPN's subacute facilities provide care to medical as well as to rehabilitative patients.

HPN's subacute program was developed in partnership with a skilled nursing facility, Shadow Mountain Transitional Care and Rehabilitation Center. Placement of the services at

this level of care presented several challenges to HPN as well as to the facility. For instance, patients admitted to a subacute level of care had more complex medical problems and required more intense care than patients who typically were cared for in a skilled nursing facility. To manage appropriately the care of the subacute patient, HPN undertook a major staff development effort to provide the facility staff with necessary skills. Additional equipment needs and staffing were evaluated, and admission criteria were developed. In return, the skilled nursing facility supports patient and caregiver education and affords family members more time with the patient, including overnight stays and weekend passes when appropriate. This practice prepares patients for their return to the community.

CASE MANAGEMENT PROGRAM

A major innovation for HPN has been its case management program, which HPN uses to evaluate, monitor, and treat members with multiple problems. A brief description of its evolution may help the reader understand why and how the current case management model works for the multiproblem patient in an HMO. A timeline is presented in Table 1, highlighting HPN's steps in the development of a case management program.

In 1985, HPN contracted with an independent home health agency, traditionally serving the fee-for-service and Medicare market, to provide case management for its members. Initially, a medical case management approach was used to care for HPN's Medicare-risk patients who were hospitalized. Soon after, Family Healthcare Services (FHS) was purchased by SHS and became the primary provider of home health services for HPN and the vehicle for delivering case management to frail elderly members in the community.

In 1986, FHS recognized that case management was lacking a social component and hired two social workers to manage the social issues such as support systems, financial management, and environmental deficits, and to help design a new model of case management for HPN. Dur-

Table 1 Health Plan of Nevada Case Management Timeline

Year	Event
1985	• Contracted with Family Healthcare Services (FHS) for case management—medical model.
1986	• Included social component to case management.
	• Established task force to design case management model.
1988	• Added complex case management for community-based clients.
1989	• Expanded case management to skilled nursing facilities and group homes.
	• Established Senior Dimensions Service Center.
1990	• Segregated hospital and alternative care management components.
1992	• Consolidated hospital and alternative care of case management components.
	• Established subacute unit and introduced case management.
	• Established case management program for AIDS patients.
1994	• Awarded grant by The Robert Wood Johnson Foundation to integrate case management in the ambulatory care setting.

ing this time, HPN established a task force to develop a case management model to better serve the needs of its Medicare-risk members who had complex medical and social problems. The task force included a family practitioner, with strong interests in geriatrics, a geriatric nurse practitioner, a social worker, a physical therapist, and then Chief Operating Officer of FHS.

After an extensive literature search and on-site visits to several model case management programs, the task force concluded that a medical/social case management system was the model that best met the needs of HPN's frail geriatric members. An outcome of this task force was the statement of philosophy and its interpretation that continues to be the foundation for

providing case management services throughout HPN today:

Philosophy

We believe that case management is a critical element of our health care delivery system which allows us to truly manage care, to avoid fragmentation of services, and use our resources in the most effective manner. The goal of case management is to provide the continuity necessary to move the client along the continuum of care towards the least restrictive, safe, cost effective environment possible.

Interpretation

In accepting the challenge of this philosophy, we understand and support all aspects of case management. Rigid, fragmented, disorganized, unbalanced health care arrangements have a negative impact on the quality of the care provided and tend to increase cost. We accept the responsibility to bring providers and members to a fuller understanding of managed care by educating them in case management principles. Appropriate care decisions are based on quality, the least amount of invasion and restriction and the best fiscal environment on a case by case basis. In the interpretation of benefits, alternatives must be available that lead to health preservation and illness prevention in a cost-effective approach.

In 1988, case management services were adopted for community-based clients with multiple and complex problems. In 1989, case management was expanded to include residents of group homes and skilled nursing facilities. Further expansion of HPN's case management program included the establishment of the Senior Dimensions Service Center in 1989 to identify high-risk cases, and to provide simple case management and the "one-stop" resource center for the Medicare-risk enrollees.

In 1990 HPN modified its case management process by segregating the hospital and nonhospital case management components. With this reorganization, case managers in the hospital functioned alongside utilization reviewers and discharge planners, each carving out a separate piece of the process; this reorganization resulted in a regression back to the classical utilization management model. Recognizing the intensity of labor, duplication of effort, service fragmentation, and increased bed days caused by this process, in 1992 HPN reengineered to consolidate case management within one department, under the leadership of a geriatric nurse practitioner. Under this new organization, the role of the institutional case manager was redefined to incorporate case management, utilization review, and discharge planning. This model has been successful and is discussed under the heading "Institutional Case Management."

March 1992 marked the opening of a network of subacute units. Case management was introduced in the subacute setting to ensure coordination of medical services, patient advocacy, and utilization management. A case management program designed to meet the special needs of the AIDS and HIV-positive population was also established in 1992 and currently functions as a separate program within Family Home Hospice, a wholly owned subsidiary of Sierra Health Services.

From 1992 to 1995 the HPN case management program continued to be refined. Policies and procedures were developed that specified types of case management and associated service levels. Specialty services were designed for high-risk pregnancies and chronic pulmonary disease. Efforts during this time also focused on building an understanding of case management services throughout the corporation. In January 1995, a separate corporate department of Case Management Services was created.

CURRENT PROGRAM CHARACTERISTICS

Case management services are offered at varying levels of intensity throughout HPN and are outlined in Table 2. For example, simple case management (Level I) is demonstrated in the Senior Dimensions Service Center where staff assist members with arrangements for

transportation and durable medical equipment. The Utilization Management Department identifies high-risk cases such as patients requiring transplants or dialysis. Home health and hospice provide a higher level of case management (Level II) by coordinating care for patients within their homes. Institutional case managers coordinate care for hospital discharge. In the ambulatory care setting, case management is provided by clinical nurses who instruct patients on disease process and medication usage.

A higher level of case management intensity is offered in the various institutional settings and through HPN's complex case management program. As the patient's needs become more complex and require intervention by professional staff, the case management services are provided by nurses and social workers specifically trained in complex case management. Levels III and IV involve medical, social, and psychological interventions and may require coordination of care across multiple sites of service and providers.

A typology of case management within HMOs was defined based on an index of intensity.[1] However, the complexity and depth of HPN's case management programs make it difficult to fit a single category. The characteristics of HPN's case management program can be better categorized by the setting in which these services are provided. Table 3 outlines the case management characteristics described within each setting: acute institutional (in-area), acute institutional (out-of-area), subacute/skilled nursing facility, custodial, and complex case management. In all settings, the case management staff performs the initial assessments on the enrollees and arranges services regardless of location.

Institutional case management

Throughout the various levels of institutional care, primary care physicians are teamed with nurse case managers. In the subacute/acute facilities, the physicians are internists; for skilled nursing facility patients, the physician is a family practitioner with extensive geriatric experience. Within the teams, clinical case managers specialize in areas such as geriatrics, medical/

Table 2 HPN Case Management Levels of Intensity

Level of intensity	Description	Examples	Provided by
Level I	Very simple One episode or contact Case finding	Arrange transportation Arrange durable medical equipment Arrange provider appointments Provide Friendly Caller services	Prior Authorization staff Member Services staff Senior Center staff Clinic Office staff
Level II	Simple One episode or contact Case finding Risk assessment Requires intervention of professional staff	Coordinate care for hospital discharge Serve as liaison between client and medical services Teach patient disease process and medication usage Coordinate community-based programs	Physicians/physician extenders Clinical RNs Institutional case managers Home health providers
Level III	Complex Short-term Medical, social, or psychological interventions Requires intervention of social worker or nurse case manager	Monitor compliance of medications Coordinate care Monitor health status Coordinate financial needs with community resources Provide risk assessment and monitor safety in home environment	Social workers Nurse case managers Home health specialty care nurses Clinical pharmacists
Level IV	Complex Long-term Medical, social, or psychological interventions Catastrophic or chronic care needs Requires intervention of social worker or nurse case manager Requires coordination of care across multiple sites of service and/or providers	Coordinate medical, social, and psychological services for complex cases such as transplant, multiple trauma, end-stage renal disease, and AIDS/HIV Assist patients with substance abuse disorders Assist terminal patients with end-of-life decision making	Social workers Nurse managers

surgery, subacute care, and terminal/hospice care. The case management team physicians become the exclusive attending physicians, responsible for the patient's care until the patient is discharged, at which time responsibility is returned to the PCP.

HPN's team approach to case management has been very successful for all parties because it has

Table 3 Characteristics of Case Management Models

Program characteristics	Institutional				Complex
	Acute institutional in-area	Acute institutional out-of-area	Subacute/skilled nursing facility	Custodial	
Location	Hospital	Corporate	Transitional care facility Long-term care facility	Transitional care facility Long-term care facility	Corporate
Case load	less than 19	20–39	20–39	100–119	60–79
Amount of face-to-face contact with enrollee	95%	0%	100%	100%	50%
Case management provided	YES	NO	YES	YES	YES
Number of case managers	20	3	7	7	10

- facilitated communication between the case manager and physician
- decreased delays in changing levels of care to the least restrictive care setting
- decreased fragmentation of care at discharge
- increased follow-through on postdischarge tests and appointments
- assisted skilled nursing facility staff in appropriate use of services, thus avoiding unnecessary transfers to emergency rooms.

Acute institutional in-area

HPN clients who are admitted to an inpatient facility have a plan of care started within 24 hours of admission. Case managers are on-site, seven days a week, to conduct initial evaluations and to develop treatment and discharge plans for the patient. Information is obtained by interviewing the patient and family, reviewing the patient chart, and consulting with the physician.

The physician/case manager teams meet every morning, seven days a week, to review their patients. During this review, they discuss the appropriate level of care, whether the patient can be in a less restrictive setting, potential home

health or complex case management needs upon discharge, and any follow-up needs at discharge such as scheduling of appointments or tests.

Acute institutional out-of-area

When a patient is hospitalized out of the HPN service area, an out-of-area case manager telephonically monitors the patient's care and coordinates discharge needs. The case manager works with the patient's family, provider, and the facility's discharge planning/UR staff to ensure the least restrictive, safe, cost-efficient setting for the patient. The case manager may be involved with arranging transportation, home assessments, case conferencing, and psychosocial, home health, or therapy services. If a face-to-face intervention is required, an on-site visit is made by a contracted case management provider in the area.

Subacute skilled nursing

A significant accomplishment of the HPN case management program was the integration of the physician/case management team with the subacute/skilled nursing facility staff. Daily rounding of the physician/case manager team and periodic assessments, based on level of care and need, contribute to the success of this program.

Custodial

In the custodial setting, the geriatric nurse practitioner supports the physician by providing medical services to the patient between physician visits. For the patient with complex issues, the geriatric nurse practitioner also serves as case manager (a model similar to that used by EverCare in Minneapolis, Minnesota). For the patient with simpler case management issues, a nurse case manager is assigned. The nurse case manager uses the geriatric nurse practitioner on a consulting basis.

Complex case management

All patients who are identified as high-risk are referred to HPN's Complex Case Management (CCM) Program. Complex case management is the coordination of care and monitoring of health status for these high-risk, complex, or catastrophic cases. Most of these patients remain in the community, the primary goal being to delay institutionalization and inappropriate access of care. Approximately 70 percent of the HPN CCM caseload is the Medicare-risk product enrollees. The CCM Program is designed to manage large or complex cases alone, or in conjunction with other divisions of SHS. Complex case managers can be either RNs with experience in case management or social workers. The complex case manager has overall responsibility for the case, regardless of setting.

Complex cases have the need for medical, social, and/or financial case management. Indicators for referrals to HPN's complex case management services include:

- *Medical* indicators such as hospital readmissions within specific time frames, noncompliance/discontinuity issues, need for specialized medical services out of the service area, or specific diagnostic groups such as AIDS/HIV, dialysis, transplant, progressive severe neurological disorders, end-stage/terminal disease process, high-risk pregnancy.

- *Social* indicators such as unsafe home environment, abuse and neglect, inability to perform IADLs, inability to access medical care on an ongoing basis, or family assistance with long-term care placement.
- *Financial* indicators such as inability to pay for long-term custodial care or medications exceeding plan limitations.

After an initial assessment by the complex case manager, which may be conducted either in person or telephonically, the frequency and type of contact are determined:

High intensity

Typically crisis intervention that requires contact until the crisis is resolved, then weekly home visits until the situation stabilizes (example: potential client abandonment by family, working on alternative placement).

Moderate intensity

Requires a home visit one to two times per month. Typically services clients with chronic "unstable conditions" such as coronary obstruction pulmonary disease (COPD) and diabetes or those more stable requiring in-person assessments such as patients with Alzheimer's disease. This intervention would also be appropriate for patients recently discharged from the hospital.

Low intensity

Requires at least monthly telephone contact. Clients may require follow-up on services that were arranged and possible Friendly Caller services. Members residing in group homes are typically served under this category. In these cases the case manager coordinates services with the group home to ensure that the member receives the appropriate medical care and necessary social services to prevent hospitalization or institutionalization.

Oversight

This level of service is provided when other case management services are involved in the case. In these instances, the case manager works closely with other care providers to offer continuity and coordination. Patients served by home health or hospitalized would fall into this category.

Table 4 describes examples of the management of different types of cases that are referred to complex case management.

Table 4 Complex Case Management Issues and Interventions

Client identified problems	Interventions
No primary care physician and chronic medical problems require ongoing medical supervision	Case manager (CM) to make initial PCP appointment and work to ensure follow-up visits.
Noncompliance with medication usage	RN CM to conduct home visit to provide education and follow-up for medication compliance on a weekly basis.
Difficulty accessing or understanding HMO system of care	CM to explain how to access the system for medical/social services and to assist with referral process. CM to serve as liaison between client and medical services, if needed.
Lack of understanding of medical problems, disease process, and medication	RN CM to teach and monitor effects of noncompliance upon body, side effects, and exacerbation of disease processes until patient is stable.
Difficulty coordinating services for multiproblem patients with psychosocial and medical needs	Team of RN CM and social worker to conduct initial comprehensive assessment and develop treatment plan that focuses on psychosocial and medical problems with appropriate interventions and follow through.
Need for coordination of community-based assistance programs and insurance benefits	Medical social worker to coordinate treatment to avoid duplication of service providers.
Financial difficulties	Medical social worker to coordinate client's financial needs with available community resources.
Need for coordination of care for organ transplant patients	RN case manager to work with "Centers of Excellence" and coordinate psychosocial, financial, and physiological services.
Drug-seeking behaviors	RN CM or social worker identifies reasons for drug-seeking behaviors and coordinates resources to assist client in treatment.
Substance abuse disorders	RN CM or social worker to identify diagnosis and refer for appropriate treatment (e.g., detoxification, treatment programs, counseling). CM to follow patient until stabilized and has adequate support system.
Terminal diagnosis	RN CM to follow patient during treatment to monitor deterioration and assist with end-of-life decision making.
Hospitalization	RN CM to coordinate care with hospital CM. RN CM to follow case after hospital discharge.
Chronic patients receiving home health services	RN CM to coordinate long-term care services with home health primary care nurse.
At risk in current home environment	Team approach of RN CM, social worker, and occupational therapist to conduct safety evaluation, develop plan of care, and follow patient until stabilized in home environment or alternate care setting.

CURRENT MODEL

Health Plan of Nevada has succeeded in both integrating case management services throughout its alternative care network and in identifying high-risk Medicare patients when they initially enroll in the HMO. However, for those members of the plan who age-in-place or develop chronic illnesses after enrollment, the need exists to work within the primary care setting to identify and serve these individuals who could benefit from case management. Often, patients are first seen by nurses or case managers in the hospital or alternative care settings in a crisis situation, inappropriately accessing care or not complying with treatment regimens.

The distribution of complex case management referral sources confirms that a large proportion of members are referred at the time of crisis (Table 5). Twenty-five percent of all complex case management referrals are initiated when patients are in the hospital, and another 20 percent are referred once they are receiving home health or hospice. Physicians are responsible for only 11 percent of the referrals to complex case management, yet the focal point of patient care is in the primary care setting. In the absence of a systematic means for referring members to complex case management from the primary care setting, the process becomes erratic and opportunities are lost for early intervention to prevent the decline of patient functional status and to assist patients in accessing services appropriately.

These findings led HPN to transition from a case management model to a care coordination model in which the primary care staff is educated in case management, and pharmaceutical services and case management are integrated into the ambulatory care setting. The intention of this model is to impact positively the quality of care provided to at-risk individuals served by an HMO.

IMPROVED CARE COORDINATION MODEL

A multidisciplinary project team was formed representing case management, clinical nursing, pharmacy, physicians, and the Senior Dimensions Service Center. Members of the team met several times to brainstorm and develop interventions that would better serve at-risk patients who would benefit from care coordination. The case management model was redefined into a more closely coordinated system that involved the entire health care team. A variety of ideas emerged relating to early, systematic identification and case management process. Some of these ideas included:

- on-site case managers assigned to the clinic setting
- training of clinic providers and staff on identification of at-risk members and availability of case management resources within all provider sites
- preventative health screening activities supported by a resource coordinator (Level 1 case manager) who would assist members with completion of questionnaires and coordination of preventive health needs
- ongoing risk assessment
- medication compliance screening
- software to test potential interactions and provide drug-specific information to patients
- pharmacy consultation
- patient education on medication usage for an older population

Table 5 Complex Case Management Referral Sources (1994)

Referral sources	(%)
Institutional case managers	25
Home health or hospice	20
Senior Dimensions Service Center	12
Physician	11
Utilization management	7
Patient or member	7
Urgent care	3
Member services	2
Mental health providers	3
Other	10
Total	100

The project team expected that these interventions would improve the quality of care by increasing provider and staff knowledge of available case management resources and increasing identification of at-risk cases after enrollment and before crises. They also anticipated that the interventions would result in proper utilization of services including hospitalization, urgent care visits, and overall expenditures.

One of eight clinic sites of Southwest Medical Associates, SHS's wholly owned medical group practice, was selected as the pilot site. Approximately 80 percent of the HMO enrollees use Southwest Medical Associates, Nevada's largest multispecialty medical group. The first intervention HPN attempted to implement was the introduction of low-level case management support to improve compliance with HPN Preventive Health guidelines. This activity required the front desk clinic staff to give to each patient a Personal Health Record form that highlights age- and sex-specific recommendations for preventive services including immunizations, cholesterol testing, breast exams, and pap and pelvic exams. Once in the examination room, the nurse reviewed the recommendations with the patient and suggested the appropriate tests, counseling, or health education classes. Patients needing or requesting classes or additional literature were referred to a resource coordinator, a case manager (Level I), who is knowledgeable in accessing resources.

Efforts to implement the intervention met with resistance and confusion from the clinic staff. The project team met again to review staff feedback on the new process. It was clear that without influencing the culture in the clinic and without "buy-in" from all levels of the clinic staff, the expectations for the project would not be met. Rather than simply applying new resources to the clinic setting, the project team decided it was necessary to truly integrate those who provide case management by making them part of the clinic team and physically locating them at the clinic site. These were the initial steps in implementing the care coordination model. It was proposed that the ambulatory care

coordination team would include the primary care provider, clinic nurse and/or nursing supervisor, office manager, case manager, social worker, resource coordinator, and clinical pharmacist. This team would be charged with coordinating the patient's care and service needs at the ambulatory care site.

To address the resistance issues expressed by the clinic staff, the project team developed an action plan. The designated "on-site case manager" spent two weeks orienting to the ambulatory care site, learning current operations. A meeting was held with the clinic's medical director to explain the project's objectives, specific interventions, advantages to the clinic, and to introduce the case management team. This was followed by a meeting with all levels of the clinic staff and providers to present the program, identify potential barriers to implementation, explain case management, review project objectives, and outline the benefits of having additional resources at the clinic site.

As part of the effort to identify potential barriers to implementation, the project team developed a staff questionnaire designed to assess the clinic staff's case management knowledge and to identify areas in which on-site case management could assist the staff with their current workload.

Moving the model to a care coordination delivery system and implementation of the ambulatory case management model began in July 1995.

LESSONS LEARNED

Although HPN is in the early stages of implementing the integration program at one clinic site, the following issues have already surfaced that may be helpful to other HMOs struggling with similar scenarios:

- Center care coordination in the primary care setting. The physician's office is the focal point of patient care and provides the greatest opportunity to intervene and therefore prevent or forestall functional decline and institutionalization of at-risk patients.

• Identify and include all disciplines who have a role in care coordination (e.g., front desk staff, physicians, nurses). Each member of the team has potential contact with the patient at different times during the office visit and each of these encounters offers another reference point from which to determine the patient's needs. Patients may tell the front desk staff about medical transportation problems that they would never discuss with a physician.

• Define the care coordination model with participation from all involved disciplines. To ensure that the model is comprehensive and addresses all of the patient's medical, social, and psychological needs, input is necessary from all areas, including mental health, nursing, social work, therapies (e.g., physical, occupational, speech), and pharmacy. This process also ensures "buy-in" from all participants.

• Communicate expectations and roles to all levels of staff that will be affected by the model. Allow opportunity to discuss and address potential barriers for implementation or misunderstandings regarding roles and responsibilities.

• Do not put resources in place until it is understood how proposed interventions will work with existing processes.

• Do not develop an organizational chart before testing the intervention. Too much attention to reporting structure can interfere with the creation of a successful model.

• Do not look at case management in isolation. All integrating components need to be considered in developing a care coordination model.

HPN continues to test and modify its evolving care coordination model. The company believes that educating the primary care staff in case management, integrating case management and pharmaceutical services into the ambulatory care setting, and conducting ongoing risk assessments will positively impact the quality of care provided to their chronically ill, multiproblem patients. The feasibility of this model is currently being evaluated by HPN under a grant from The Robert Wood Johnson Foundation. Should the results prove positive, HPN will be expanding its study to include additional clinic sites as well as network providers.

REFERENCE

1. Pacala, J.T. et al. "Case Management in Health Maintenance Organizations, Final Report." In *Chronic Care Initiatives in HMOs.* Washington, D.C.: Group Health Foundation, 1994.

A Look at the Newest Ethical Issues in Workers' Compensation

Anne Llewellyn

Case managers are being used in almost every aspect of health care today. Historically, we are mature health care professionals, many trained in a primary field during a time when the rules were strict but not as confusing as today. Fee-for-service medicine allowed us as health care workers to care for clients in an unrestricted manner. We did not have to ask, "What is your health care plan, is this service covered, and are the providers on your plan able to implement this service?"

Today, the rules are more complex and we face issues that are difficult for us to understand. In order to practice effective case management, we must understand ethical principles and incorporate them into our daily practice.

I recently closed my first workers' compensation case, which I had worked on for three years. As I was doing the final report, I thought back on the beginning of this case and how it developed, as well as what impact I had.

The client was a 67-year-old man who was injured in an auto accident when he was returning to his job after a meeting with his employer regarding his upcoming retirement. The client was broadsided and ejected from the car. He suffered a closed head injury among other internal injuries. He survived, but was left in a persistent vegetative state.

Inside Case Management 1997; 3(10): 5–7
© 1997 Aspen Publishers, Inc.

The challenge of this case was working with all of the providers and the various opinions and goals each had for the client.

I was the advocate for the client and worked with the wife to help her deal with the loss of her husband, as well as advocate cost-effective care. I educated the wife about her husband's overall and changing condition, and encouraged the team as the client moved along the continuum of care to foster the support that the client and his wife needed to deal with this catastrophic situation.

The outcome of this case was that we as a team were able to give the wife the autonomy and respect to care for her husband as best she could until his death, in the setting and manner that gave her the dignity she desired for her husband.

Autonomy is defined by the Ethics Statement of the Case Management Society of America (CMSA) as a "form of personal liberty of action when the individual determines his or her own cause of action in accordance with a plan chosen by himself or herself." The role of the case manager as client advocate comes from this principle. This principle focuses on the needs of the client, as perceived by the client, which are pre-eminent.

CMSA as a national organization has said that the field of case management is made up of multidisciplinary professions. Case managers of today must first adhere to the code of ethics for their profession of origin.

Those of us who work in workers' compensation case management can refer to the ethical principles from the recent CMSA Ethical Statement and apply them to the issues we are facing in our practice. In addition to autonomy, these principles are beneficience, nonmaleficence, justice, and veracity.

BENEFICENCE

Beneficence is "the obligation or duty to promote good, to further a person's legitimate interest, and to actively prevent or remove harm." This principle is an attempt to balance paternalism and promote self-determination. In workers' compensation, paternalism is something that we must be on guard to avoid. At times, due to the laws that govern workers' compensation, the client can become like the child, and the professionals who are charged with managing the case become similar to a parent.

I recently was at a conference where a vocational specialist asked a panel comprised of two attorneys and two judges the following question: "Is it appropriate for the plaintiff's attorney to sit in while a client is being tested by the vocational specialist?" A judge replied that if the attorney does not disrupt the testing, it is his right to sit in on the testing.

This comment surprised me. When and how did we evolve to this point in healthcare, when a client is not allowed the privacy needed to take a test designed to assist the professionals in gaining insight on how to assist the client to overcome a work injury? Where is the trust in our industry or the respect for the client?

NONMALEFICENCE

Nonmaleficence means refraining from doing harm to others. The realization of this principle in case management practice involves an emphasis on quality outcomes. This principle raises the question "What is a quality outcome?" In the field of workers' compensation, sometimes the outcome may be return-to-work for a client, or helping the client adjust to a situation where he or she will need to learn a new skill as a result of an injury, or learn how to accept and go on with a disability.

I once had a client who was a block mason. He loved his work. Unfortunately, he hurt his back and it was doubtful that he would return to his line of work. The man was devastated by this and really wondered how he would now support his family since being a block mason was the only work he knew.

As I worked with him along with the rehabilitation team, I realized what an injury could do to someone emotionally as well as physically. Once he completed his rehabilitation program, the client decided to move his family to another area of the county where he had a friend who could help him get work in a field offering a lighter type of work. I never found out how he did, but I feel that the coping and functional ability skills he learned from me and the team allowed him to go on with his life.

JUSTICE

Justice is defined as maintenance of what is right and fair. This is a concept that, as managed care comes more into the mainstream of healthcare, we are dealing with more and more. Many people see managed care as a way of giving them less than what is needed to adequately care for them for the sake of profit, and they are outraged.

Our challenge as case managers is to educate the public that managed care should give the client what is needed, when it is needed. We must work at restoring trust in the system. This can only be done through education of the consumers about their rights and through open communication among providers, the patients, and payers.

I recently had a client and his wife express to me their concern that the physician they were seeing was treating them differently because they were in a managed care workers' compensation plan. They told me that they had good insurance and did not want less care because this was a job related injury. I explained to them that they were seeing this physician because he was experienced in the specific injury incurred by the client, and that he had a very good reputation. I also encouraged them to talk with the physician regarding this concern.

During the examination, they did not bring the issue up. I felt that it was important to discuss the issue with the physician and not avoid the topic. I asked the doctor to address their concerns. He was able to do this in a very professional manner. Because workers' compensation can be very adversarial, the case manager can be the professional to ask the difficult question and listen to all sides in order to diffuse a potentially volatile situation.

We must restore trust in the system by being prompt with obtaining authorizations, communicating to all parties, and implementing treatment once the authorization is received. We must ensure progress is being made and, if not, talk to the physician and recommend alternatives. We must move the case along, but not at a speed that would not allow time for healing.

VERACITY

Veracity means truth telling. Trust is essential in the practice of case management. In order to develop trust, we must build a relationship with the client, providers, and payers.

Telling the truth is essential to building relationships. Even if you make a mistake, by telling the truth you will be ahead in the end. We all make mistakes, but if we cover up those mistakes, trust is lost.

Ethical principles have always guided case managers. By using negotiation skills, critical thinking, and the background of clinical knowledge, case managers ignite the ethical concepts that guide us and are applicable to our cases, our profession, and our everyday lives.

REFERENCES

1. Case Management Society of America. Proposed CMSA statement regarding ethical case management practice. *J Care Management.* 1995; (1):332.
2. Saulo, M., EdD, RN, and Wagner, R., MA, MDiv. How good case managers make tough choices: Ethics and mediation. *J Care Management.* 1996; (2):83.
3. Kidder, R.M. *How Good People Make Tough Choices.* New York: William Morrow and Company. 1995; 12–23.

PART II

The Case Manager's Universe

A Case Study of Nursing Case Management in a Rural Hospital

Wanda Anderson-Loftin, Danette Wood, and Linda Whitfield

Candler County Hospital is the primary access for many residents of Candler and surrounding counties. Like many other small rural hospitals, it is struggling to survive in a climate of spiraling health care costs, decreasing reimbursement, declining use, and increasing fiscal constraints. Nursing case management has been instrumental in decreasing costs, increasing quality, and redesigning the RN's role.

THE PROBLEM

Candler County Hospital is a non-profit, acute care, 60-bed hospital located in a nonmetropolitan statistical area of southeast Georgia. The case mix is not unusual for small rural hospitals in that it is composed of large percentages of vulnerable populations. Sixty-six percent of the patients are elderly, 85 percent are on Medicare or Medicaid, and 5 percent are uninsured. Statistics are unavailable on the percentage of minorities, however, it is estimated to be a significant number. Poverty increases the vulnerability of many of these patients; the median per capita income in Candler County is $12,578.[1]

The high cost of health care is a problem nationwide.[2] However, several factors that contribute to the high costs of care at Candler County are endemic to small rural hospitals.[3] The poor general health status of the older person, the poor, and minorities[4] and their increased incidence of complications are associated with an average length of stay that is greater than the national average. Cost shifting is not possible given this case mix. Furthermore, expensive emergency department care is substituted for primary care on evenings and weekends when physicians' offices are closed.

These problems are compounded by the problems of decreasing reimbursements, declining use, maintenance of quality, and the inability to attract and retain health professionals. In 1992, nursing case management was implemented to decrease costs and improve quality. Case management has also served as the vehicle for redesigning the RN's role[5] to more fully utilize knowledge and skills and consequently attract and retain RNs.

NEW ENGLAND MODEL OF NURSING CASE MANAGEMENT

The New England model[6] of nursing case management was used as a framework for developing case management at Candler County Hospital. In this model, the purposes of case management are to achieve standardized outcomes within designated lengths of stay with appropriate use of resources, while promoting professional development and satisfaction of RNs. Case management is conceptualized as a process and a role enacted by a nurse case manager. The nurse case manager manages and evaluates the

Nurs Admin Q 1995; 19(3): 33–40

care of high-volume, high-cost, high-risk patients across all hospital settings for an entire episode of care.[7]

Case management is generally embedded within a system of managed care in the New England model. At the Candler County institution, however, case management was implemented without a system of managed care in place. In the common usage of the term, managed care refers to organizations such as health maintenance organizations (HMOs) or preferred provider organizations (PPOs) whose goal is to achieve maximum value from the resources used.[8] In the New England model, managed care is a method of organizing unit-based care to achieve standard outcomes, within a designated length of stay, with appropriate use of resources.[6] The difference in managed care and case management in this model is that managed care focuses on the care of individual, high-volume patients while they are on a specific unit, and the focus of case management is on aggregate, high-risk, high-cost patients across all settings for an entire episode of care.

Case management plans, critical pathways, and Care Maps[9] are tools used in managed care to achieve desired outcomes. Case management plans are analogous to multidisciplinary care plans. These plans outline the desired outcomes for patients of a particular diagnosis-related group (DRG) and specify the amount and sequence of resource utilization necessary to achieve outcomes. Critical pathways are an abbreviated one-page version of the case management plan and describe critical interventions and activities that must occur within a given timeframe to achieve desired outcomes.[7] Care Maps go beyond traditional critical pathways in that Care Maps contain standard outcomes as quality indicators in addition to key, multidisciplinary interventions graphed against a timeline.[9]

At Candler County Hospital, the nurse case manager uses the tools of managed care not only as an effective method for improving quality and decreasing costs, but also to facilitate utilization review and pattern a new design for the RN work role.

THE PLAN

Fear of hospital closure and the resultant impact on the health of the community motivates many administrators in rural hospitals to seek innovative strategies for preserving community health care.[10,11] The director of nursing at Candler County Hospital envisioned case management as such a strategy.

The idea

The idea for case management was born of three precipitating factors. The first was the prolonged length of stay previously described. The second factor was the buzzword, case management, which appeared frequently in nursing and hospital literature. The third factor was an RN on staff who was approaching graduation as a clinical nurse specialist in rural community health at nearby Georgia Southern University. This RN had been employed as a critical care nurse, but also worked in the emergency department or as house supervisor as needed. The clinical skills of this nurse were exemplary and she had earned the respect of the medical and nursing staffs. These factors were the catalysts for action.

In June of 1992, the hospital administrator was consulted concerning the feasibility of creating a position for case manager. Being a proactive leader and a proponent of providing individuals every opportunity to reach their potential, he readily approved the concept and the necessary finances.

Identifying the patient population

Identification of the patient population was a part of the initial phase in establishing case management. The 10 DRGs that had the highest volume of hospital admissions were identified from computerized data. It is significant to note that pneumonia, which is the highest volume DRG admitting diagnosis at Candler County Hospital, also predominantly affects the older patient. For example, an unpublished study completed in 1994 revealed that 71 percent of the patients admitted with pneumonia were over 60 years old and 53 percent were over 70 years old. Furthermore, the older patient has more chronic illnesses, which prolongs the length of stay. These facts help explain why the length of stay at Candler County Hospital is higher than the national average.

Gaining physician support and ownership

The physicians at Candler County Hospital are usually supportive of new ideas to improve care. These ideas must be clearly and concisely presented by a knowledgeable individual who seeks and uses their input, and implementation of the idea cannot place unrealistic demands on their time. Therefore, education and training of the nurse case manager in case management and patient care standards were deemed critical in gaining physician support. The nurse case manager worked with the utilization review department for six months to learn Medicare, Medicaid, and private insurance patient care standards. An intensive independent study of case management was undertaken and sample critical pathways, based on current nursing and medical knowledge,[12] were developed to present to the medical staff.

In November 1992, case management was presented as an option to the medical staff. A detailed explanation was given and sample critical pathways were demonstrated. The physicians freely discussed the advantages and disadvantages of this type of patient management. After assurance that patient management could be individualized as necessary, the medical staff expressed their acceptance and willingness to support this patient care concept. Although the concept originated with nursing administration, physician acceptance was critical for success of the project.

Developing critical pathways

Having gained physician support, critical pathways for the 10 DRGs that had the highest volume of hospital admissions were developed by the nurse case manager. This was contrary to the multidisciplinary process recommended in the New England model for the following reasons. Physician case loads at this institution are extremely heavy. This is due in part to the shortage of health care personnel in this area and also due to the large numbers of chronically ill patients who require more frequent medical interventions and treatment. None of the physicians felt that they had adequate time to be active participants in the development of the critical pathways. Time constraints were also a problem with other disciplines. In small hospitals such as Candler County, health care personnel wear many hats, and other disciplines felt that numerous meetings would hinder direct care responsibilities. Limited availability of some disciplines, such as social work, also hindered a multidisciplinary planning process. There is a part-time social worker at Candler County who is available for high-priority patient needs; a paraprofessional carries out the daily routine social work functions. Therefore, after an exhaustive literature review, in addition to working with Medicaid, Medicare, and insurance standards, the nurse case manager designed the basic critical pathways that incorporated the care necessary for all disciplines. These plans were critiqued by physicians, nurses, and other members of the health care team and appropriate changes were made.

IMPLEMENTATION

Case management is implemented when a patient is admitted to the hospital. Ideally, this is done within 24 hours of admission. The admission diagnoses, as substantiated by clinical and diagnostic data, are used for the selection of the specific critical pathway. There are times when a combined critical pathway is necessary. Infrequently, an incorrect critical pathway is chosen, and a change is made when this is determined. The critical pathway is placed on the chart for easy access. Physicians continue to change their treatments according to present developments in health care and these changes are reflected in updated critical pathways. Physicians will communicate these changes directly on the pathways. In this way, the pathways are continually individualized and refined.

The nurse case manager concurrently monitors patient care while the patient is in the hospital. The nursing staff's input about patient condition and nursing care suggestions is sought and used. Dialogue among the case manager, nursing staff, and other disciplines is constant. Informal education sessions are ongoing as the staff continues to learn about public and private payment sources and how their requirements affect medical and nursing care. An after-discharge review is sometimes necessary to follow up with problems.

All patient care may not follow critical pathways. Deviations from pathways are termed variances. Variances, in the Candler County case management project, include patient factors, physician factors, and system failures and are addressed under a program of continuous quality improvement (CQI).

Although all physicians supported the concept of case management, all do not case manage their patients. This fact was somewhat disappointing. However, case management is entirely voluntary at our institution, and the physician's decision is respected.

INTEGRATING CQI

The hospital began the transformation process to CQI in 1992 by educating several managers in Deming's[13,14] concept of quality enhancement. Therefore, early in the development of case management CQI was incorporated into the plan.

Case management plans are used as a component of CQI. Data are evaluated against standard outcomes established by the case management plan. These outcomes are the criteria for care in the CQI plan. Thresholds are established by a multidisciplinary committee for acceptable levels of compliance with standards. Variances are monitored concurrently and the emphasis is to deal with variances as they occur. If a pattern of problems can be established, investigation and

corrective action are initiated. Issues that are not resolved and involve physician responsibilities are referred to the peer review committee for follow-up.

INTEGRATING UTILIZATION, PHARMACY, AND THERAPEUTIC REVIEW

In the evolution of case management at this facility, utilization review was integrated into the process. The critical pathway was revised to include Medicare, Medicaid, and insurance guidelines for patient admission severity of illness and patient treatment intensity of services. To decrease some departmental reviews, the nurse case manager assumed responsibility for utilization review, thereby decreasing costs. Because medication treatment is an integral part of the patient recovery process, a section was added to allow pharmacy and therapeutic reviews to be done while using the same forms and review process.

REDESIGNING THE RN WORK ROLE

Nursing case management has proven an effective method of redesigning the RN work role, creating a work excitement, and retaining a highly qualified, master's-prepared nurse. Moreover, the nurse case manager role has high potential as a recruitment tool for other RNs in the near future. Candler County, like other rural areas,[3] has difficulty attracting and retaining RNs. Because of the nursing shortage, the RNs function primarily in specialty areas and management or supervisory positions. Licensed practical nurses form the stable core of direct patient care providers as in most other small rural hospitals.[15] Creation of the case manager role provided an opportunity for high-volume, high-risk patients to have their care planned, managed, and evaluated by a highly educated and experienced professional nurse. Besides performing the case manager role, the nurse case manager also acts as quality assurance coordinator and utilization review nurse. By combining these positions with the case manager position, the nurse administrator was able to justify the funding for the clinical nurse specialist case manager position. Moreover, a cost savings in budgeted full-time equivalents was realized in the process.

The nurse case manager also acts as nurse researcher. Findings reported in this paper were the result of a study conducted by the nurse case manager and support the benefits of case management to the institution over the last two years.

RESULTS

The investigation reported here was conducted between November 1992 and February 1994. The objectives were to describe and analyze the influence of case management on cost data such as length of stay and to describe and analyze the influence of age, socioeconomic status, physician, and time of year on length of stay of case managed patients.

The total population of 768 patients case managed during the time interval of this investigation was included in this retrospective study. Patients in the study were classified according to the DRG groups in the box.

The most significant result was achieved in decreasing the length of stay. Comparison data of the length of stay before and after implementation of case management are shown in Figure 1. The average length of stay was 8.2 days be-

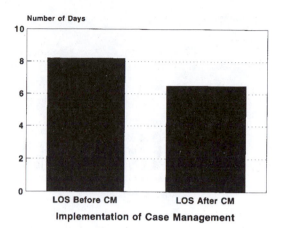

Figure 1. Influence of case management on length of stay.

fore implementation of case management and 6.5 days after implementation. The overall reduction in average length of stay was 1.7 days.

Age was a major influence on length of stay as shown in Figure 2. Patients 63 years and older accounted for 67 percent of the patient stays longer than the national average of 7 days. Seventeen percent of extended stays were by patients 73 to 77 years of age. These extended stays represent a considerable amount of unreimbursed care and are a major factor in increased costs, considering that 50 percent of all patients admitted are 63 years or older.

Socioeconomic status, as represented by insurance status, was analyzed and the differences in lengths of stay compared. The privately insured patient group had the lowest percentage of extended stays at 10 percent. This patient group is generally comprised of the young to middle-age group in the middle to upper socioeconomic class. The group with the highest percentage of extended stays, 53 percent, was patients receiving combined Medicare and Medicaid. This group of patients represent the debilitated, impoverished older people who are in nursing homes. In the group receiving Medicare, 50 percent of the stays were extended. This group of patients are generally the independent older people who live in their own home. It is no surprise that younger, privately in-

---

Case Managed DRGs

DRG 014, cerebral vascular accident
DRG 087, pulmonary edema
DRG 089, pneumonia
DRG 121, myocardial infarction
DRG 278, cellulitis
DRG 294, diabetes mellitus
DRG 316, end stage renal disease
DRG 321, urinary tract infection
DRG 416, sepsis
DRG 296, dehydration

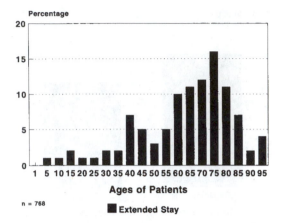

Figure 2. Patient stays longer than seven days according to age.

sured patients are able to be discharged within the targeted length of stay more frequently than the older individual. Neither is it a new notion that financially independent older people fare better healthwise than impoverished older people. However, it is significant to note that because 66 percent of the patients at this hospital are older and 85 percent are on Medicare or Medicaid, high extended stays, coupled with declining reimbursements in these two insurance programs, place great financial strain on an already stressed system. For example, Medicaid reimbursement was capitated at $2,483 during the time of the study.

Length of stay was analyzed by individual physicians for percentage of extended stays compared to length of stay within DRG criteria. The data showed that the range of extended stays, by physician, was 30 to 50 percent. More clearly, physician Y had the lowest percentage of patients with extended stays at 30 percent and physician X had the highest percentage of patients with extended stays at 50 percent. These results were generally uninterpretable because of the differences in individual physicians' case mix.

Length of stay by month was examined for patterns of extended stays related to seasonal variations. No patterns were discernible. The month with the lowest percentage of extended stays was February 1994. The month with the highest percentage of extended stays was July 1993. It is anticipated that a longer period of study will show trends not apparent in this 16-month study period.

CONCLUSION

Nurse case management has been shown to reduce costs of care and has spawned a visionary idea about how to improve patient care services to the community. Nursing case management at this institution has been associated with an initial decrease in the length of stay by 1.7 days. This decreased length of stay represented an estimated cost savings of $65,932 across the 16-month period of study. The need to extend case management beyond the walls of the hospital is apparent from the large percentage of older patients who have extended stays. Many of these patients are the impoverished older persons admitted and discharged from nursing homes in the area. Therefore, a case manager role that crosses both hospital and community settings is needed. If lengths of stay can be decreased in this population, the cost saving realized would justify the additional case manager position even without direct reimbursement for case management activities. With hospital–nurse-physician collaboration, extended case management services could be billed through physicians' offices. Physicians would benefit by decreased telephone calls from patients and families, increased patient satisfaction, and decreased patient emergencies. Nurses would be directly reimbursed for case management services through physician billings. Thus, hospital expenses for services provided but generally not billable are defrayed. Unnecessary hospitalizations would be prevented, and early intervention by case managers would mean that patients whose admission was necessary would be admitted at a lower acuity. The extension of the case manager role from hospital to community would provide a new role for RNs and serve to attract and retain professional nurses in the rural area. The benefits of this redesigned work role will be even more apparent as we continue to move toward a capitated health care environment in which the reward lies in keeping patients well and out of the hospital.

REFERENCES

1. Bachtel, D.C., and Boatright, S.R., eds. *The Georgia County Guide*. 11th ed. Athens, Ga.: University of Georgia College of Agricultural and Environmental Sciences and U.S. Department of Agriculture, 1993.

2. Feldstein, P.J. "Measuring Changes in the Price of Medical Care." In *Health Care Economics*. 4th ed. Albany, N.Y.: Delmar Publishers, 1993.

3. Parker, M., et al. "Issues in Rural Case Management." *Family and Community Health* 14, no. 4 (1992): 40–56.

4. Miller, M.K., Stokes, C.S., and Gifford, W.B. "A Comparison of the Rural-Urban Mortality Differential for Deaths from all Causes, Cardiovascular Disease and Cancer." *Journal of Rural Health* 3, no. 23 (1987): 23–34.

5. Sowell, R., and Fuszard, B. "Inpatient Nursing Case Management for Rural Hospitals: A Case Study." *The Journal of Rural Health* 5, no. 3 (1987): 201–15.

6. Etheredge, M.L.S. *Collaborative Care: Nursing Case Management*. Chicago, Ill.: American Hospital, 1989.

7. Zander, K. "Nursing Case Management: Strategic Management of Cost and Quality Outcomes." *Journal of Nursing Administration* 18, no. 50 (1988): 23–30.

8. Hicks, L., Stallmeyer, J.M., and Coleman, J.R. "Nursing Challenges in Managed Care." *Nursing Economics* 10, no. 4 (1992): 265–75.

9. Hampton, D.C. "Implementing a Managed Care Framework Through Care Maps." *Journal of Nursing Administration* 23, no. 3 (1993): 21–27.

10. Bindman, A.B., Deane, D., and Lurie, N. "A Public Hospital Closes: Impact on Patient's Access to Care and Health Status." *JAMA* 264 (1990): 2899–2904.

11. Mick, S.S., and Morlock, L.L. "America's Rural Hospitals: A Selective Review of 1980's Research." *The Journal of Rural Health* 6, no. 4 (1990): 437–62.

12. Larson, E.B., and Eisenburg, M.S. *Manual of Admitting Orders and Therapeutics*. 2d ed. Philadelphia, Pa.: W.B. Saunders, 1987.

13. Deming, W.E. *Quality, Productivity, and Competitive Position*. Cambridge, Mass.: Massachusetts Institute of Technology Center for Advanced Engineering Study, 1982.

14. Deming, W.E. *Out of the Crisis*. Cambridge, Mass.: Massachusetts Institute of Technology Center for Advanced Engineering Study, 1986.

15. Fuszard, B., et al. "Rural Hospital of Excellence: Part I." *Journal of Nursing Administration* 24, no. 1 (1994): 21–26.

Population-Based Case Management

Faiga J. Qudah and Melissa Brannon

With the current changes in the financing and delivery of health care, new arrangements for organizing, providing, and paying for care have emerged. One need only to read about the number of hospital mergers that have occurred and the provider networks that have formed. Pressures to contain cost have moved payment arrangements from price discounts to case reimbursements and now to capitated payments.[1] Price discount is volume sensitive, and higher utilization rates (i.e., more admissions, procedures, tests, etc.) generate higher revenue.

Case reimbursement is similarly volume sensitive. Higher admission rates generate higher revenue, but only if the cost per adjusted discharge is less than the revenue per case. Capitated payment places the provider (a hospital or physician) at financial risk. In capitated arrangements, a financing organization, such as an insurance plan, pays a fixed amount per member per month (PMPM) to the provider, who assumes the risk for utilization or the cost of providing care. Although capitation has yet to become the most common payment arrangement, provider organizations have begun to organize themselves into provider networks poised to accept this financial risk. As a result, more providers are forming or becoming parts of integrated systems to increase their access to covered lives within the market.[2] The focus of efforts to improve health care has shifted from providing acute care to managing care across a continuum. Case management programs offer strengths and weaknesses in meeting the goal of managing care.

While traditional case management programs have proven to be effective in coordinating care and services, most deal with separate components of care and not the full continuum.[3,4] The result is fragmentation and duplication of processes. Inpatient case management, for example, deals with the inpatient stay and may include prehospital needs and early discharge but rarely addresses the events causing the acute episode or the ongoing needs of the patient.[5] Insurance-based case management usually focuses on utilization review, specialist referrals, and precertification. Community-based case management programs often do not include the acute or hospitalization phase. The success of integrated systems depends on their ability to coordinate care and utilize resources to proactively manage health. Population-based case management provides a differentiated, focused approach to managing health across the full continuum. The purpose of this article is to expand

The authors would like to thank Steve Mason, Executive Vice President, and to acknowledge the Research and Development Department, the Wellness and Prevention Department, and the Integrated Care Management Department at Harris Methodist Health System for their work and collaboration in the continuing development of IHM.

Quality Management in Health Care 1996; 5(1): 29–41

current thinking about case management so that implementation of new case management programs will be seen as key to the success of fully integrated systems.

INTEGRATED FINANCING, MANAGEMENT, AND DELIVERY

An efficient integrated health system has three principle components: financing, management, and delivery. The relationship of these three components is critical to providing the most appropriate and cost-effective health care to a defined population. A defined population may be a geographically distinct community, a demographic or payer segment within such a community, a group of covered lives within a provider or practice site, all the patients admitted to a hospital, or a diagnosis group within any of these collections of people.

In the past, patients requiring acute care services provided by hospitals made up the health care population.[6] In today's world of managed health care, integrated health systems look at the health care population in terms of covered lives.[7] These covered lives come through insurance platforms such as a health meintenance organization (HMO) or other payer groups and make up the financing component of an integrated system. The goal is to service the optimal number of covered lives required to reach operational and economic efficiency.

The covered lives receive care through a network of providers that make up the delivery component of the integrated system. This network of providers includes physicians, hospitals, pharmacies, and ancillary health care providers such as home health services and ambulatory care centers. The delivery component creates a provider network around a set of negotiated contracts that are market driven and render value through high customer satisfaction, superior outcomes, and competitive cost.

At the core of an integrated system is the management component. Managing the health of these defined populations is equivalent to managing the assets of integrated systems. The goal here is to create a continuous improvement management process and implement a care delivery model to produce the best return on the investment—the best health possible for the members. The new care delivery models are accountable for reducing costs, improving outcomes, increasing accessibility, and maintaining profitability.

INTEGRATED HEALTH MANAGEMENT: A CARE DELIVERY MODEL

Integrated health systems (IHSs) like Harris Methodist Health System (HMHS) are well positioned to reform health care delivery. Harris Methodist Health Plan offers a diverse range of products, from an HMO to a point-of-service indemnity product to life insurance, and HMHS is the largest fully integrated health care system in north Texas, serving 250,000 members and nearly 2,000 employers. The regional network includes more than 3,000 private practice family doctors and specialists, more than 50 hospitals, and more than 600 pharmacies. In addition, HMHS owns and operates seven hospitals, all of which earned Joint Commission on Accreditation of Healthcare Organizations accreditation with commendation in 1995. Two HMHS hospitals were named among *Modern Healthcare*'s Top 100 Hospitals in America, and the Harris Methodist Fort Worth Emergency Department Redesign Team recently won the *USA Today* Quality Cup for improving emergency care. The health plan's success is based on the partnerships developed with employers and employees, doctors, hospitals, and pharmacies.

Because integrated systems control the financing, management, and delivery of an array of health services and products, they provide customers with the most appropriate, most cost-effective, and highest possible quality of care available in their market segments. HMHS has developed a set of processes to manage its financing and delivery components and thus realize the full potential of integration. One of these processes is integrated health management (IHM), a care delivery model with a systemwide focus on managing the health of a defined population through wellness promotion, illness prevention, and care coordination across a full continuum (see the appendix for a sample IHM plan).

Before becoming an integrated system, HMHS was a system of hospitals that treated acute and chronic diseases of inpatients and outpatients. Its evolution into an integrated system with its own financing arrangement and delivery network forced it to develop a new mindset—basically to shift from managing illness to managing wellness (Figure 1). The focus is now on managing the health of a population rather than on episodes of illness and hospitalizations. The point of management will shift from hospitals to primary care providers and from utilization review to ongoing care management to provide access and accountability across the continuum of health. Success will be measured by overall system performance (rather than individual provider performance) and the ability of the system to collectively meet the needs of the population.

Prevention, early intervention, and care coordination across a full continuum are the primary

objectives of the IHM care delivery model. Six levels of activity serve as the foundation for IHM (Figure 2). Each level has an element of strategy development that requires interface between the financing and delivery components. Level 1 encompasses population needs assessment; Level 2, resource allocation and alignment through network design; Level 3, health planning through priority segment plan development; Level 4, wellness and prevention; Level 5, care management; and Level 6, case management. The role of case management is expanded to include population management, a strategic activity that, as part of an overall delivery model, can improve the community's health and achieve targeted outcomes. Below, after a brief description of each level of the IHM model, specific case management strategies are discussed.

Population needs assessment

At Level 1, population managers collect data to assess the needs of the population. The population to be served is defined and segmented based on possible management criteria, such as

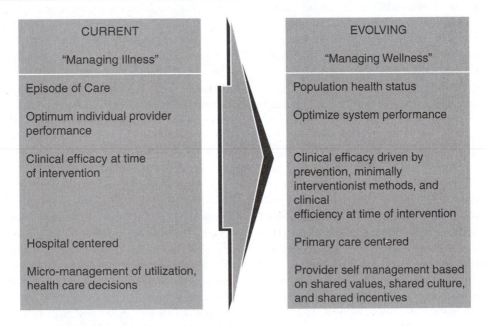

Figure 1. The shift in the health care delivery paradigm.

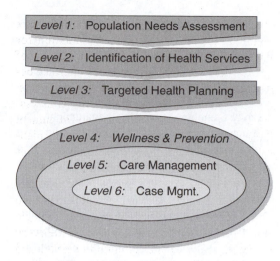

Level 1: Population Needs Assessment

Level 2: Identification of Health Services

Level 3: Targeted Health Planning

Level 4: Wellness & Prevention

Level 5: Care Management

Level 6: Case Mgmt.

Figure 2. The six levels of the integrated health management model.

type of health insurance product, health plan, physician group, hospital, customer, payer, or major employer account. Data are collected using a variety of instruments and techniques to identify

- health history (e.g., ICD-9 Claims-Based Paid Population Segmentation System [ICPSS]),[8]
- utilization patterns (e.g., admissions per thousand, days per thousand, average length of stay, pharmacy cost per member per month, etc.), and
- risk factors (e.g., health risk assessments, public health statistics, etc.).

It is important at this stage to identify goals and expected outcomes with providers and/or client groups. This will affect how the population segments are managed and prioritized. Goals are also used to determine resources needed to accomplish related goals. A gap analysis using national benchmarks and standards helps identify opportunities and actions and a Pareto analysis helps focus on and prioritize key strategic areas.

Network design, resource allocation, and alignment with goals

Population managers then work with the health plan, community managers, and providers to figure out a benefit and network design that will meet the needs of the population. They use an analytical framework to determine types and levels of health services needed and distribution points for these services. A gap analysis compares current available resources and skills with those required to meet the needs of the defined population or segments within. As part of Level 2, the performance patterns of providers within the delivery network are profiled for key quality and cost-effectiveness measures. For example, the referral patterns of primary care physicians are evaluated to determine both the frequency and type of referrals made. Any services required to meet the needs of designated population segments are also analyzed to determine capacity and accessibility. For example, having an adequate number of nursing home beds is important, but equally important is the quality and geographic location of those beds within the community. At Level 2, products and services are tailored to the needs of a defined population and cost-benefit analysis is used to allocate and align resources.

Strategic and targeted health planning

At Level 3, population managers develop a strategic health plan for the population. A comprehensive list of interventions and expectations is developed. Root causes are identified and specific approaches to accomplishing changes are developed, including potential problem assessment and contingency plans. An impact-effort analysis is used to help prioritize actions based on their potential impact on outcome measures and the likelihood of performing them successfully with available resources. For example, if utilization of physical therapy treatments is higher than the target or a national benchmark, is there an associated impact on the surgical rate of orthopedics or readmission of orthopedic surgical cases that justifies the utilization rate of physical therapy? Validating priorities and performing a cost-benefit analysis of resources used by the target population segments provide the information necessary to develop action plans that include wellness and prevention, case management and benefit network design.

Wellness and prevention

Level 4 comprises targeted wellness and prevention and also health promotion and demand management. Case managers work with wellness and prevention staff to identify appropriate referrals for both areas. At this level, initiatives are implemented using wellness and prevention programs to target individuals with varying health conditions and health behaviors at the earliest possible point on the health continuum. The population is triaged according to the results of the health risk assessment, and interventions are designed based on the presence of urgent, high-risk, and low-risk conditions or behaviors. The goal is to refer urgent and high-risk individuals for early proactive case management and wellness and prevention programs. Demand management programs provide decision support and information at the point where a consumer is making a decision about how to enter the health care system. A telephone clinical triage system helps consumers make informed decisions to access the right care at the right time and use the right resources. It can have a tremendous impact on the cost and quality of health care. Unnecessary emergency department visits can be reduced by up to 90 percent and unnecessary physician office visits can be reduced by 40–60 percent.

Another Level 4 goal is to educate and motivate the targeted population or certain segments to take responsibility for their health and the quality of their lives. The desired outcome is healthier and better educated people who share the demand for appropriate and cost-effective health care services. It is important to understand that Level 4 is not solely an education process but a transition process as well. Programs delivered at this level are designed to encourage individuals within the population to set goals and make commitments to improve their own health, reduce the risk of future health problems, and accept accountability for self-care.

Care management

Level 5 encompasses care management. The care management process is coordinated across a full continuum, as illustrated in Figure 3. It is an ongoing process in which a population manager establishes systems to evaluate the health status of the population and monitor the outcomes achieved and resources used. The population manager serves as the chief strategist for managing health, setting the strategic plan of care, coordinating the care delivery, and evaluating the plan of care for a defined population.

Unlike traditional case management, where the goal is to manage a single episode or illness in an acute care setting, care management is intended to prevent or reduce the possibility of an acute episode of illness by monitoring an individual's health needs and identifying behavior patterns that put the individual at risk. To accomplish this goal, the population manager is held accountable for monitoring the health of individuals in a designated population segment, identifying variances from established norms or targets, determining the root causes of these variances, and coordinating the development of specific action plans with a multidisciplinary team. Health status information is reviewed on an ongoing basis to help in reevaluating needs at Levels 1 and 2 and redesigning plans. One of the goals of the care management processes is to identify and refine case management triggers that allow high-risk individuals to be referred earlier in the continuum, when prevention will have the greatest impact.

Case management

Level 6 encompasses case management. Acute, episodic case management is linked with ongoing case management across the full continuum of health care. Case managers are assigned to members by primary care physicians and are responsible for managing health, illness

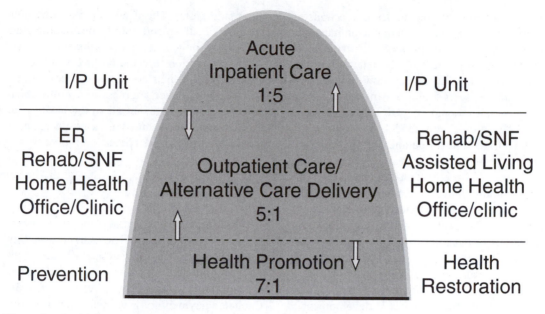

Figure 3. The full continuum of care.

prevention, and coordination of care and services, including during acute episodes or hospitalizations. They may coordinate with hospital-based case managers and use specialty case managers as resources or manage care independently, but they always maintain accountability across the continuum.

The initial Level 6 goal is early identification of high-risk individuals with complex conditions that will likely result in a deterioration of health or an acute episode or that will respond positively to ongoing coordination of care and services. The next goal is to quickly arrange for each patient the most appropriate provider and level of care, thereby reducing the risk of further complications. The final goal is to facilitate a seamless and timely transition through each level in the continuum or to maintain the best possible level of health. These goals are accomplished through collaboration between the financing and delivery components of an integrated system, including the formation of a multidisciplinary ad hoc team to implement the care plans and possibly the development of practice guidelines for prevention as well as disease management.

The role of the case manager in an integrated system is to develop and manage a comprehensive plan of care throughout the continuum in a way that takes advantage of all the resources an integrated system has to offer. This means new challenges for coordination of service and communication between providers, payers, facilities, and clients. The barriers of service setting, provider category, and financing source are removed, making it possible to impact health across the continuum. By building on their existing skills and knowledge; developing new competencies for transition management, wellness and prevention, and multidisciplinary decision making; and expanding their clinical expertise to include all phases of disease management, case managers in an integrated system can become an essential cornerstone to its success.

IMPLEMENTING IHM: A COLLABORATIVE PROCESS

The development and implementation of IHM as a care delivery model has taken HMHS through a massive learning experience in the last few years. The process continues to evolve. As an organization that has undergone a transformation from a hospital system into an integrated financing, management, and delivery system, HMHS had to recreate itself—redefine its mission and vision, develop a new management structure, revise its strategic plan, and commit to a new organizational culture. The development of a new care delivery model was an important factor in this transformation. During the development, essential components were identified, including (1) agreement on common definitions; (2) common clinical and financial information systems, a variance monitoring process, and database development; (3) multidisciplinary coordination; (4) integration with the system's continuous improvement process; (5) a centralized organizational structure for the coordination of care across a full continuum; (6) development of clinical guidelines; and (7) development of wellness and prevention programs.

A new management structure for case management

HMHS developed an organizational structure that centralized the care and case management infrastructure at one level of organization. The case management, utilization review, and discharge planning functions at the HMHS hospitals now report to the integrated care management (ICM) department at the system level. Hospitals have traditionally approached management through utilization review, discharge planning, and patient care services using critical pathways.[9] This was the case at the HMHS hospitals. Each of these functions operated independently of each other. With HMHS's transformation into an integrated health system, it was essential to integrate care delivery. This meant that acute or episodic case management had to be linked with ongoing care management on the financing side and that any handoff from either side had to be coordinated. It also meant that financing and provider side incentives had to be aligned and that both sides had to be held accountable for admission rates (to control health plan costs) and lengths of stay (to control pro-

vider side costs). The ICM department became the hub of all episodic and nonepisodic care planning, monitoring, and coordination of care for the population served. For the HMHS hospitals, this meant their entire hospital population, regardless of payer source; for the physician practice groups, it meant all of the health plan members they had; and for the health plan, it meant all of its enrolled lives.

A new partnership with physicians and hospitals

Physicians and hospitals are at different stages of consolidation. The market is getting ready for physician capitation. With incentives now becoming more closely aligned, IHM has become more valued by physician groups. Capitated payment for a defined number of covered lives provides a powerful incentive to assess needs and determine appropriate programs and required services.[10] To be successful in a capitated market, physicians would have to manage their population of covered lives proactively and embrace wellness and prevention as their goals. IHM teams are now assigned to major physician economic groups within the delivery network. The population managers and case managers are relocated in the offices of some of these physician groups and work as a team with utilization management nurses assigned to one or two hospitals that the physician groups designated as their admission sites.

IHM teams have forged partnerships with physician groups and helped them incorporate IHM into their practice. Together, they have worked toward the creation of a comprehensive medical management program that includes the development of policies and procedures for the groups' utilization management; the implementation of a specialty referral process; the application of criteria for medical necessity and appropriateness; the implementation of an on-site precertification and utilization review process; the analysis of group and individual practice patterns, including referral patterns; a profiling of the groups' populations through the collection of health risk assessment (HRA) information; and an analysis of utilization rates. The impact of these IHM teams is significant. Indeed, they have affected not only the management of the health plan's covered lives but also the entire clientele of the physician groups.

Results

The collaborative relationship between the health plan and the physician groups helped reduce the health plan's commercial HMO utilization rate from 72 admissions per thousand covered lives to 52 admissions per thousand in a 15-month period. Similarly, during 11 months of case reimbursement, the average length of stay dropped from 4.30 to 3.66. In the senior health plan, a Medicare risk product operational only since March 1995, an aggressive population-based case management program pushed the admission rate from 369 per thousand covered lives down to 196 and bed days from 1,669 per thousand covered lives down to 1,249 by the end of 1995. The latest year-to-date average is 191 admissions and 1,076 days per thousand covered lives, and the average length of stay is currently 5.63, down from 6.20 at the end of 1995.

• • •

Population-based case management is still in the beginning stages. Forming new partnerships with physicians and hospitals to help manage the health of covered lives in the Harris Methodist Health Plan has opened the door to the future. That future is one that allows an integrated health system like HMHS to move and grow in response to changes in the marketplace and the social issues affecting the communities around it. Its success as an integrated system will depend on its ability to impact the health not just of its enrollees but others who are in need of care. If it is able to achieve such an impact, HMHS will have fulfilled its mission, which is "to improve the health of all people in each community we serve."

REFERENCES

1. Health Care Advisory Board. *The Grand Alliance: Vertical Integration Strategies for Physicians and Health Systems.* Washington, D.C.: The Advisory Board Company, 1993.

2. Health Care *Advisory Board. Hospital Networking, Strategy Briefing for Chief Executives.* Washington, D.C.: The Advisory Board Company, 1995.

3. Satinsky, M. *An Executive Guide to Case Management Strategies.* Chicago, Ill.: American Hospital Association, 1995.

4. Mullahy, C.M. *The Case Manager's Handbook.* Gaithersburg, Md.: Aspen Publishers, 1995.

5. Stevens, R. *In Sickness and in Wealth: American Hospitals in the 20th Century.* New York, N.Y.: Basic Books, 1989.

6. Maculate, J., and Shlala, T. "Case Management Can Reduce Cost and Protect Revenues." *Healthcare Financial Management* 49, no. 4 (1995): 64–70.

7. Health Care Advisory Board. *Vision of the Future.* Washington, D.C.: The Advisory Board Company, 1993.

8. Ghate, B., and Rushing, S. "ICPSS-ICD9 Claims Based Population Segmentation System." Harris Methodist Inc., Research Development Department, 1996

9. Bergman, R. "Reengineering Health Care." *Hospitals and Healthcare Networks* 68, no. 3 (1994): 28–36.

10. Shortell, S., Gillies, R., and Devers, K. "Reinventing the American Hospital." *Milbank Quarterly* 73 (1995): 131–60.

Sample Integrated Health Management Plan for Cardiovascular Health

The following provides an illustration of IHM focused on cardiovascular health management for a fictitious company, Industrial Products.

Level 1: Assess needs of population

- Segmentation strategy
  - A case management strategy will be developed to manage the cardiovascular health of members at Industrial Products.
- Mutual goals
  - Decrease overall utilization of health care services.

- Specific measurable targets include (1) reduction of PMPM medical costs; (2) reduction of days per 1,000.
- Health history
  - Industrial Products has 7,500 employee members. The majority are male, blue-collar workers between the ages of 45 and 60.
  - ICPSS Pareto analysis shows that 14.6% of Industrial Products' employees accounted for 80.9% of the entire population's illness defined by claims paid in fiscal year 1995 (see Figure A1).

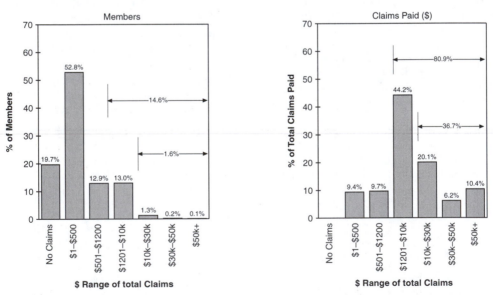

Figure A1. Data on percentage of members by range of total claims and on percentage of total claims paid by range of total claims.

—Five key disease categories accounted for a total of 44.4% of all illness at Industrial Products in fiscal year 1995 (see Figures A2, A3, and A4).

- Utilization patterns
  —There is a gap of 4 admissions per 1,000 above national utilization benchmarks. This variance is all related to the five key disease categories. The average length of stay for the population is on target.
- Risk factors
  —Health risk assessments reveal the areas for highest risk for health problems are cardiovascular and cancer risk.
  —Lifestyle behaviors related to these conditions for this population include smoking, high-fat diet, and sedentary lifestyle.
  —The readiness-to-change survey shows that 25% are at a stage ready to change.

Level 2: Network design, resource allocation, and alignment with goals

- Gap analysis of current skills and resources needed indicates there is an overage of acute care beds, locations of services are adequately dispersed, and there are adequate types of services and physicians.
- Fourteen physicians vary greater than 50% from targeted PMPM goals for under- or overutilization (see Figure A4). Ninety-six percent of this variance is accounted for by admissions or procedures in the five key disease categories.

Level 3: Strategic and Targeted Health Plan

- Action plan
  —Review trends and patterns of 21.3% (975) of members that account for 44.2% of claims.
  —Refer the 1.6% (120) of members that account for 36.7% of claims to case management to review individual cases and determine appropriateness for case management.
  —Identify any new case management triggers based on review of practice patterns and trends or review of individual cases.
  —Identify root causes of top five disease categories.

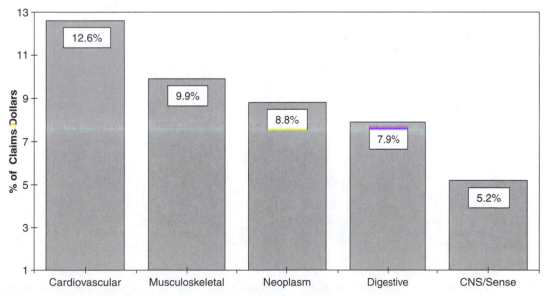

Figure A2. Percentage of claims dollars by ICD-9 disease category.

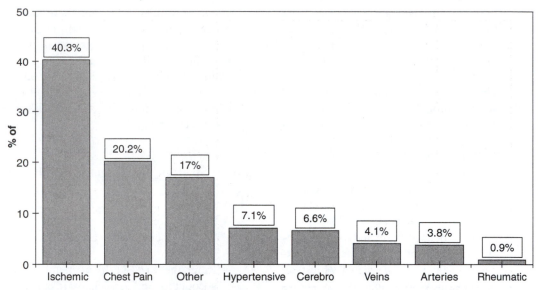

Figure A3. Percentage of claims dollars by cardiovascular subcategory.

- Cardiovascular disease accounts for the largest percentage of claims paid.
- Ischemic cardiovascular disease is the highest category within cardiovascular (40.3%) (see Figure A3).

- Chronic ischemia and acute myocardial infarctions represent a total of 92.5% of all ischemic disease (see Figure A4).
  —Investigate practice patterns with the 14 physician outliers with variance greater

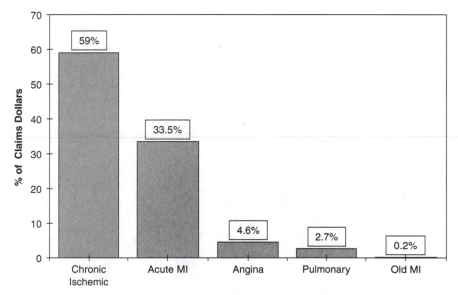

Figure A4. Percentage of claims dollars by ischemic subcategory (ischemic is itself a subcategory of cardiovascular).

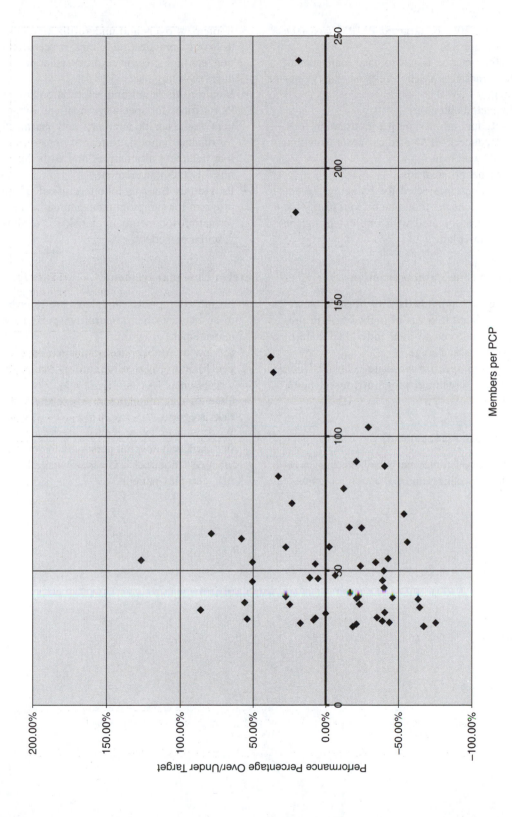

Figure A5. Physician performance data.

than 50% of targeted PMPM cost (see Figure A5).

- Refer practice issues to case management for practice guideline review or development.
- Expected outcomes
  —Reduce admissions per thousand by four.
  —Reduce PMPM medical costs to within 5% variance.
- Cost-benefit analysis
  —Savings projected for reducing the admissions per thousand by four justify the cost associated with implementing the action plan.

Level 4: Wellness and prevention

- Refer the individuals with lifestyle behaviors related to areas of highest risk to programs tailored to their individual state of readiness to change.
- Develop specific worksite offerings (i.e., mobile screening, programs, health fairs, etc.).

Level 5: Care management

- Monitor outcomes and behaviors changes related to wellness and prevention programs.

- Implement over- and underutilization controls (e.g., practice guidelines, precertification, etc.) for specific cardiovascular procedures over targets.
- Monitor utilization and referrals on site at PCP offices for specialty, inpatient, outpatient, home health, ancillary, and pharmacy for related diagnosis to identify cost-effective treatment alternatives and early referrals for case management.
- Provide 24-hour telephone clinical triage program for symptom management and information for members at risk for cardiovascular episodes.

Level 6: Case management

- Ensure appropriate candidates are referred to an acute ischemic cardiovascular case management program.
- Review or establish case management triggers for early, aggressive cardiovascular intervention.
- Case manage members in urgent and high-risk categories.
- Work with PCPs, specialty physicians, office staff, and hospital personnel to develop practice guidelines and case manage high-risk, complex patients.

Telephonic Nursing: Empowering Patients at Risk for Preterm Birth

Marianne E. Weiss and Annette K. Adams

As health care systems search for cost-effective mechanisms for reducing the need for acute care services, innovative programs targeting health promotion and disease prevention for at-risk clients are being implemented and tested. There has been considerable interest in developing models of care to promote reduction in the incidence of preterm birth. The U.S. preterm birth rate of over 10% of births (Adams, 1995) is high among developed countries (Morrison, 1990). The birth of a preterm infant has enormous human and economic costs to the family and the health care system in both the short and long term. Preterm delivery is the most significant contributor to perinatal morbidity and mortality, accounting for 10% of all births and 75% of perinatal deaths (Creasy, 1994). The incidence of respiratory distress, patent ductus arteriosus, and necrotizing enterocolitis are inversely related to gestational age at birth.

Efforts directed at preventing preterm birth have included education about risk reduction and early detection, home surveillance with home uterine activity monitoring (HUAM) to support early detection, and development of protocols and testing of new pharmacological agents for hospital-based and home treatment of preterm labor symptoms. Despite these efforts the preterm birth rate continues to rise.

The literature on the effectiveness of preterm birth prevention efforts is contradictory. Some education-based prevention programs and programs offering frequent provider contact have produced promising results while others have not supported these approaches (Andersen, Freda, Damus, Brustman, & Merkatz, 1989; Bryce, Stanley, & Garner, 1991). Results of testing of the efficacy of home uterine monitoring have also been contradictory (Collaborative Group on Preterm Birth Prevention, 1993; Mou et al., 1991; Nagey, Bailey-Jones, & Herman, 1993). The weight of evidence does not at this time support the use of HUAM for monitoring of patients at risk for preterm labor (U.S. Preventive Services Task Force, 1993). Several studies have addressed the importance of nurse contact as a key feature of home management programs for preterm birth prevention (Hill et al., 1990; Knuppel et al., 1990; Watson et al., 1990). In fact, the increase in nursing services associated with HUAM may be the factor that positively impacts patient outcomes. Models are currently being tested that use an approach incorporating telephonic nursing care to virtually eliminate the need for HUAM.

Development and testing of new models for management of the at-risk patient population is imperative in the emerging era of health care. Case management has been proposed as a mechanism for providing quality health care, decreasing fragmentation, enhancing the client's quality of life and containing costs (American

Nurs Admin Q 1995; 1(3): 58–64

Nurses Association, 1988). Several models for case management have been explored, including health plan-based case management/utilization management (Henderson and Wallack, 1987), clinical nurse specialist case management (Gibson, Martin, Johnson, Blue, & Miller, 1994), and case management by the primary nurse (Zander, 1988). All are focused on quality and cost control accomplished by timely and appropriate use of resources and coordination across the continuum of care.

TELEPHONIC CASE MANAGEMENT

The era of managed health care has created the need for innovative strategies for meeting client's health care needs. Increasingly, patient care is being shifted from hospital to home. Home health care, although less expensive than hospital care, still requires substantial expenditures of providers' resources. In some cases, patients require frequent short contacts with providers for monitoring of health status, teaching, and coordination of care. Often, these are patients who are at risk for a major illness event or who have recently been discharged and are at risk for a subsequent event. Telephonic nursing care may offer a cost-effective alternative for selected patient groups. Through regular contact with a nurse, the patient's health status can be monitored, focused teaching can occur, and care needs can be coordinated. The focus of these regular contacts is risk reduction, risk identification and management, early recognition of prodromal symptoms, and timely home-, office-, or hospital-based intervention as needed.

Studies of telephone follow-up programs for post-hospitalization management have demonstrated that telephone contact has a significant effect on compliance with treatment recommendations, as well as improved physical and psychological outcomes (Maisiak, Koplon, & Heck, 1990; René, Weinberger, Mazzuca, Brandt, & Katz, 1992; Weinberger, Tierney, Booher, & Katz, 1991). It has been postulated that the mechanisms associated with these improved outcomes are social support and provision of information. In a study of patients with osteoarthritis (Weinberger et al., 1991) 79% of patients reported at least one positive action as a result of the telephone contact program. Specific outcomes included asking the physician more questions, greater compliance with physician's orders, and feeling more in control of their disease condition. These results suggest that a key element of the telephone contact program is client empowerment.

Telephonic case management for preterm birth prevention

The birth of a preterm infant has enormous human and economic costs to the family and the health care system. Perinatal and neonatal costs associated with preterm birth can result in huge losses for managed care programs. Preterm birth prevention programs have typically focused on primary prevention and health promotion through risk screening and education. The high-risk patient receives closer medical follow-up and admission for labor suppression when preterm labor occurs.

Telephonic case management of the perinatal patient at high risk for preterm labor has been proposed as a cost-effective proactive strategy for preventing catastrophic health outcomes and expenses associated with inappropriate use of in-home uterine activity monitoring technology and long-term intensive care of the preterm neonate.

Telephone case management programs are being developed in hospital, outpatient, and insurance settings. Kotula (1994) described the role of the perinatal case manager as coordinating medical, social, and funding resources to extend the pregnancy to the most optimal outcome for mother and infant. Specifically, the case manager promotes communication about the treatment plan; increases the client's self-care abilities and stress management/coping strategies through education; promotes effective and timely use of family, community, and health care resources while minimizing or preventing hospitalization; and promotes development of care systems to facilitate access, decrease cost, and improve quality of care.

Telephonic nursing care

The case manager role includes components of systems development and direct patient care. Zander (1988) has advocated for a case management approach by the primary nurse. Extending this concept to preterm birth prevention efforts, direct nursing care services are provided telephonically. Telephonic perinatal nurses (TPNs) conduct assessments, identify patient problems, implement nursing interventions, and evaluate patient outcomes. Benner (1984) has described seven domains of nursing practice:

1. the helping role,
2. the teaching-coaching function,
3. the diagnostic and patient-monitoring function,
4. effective management of rapidly changing situations,
5. administering and monitoring therapeutic interventions and regimens,
6. monitoring and ensuring the quality of health care practices, and
7. organization and work-role competencies.

All of these role dimensions are evident in the role of the TPN. In the helping role, the TPN develops an ongoing relationship that forms the basis for supporting, guiding, and empowering the patient in managing the experience of being high risk. In the teaching-coaching function, the TPN individualizes teaching to the patient's specific needs, cultural background, and life situation. Patient monitoring and diagnosis of changing responses are key aspects of the role of the TPN. Prodromal symptoms of preterm labor may be evident days to weeks prior to the onset of true preterm labor and are often evident not by a single symptom but a pattern of subtle, nonspecific symptoms that together suggest impending preterm labor.

When preterm labor symptoms develop, patients need immediate access to the TPN for advice, support, and assistance with access to therapeutic intervention. The TPN service must be available on a 24-hour basis. Application and monitoring of specific home interventions is a key role of the TPN. The TPN monitors contraction patterns of patients on oral tocolytic regimens, makes recommendations for rest and activity, and instructs and encourages patients about appropriate fluid intake. A difficult task for clients at risk for preterm birth is integration of lifestyle changes into daily decisions. The TPN provides information and support during decision making about appropriate activities, engages family participation in household tasks, asks for help, stress management, child care issues, and plans for travel.

Prioritizing patient needs is a key aspect of work role competencies of the TPN. With changing symptom profiles, the TPN, who may manage a caseload of 30 to 50 patients with whom she or he is in frequent contact, must adjust contact schedules to meet the immediate demands of her or his client group. Coordination of care with other health team members and monitoring the quality of care processes and outcomes are role functions that place the TPN in a pivotal role in care management of the client at risk for preterm birth.

Because of the subtleties of preterm labor symptomatology, assessment and intervention are ongoing and require critical analysis and decision making. The expert nurse as described by Benner (1984) uses intuitive skills developed through extensive experiential learning to rapidly grasp the client situation. Synthesizing information from past telephone contacts and current assessment information, the TPN is able to determine the patient's current status and determine the need for intervention, support, or education. Although telephonic nursing programs typically operate with prescribed protocols for responses to patient symptoms, the TPN uses highly advanced skills to interpret the nature and meaning of the subtle and often nonspecific presentation of preterm contraction symptomatology. The TPN must be able to make critical decisions about whether the symptom pattern reflects a uterine contraction pattern that can be managed through the implementation of specific self-care measures in the home or whether the patient requires immediate hospital-based assessment and intervention. The ability to make appropriate choices affects not only patient outcome, but also resource use in a cost-conscious managed care environment.

Although the role of the TPN is highly defined in terms of protocols for symptom management and teaching for risk reduction, active engagement of the patient in adhering to treatment recommendations and in implementing health promoting behavior change is a key factor in the success of preterm birth prevention efforts.

HEALTH PROMOTION

Pender's (1987) Health Promotion Model identifies cognitive-perceptual factors and modifying factors that affect the individual's or family's participation in health promoting behaviors. Knowledge of the interaction of these factors is important to structuring health promotion interventions for individuals and client populations. Preterm birth prevention programs are designed to educate and support clients in engaging in health promoting and health protecting behaviors. Specifically, the program focuses on general health promotion, specific risk reduction strategies, and early recognition of symptoms of preterm labor with active care-seeking and ease of access to health services.

Cognitive perceptual factors that may have a positive effect on personal health include placing a high value on health, having a sense of control over one's health and a strong sense of self-efficacy in effecting health status changes, having a general positive feeling about one's health, believing in the benefits of health-promoting behaviors, and having the ability to overcome barriers of availability, convenience, or difficulty in implementing health-promoting behaviors. Modifying factors include demographic, biological, interpersonal, situational, and behavioral characteristics of the individual that may influence the likelihood of engaging in health promoting behaviors (Pender, 1987). In a study by Weiss, Saks, and Harris (1995), women who had placed a high value on health during pregnancy and had engaged in specific behaviors to support a healthy pregnancy intensified their efforts (increased rest periods, stress reduction, precautionary contact with provider) when faced with the possible onset of preterm labor symptoms.

The TPN assesses each of the variables previously listed to determine the likelihood of engaging in health promoting behaviors, adhering to the treatment plan, and accessing health care services when symptoms occur. Focused education can be initiated to target such areas as the benefits of health promoting behaviors (such as increased fluid intake and activity modification) on neonatal outcomes. The TPN can also identify solutions to poor compliance such as modification of the work environment, planning and scheduling, and transportation issues.

To obtain the benefits of positive health behaviors, a sustained effort must occur. Preterm birth prevention requires a sustained commitment on the part of the patient and family to adhere to a treatment plan for a prolonged period (up to 20 weeks). Patients who are empowered to be active participants in their care navigate the course of high-risk pregnancy with greater commitment and in better control of the emotional and physical developments associated with high-risk pregnancy.

EMPOWERMENT

Rappaport (1984) has defined empowerment as a process by which people gain mastery over their own lives. Gibson (1991) further specified that empowerment is a social process of reorganizing, promoting, and enhancing clients' abilities to meet their own needs, solve their own problems, and mobilize the necessary resources to feel in control of their lives. Women experiencing preterm labor view it as a life-threatening event for their infant. Once the crisis has subsided, women face an uncertain period of living at home with activity limitations that create personal and family disorganization. There is a feeling of loss of control and powerlessness (Loos & Julius, 1989; Stainton, Harvey, & McNeil, 1991). Yet, the choices these women make affect their personal health and that of their infant and family. Empowerment requires assertion by the client of the right to make one's own decisions and experience the consequences. The health care provider's role is providing information, ease of access to care and services, reinforcement, and support.

The relationship between the TPN and the client is interdependent. There is a reciprocal exchange of information. The TPN calls the client on a regular basis to inquire about symptoms, to monitor over time developing symptom patterns, and to educate about and reinforce appropriate health behaviors to reduce the risk of preterm labor or to manage prodromal symptoms. The client's responsibility is to contact her preterm birth nurse if she experiences or has questions about her symptom pattern. Through preterm birth prevention classes and individual client contacts, the TPN encourages the dual responsibility for case manager (TPN)/client contact. Some patients accept this responsibility easily. For others, it is a progressive empowerment.

Connelly, Keele, Kleinbeck, Schneider, and Cobb (1993) described four levels of client empowerment: participating, choosing, supporting, and negotiating. Although these levels were originally described for patients with mental illness, they describe well the progression from dependency to interdependence in women at risk for preterm birth.

Participating involves increased levels of active involvement in the processes of care. This may be evidenced by more curiosity about clinical progress, greater adherence to the provider's recommendations for activity level, and more openness to support and assistance from friends and family. Participation by the client and supportive family members in preterm birth prevention classes is encouraged by the case manager. Clients at home on monitoring or home therapy are encouraged to ask questions and to initiate telephone contact as needed with the TPN.

Maria's nurse first contacted her in the hospital following suppression of preterm labor at 26 weeks. During the next 6 weeks, the preterm birth prevention program nurse called Maria three times per week. During that time, Maria experienced two additional episodes of preterm contractions. Each time, she called the TPN to validate her symptoms and her decision to go to the hospital for assessment. At 32 weeks' gestation, Maria told the TPN that she was having contractions and also didn't feel well. Although the TPN could not obtain more specific information, Maria was very clear that something was different and that she needed to be evaluated. On admission, she was diagnosed with HELLP (hemolysis, elevated liver enzymes, low platelet count) syndrome.

Choosing involves making personal choices and experiencing the consequences of those choices. Empowerment is personal freedom to make choices about one's behavior while accepting personal and social responsibility for the consequences. Choices can only be as good as the information provided to make an informed decision and the degree of self-control of the individual to make cognitive rather than emotionally driven choices.

Sandy had experienced an episode of preterm labor 3 weeks earlier. She had no family or friends to offer support, since she had just moved to the area. Her relationship with her boyfriend was tenuous, as was her relationship with his mother. During a regularly scheduled telephone contact, the preterm birth case manager noted an increase in the level of prodromal symptoms. The case manager explored what had changed in Sandy's situation. Sandy admitted she was no longer taking her Terbutaline. Her boyfriend's mother had told her it would "cause her baby to have headaches when it grew up." After further discussion with the case manager, Sandy decided she would take the medication and try to explain it to her boyfriend's mother. She risked loss of support at a time when she was very vulnerable but made what she believed was the responsible choice for her baby. The case manager discussed strategies that Sandy might use in approaching her boyfriend and his mother.

Supporting involves the process of moving beyond the individual's internal world to sharing the experience with others and by doing so, giving and receiving of mutual support. Many women at this stage feel frustrated and isolated with their dependence on others. This stage of empowerment involves identification of those areas where a contribution can be made to others in return for the assistance needed. Families need to clearly define what contributions to family life can be made by each member given the constraints of the current health care demands. Being at risk for preterm labor then becomes a family experience, with each member providing support for the others. Fleury (1991) described social support systems as key elements in client empowerment potential. Families can be facilitators of change or they can create barriers to health-promoting changes through construction of boundaries for behavior that decrease the client's sense of autonomy and responsibility.

Pamela had prodromal symptoms for preterm labor periodically since 19 weeks' gestation. At 28 weeks' gestation, she was being treated aggressively with oral tocolytics and twice weekly steroid injections. She was tired and frustrated, with the steroid injections compounding her mood. The TPN explored Pamela's feelings and together they identified her feelings of needing more support coupled with her frustrations with feelings of dependence resulting from prescribed activity restrictions. The TPN offered a number of suggestions based on what other couples had done in similar situations. That evening Pamela had a long discussion with her husband, Sam. The couple decided that Sam would rearrange his work schedule to spend more time at home. Sam would learn how to give the injections, reducing the need for extra visits by the home health nurse. They also identified that Pamela could assist Sam with certain aspects of the work he did at home.

Negotiating within the family unit and with health care providers occurs in the fourth stage of empowerment. In this stage the woman and her family work collaboratively with the health care team. Discussion regarding health care needs is initiated by either party and is discussed openly. The provider relinquishes the need to control the client's decision making, recogniz-

ing that the client and family have the right and are able to make responsible decisions. Cooperation between client and provider is the hallmark of this stage.

Elena was a primigravida with a bicornuate uterus and a history of hypertension. She had recently been hospitalized with preterm labor. Although she continued to be symptomatic, she was able to remain at home on nifedipine with daily nursing contact. At her integrated perinatal and internal medicine appointment at 29 weeks' gestation, her internist wanted to decrease the nifedipine. Elena informed the internist that she did not want the dosage decreased because the tocolytic effect was too important to lose at this critical time. Further discussion with her obstetrician supported her views.

PREVENTING PRETERM BIRTH

Telephonic nursing, including aspects of both direct care and case management, is a component of an overall strategy to prevent preterm birth. Key aspects of this strategy include:

1. General health education during pregnancy.
2. Preterm birth prevention education for all pregnant women. This includes availability of printed materials in providers' offices and content presented in prenatal classes.
3. Use of a risk assessment tool for screening patients at risk for preterm labor. Every pregnant woman should be screened. These tools will detect 40% to 60% of women who will deliver preterm.
4. In-depth education on risk reduction and early detection of symptoms for women at risk for preterm labor.
5. Nursing case management and frequent monitoring to promote risk reduction and early recognition of symptoms in at-risk clients.
6. Education of ambulatory medical, nursing, and ancillary personnel about recognition and management of preterm labor.
7. Development of policies and procedures for telephone and in-person triage of pa-

tients who call office, urgent care, or hospital units.

8. Development of referral mechanism to preterm birth prevention education and case management programs.

Preterm Birth Prevention Programs focus on both the individual patient and the patient population as an aggregate. Because 50% of women who experience preterm labor have no risk factors prior to the first preterm labor event, programs that only target women at risk will fail to have maximum impact on perinatal outcomes. Therefore, preterm birth prevention efforts address both primary and secondary levels of prevention. Primary prevention is targeted toward increasing the general health of the population and thereby reducing the risk of preterm labor and birth. General health promotion strategies, such as nutrition education and prevention of sexually transmitted diseases, target specific risk factors for preterm birth. Specific health protection recommendations, such as increasing fluid intake during hot summer weather and seeking immediate treatment for urinary tract infections, may prevent the onset of preterm labor in susceptible women.

Secondary level prevention targets clients at risk for disease. Fifty percent of women who deliver preterm infants have identified risk factors. Of women who are identified as being at risk through standard prospective risk screening, one fourth to one third will actually deliver preterm (Holbrook, Laros, & Creasy, 1989). This group needs a more intensive specialized approach to reducing risks and monitoring symptom progress. Individualized plans of education, support, and monitoring can be readily accomplished using a telephonic nursing approach. Further, in a case manager role, the TPN interfaces with the perinatal team in both the ambulatory and inpatient settings to develop mechanisms for appropriate and timely access to care for assessment and treatment at the onset of preterm labor.

• • •

Telephonic nursing is a strategy currently being tested as a method of providing direct care and case management services to clients at risk for preterm delivery. This strategy will only be as successful as the TPN is in promoting client empowerment. The empowered client will participate in the treatment plan, make informed decisions that are right for her personal and family situation, and take responsibility for engaging in health-promoting behaviors that support a positive birth outcome.

REFERENCES

Adams, M.M. (1995). The continuing challenge of preterm delivery. *Journal of the American Medical Association, 273,* 739–740.

American Nurses Association. (1988). *Nursing case management.* Kansas City, MO: ANA.

Andersen, H.F., Freda, M.C., Damus, K., Brustman, L., & Merkatz, I.R. (1989). Effectiveness of patient education to reduce preterm delivery among ordinary risk patients. *American Journal of Perinatology, 6,* 214–217.

Benner, P. (1984). *From novice to expert: Excellence and power in clinical nursing.* Menlo Park, CA: Addison-Wesley Publishing Company.

Bryce, R.L., Stanley, F.J., & Garner, J.B. (1991). Randomized controlled trial of antenatal social support to prevent preterm birth. *British Journal of Obstetrics and Gynecology, 98,* 1001–1008.

Collaborative Group on Preterm Birth Prevention. (1993). Multicenter randomized, controlled trial of a preterm birth prevention program. *American Journal of Obstetrics and Gynecology, 169,* 352–366.

Connelly, L.M., Keele, B.S., Kleinbeck, S.V.M., Schneider, J.K., & Cobb, A.K. (1993). A place to be yourself: Empowerment from the client's perspective. *Image, 25*(4), 297–304.

Creasy, R.K. (1994). Preterm labor and delivery. In R.K. Creasy and R. Resnik (Eds.). *Maternal-fetal medicine* (3rd ed.). Philadelphia, PA: W.B. Saunders.

Fleury, J.D. (1991). Empowering potential: A theory of wellness motivation. *Nursing Research, 40,* 286–291.

Gibson, C.H. (1991). A concept analysis of empowerment. *Journal of Advanced Nursing, 16,* 354–361.

Gibson, S.J., Martin, S.M., Johnson, M.B., Blue, R., & Miller, D.S. (1994). CNS-directed case management: Cost and quality in harmony. *Journal of Nursing Administration, 24*(6), 45–51.

Henderson, M.G., & Wallack, S.S. (1987, January). Evaluating case management for catastrophic illness. *Business and Health,* pp. 7–11.

Hill, W.C., Fleming, A.D., Martin, R.W., Hamer, C., Knuppel, R.A., Lake, M.F., Watson, D.L., Welch, R.A., Bentley, D.L., Gookin, K.S., & Morrison, J.C. (1990). Home uterine activity monitoring is associated with a reduction in preterm birth. *Obstetrics and Gynecology, 76(1) supplement,* 12S–18S.

Holbrook , R.H., Laros, R.K., & Creasy, R.K. (1989). Evaluation of a risk-scoring system for prediction of preterm labor. *American Journal of Perinatology, 6,* 62–68.

Knuppel, R.A., Lake, M.F., Watson, D.L., Welch, R.A., Hill, W.C., Fleming, A.D., Martin, R.W., Bentley, D.L., Moenning, R.K., & Morrison, J.C. (1990). Preventing preterm birth in twin gestation: Home uterine activity monitoring and prenatal nursing support. *Obstetrics and Gynecology, 76(1) supplement,* 24S–27S.

Kotula, C. (1994). High risk pregnancy. *Continuing Care, June, 1994,* 16–19, 28.

Loos, C., & Julius, L. (1989). The client's view of hospitalization during pregnancy. *JOGNN, 18,* 52–56.

Maisiak, R., Koplon, S., & Heck, L.W. (1990). Subsequent behavior of users of an arthritis information telephone service. *Arthritis and Rheumatism, 33*(2), 212–218.

Morrison, J.C. (1990). Preterm birth: A puzzle worth solving. *Obstetrics and Gynecology, 76(1) supplement,* 5S–12S.

Mou, S.M., Sunderji, S.G., Gall, S., How, H., Patel, V., Gray, M., Kayne, H.L., & Corwin, M. (1991). Multicenter randomized clinical trial of home uterine activity monitoring for detection of preterm labor. *American Journal of Obstetrics and Gynecology, 165,* 858–866.

Nagey, D.A., Bailey-Jones, C., & Herman, A.A. (1993). Randomized comparison of home uterine activity monitoring and routine care in patients discharged after treatment for preterm labor. *Obstetrics and Gynecology, 82,* 319–323.

Pender, N.J. (1987). *Health promotion in nursing practice* (2nd ed.). Norwalk, CT: Appleton & Lange.

Rappaport, J. (1984). Studies in empowerment: Introduction to the issue. *Prevention in Human Services, 3,* 1–7.

René, J., Weinberger, M., Mazzuca, S.A., Brandt, K.D., & Katz, B.P. (1992). Reduction of joint pain in patients with knee osteoarthritis who have received monthly telephone calls from lay personnel and whose medical treatment regimens have remained stable. *Arthritis and Rheumatism, 35*(5), 511–515.

Stainton, M.C., Harvey, S., & McNeil, D. (1991). *A phenomenological study of the high risk perinatal situation.* Calgary, Alberta: University of Calgary and Foothills Hospital.

U.S. Preventive Services Task Force. (1993). Home uterine activity monitoring for preterm labor: Review article. *Journal of the American Medical Association, 270,* 371–376.

Watson, D.L., Welch, R.A., Mariona, F.G., Lake, M.F., Knuppel, R.A., Martin, R.W., Johnson, C., Bentley, D.L., Hill, W.C., Fleming, A.D., & Morrison, J.C. (1990). Management of preterm patients at home: Does daily uterine activity monitoring and nursing support make a difference? *Obstetrics and Gynecology, 76(1) supplement,* 32S–35S.

Weinberger, M., Tierney, W.M., Booher, P., & Katz, B.P. (1991). The impact of increased contact on psychosocial outcomes in patients with osteoarthritis: A randomized, controlled trial. *The Journal of Rheumatology, 18*(6), 849–854.

Weiss, M., Saks, N.P., & Harris, S. (1995). Resolving the uncertainty of preterm labor symptoms: Recognizing and responding to the possibilities. Submitted for publication.

Zander, K. (1988). Nursing case management: Strategic management of cost and quality outcomes. *Journal of Nursing Administration, 18*(5), 23–30.

In Case Management, Who's Watching the Store? Implementing Practice Parameters and Outcomes

Kathleen Moreo

As the practice and the profession of case management bend around the curve and head into the next century, case managers are being held accountable for long-standing claims of quality, cost-effective care coordination. Toughened managed care and workers' compensation carriers are implementing blended managed care programs with a hands-on approach to cutting costs.

Plaintiff and defense attorneys alike are challenging case managers to definitively state their qualifications and their merit in cumbersome health care litigation. Physicians are questioning the recommendations of case managers and challenging case management decisions not yet rooted in a standard of care. The purchasers of health care services—consumers—are becoming more savvy in their pursuit of the very best product for the very best price.

Interdisciplinary teams are struggling to accept the case manager as being central to the coordination of care, offering new age, multiple team-leader approaches in place of traditional case management models.

It is difficult to think in terms of *traditional* when dealing with such a young profession. Case managers have claimed to be *evolving* for at least the past 10 years—*traditional* implies a maturity unclaimed in this profession. In many ways, however, we have repeatedly professed

and practiced a traditional role and function within the health care delivery system. This role has been to:

- seek out and address funding, treatment options, and coordination of services;
- advocate for the client/family in an appropriate manner conducive to the processes of the pay source;
- negotiate with all parties in a fair and equitable manner;
- promote communication among all parties; and
- develop, monitor, and manage a reasonable, achievable care plan.

These criteria are understood and accepted between the pay source and the case manager. In addition, the case manager is often evaluated according to the following questions:

- Were realistic objectives established and met?
- Do the case notes correspond with the billable hours?
- Is the length of time billed appropriate for the activity?
- Have cost savings issues been identified, coupled with appropriate negotiations?
- Have services been delivered in an ethical, timely, and well executed manner?
- Did closure occur at an appropriate time, or is clear documentation presented for ongoing active case management?
- Did the case manager follow policy and procedure?

Inside Case Management 1997; 3(10): 7–8

That was then and this is now. Before the ink dries on the traditional case manager's proposal, intended services are now being critically analyzed and scrutinized, with one theme evident: The time has come to incorporate practice parameters and outcomes in case management. In other words, we can't just talk about it anymore.

DEVELOPING STANDARDS

The case managers' professional organization began to address these issues in 1994 with the publication of the Case Management Society of America's (CMSA) Standards of Practice for Case Managers. An 8,000-member active association representing case managers nationwide, CMSA strongly supports practice guidelines as one way to ensure that case management is being performed by qualified individuals. These standards have become paramount within the health care industry and are currently being used in health care delivery models, job descriptions, publications, legal proceedings, and universities.

Developing standards is an important step toward defining practice parameters that represent excellence in the profession.

MEASURING OUTCOMES

Certainly, practice parameters in the current health care delivery system will be measured by outcomes, but here our profession is also sorely lacking. For the past few years, we have struggled to define qualitative measurements in a decidedly quantitative system.

A few delivery systems have successfully incorporated outcomes measures, and their reports have been overutilized to the point of great redundancy. We have yet to see a user-friendly, simplified computer software system that can develop our outcomes studies in a way that makes sense. If we had such a system, it could replace most of our marketing efforts.

Case managers struggling to meet the demands of outcomes studies within their caseload often rely on qualitative outcomes reports, using such descriptive language as "patient length of stay decreased significantly," "client satisfac-

tion is within excellent range," "recommend data collection to validate," and the classic statement, "case management intervention yielded substantial cost savings."

These reports aren't turning new proposals into contracts. Case management professionals are now being called upon to match outcomes quality with equally high standards of measurement to accurately define, in quantitative terms rather than qualitative terms, the overall impact of care on our clients.

THE CENTER FOR CASE MANAGEMENT ACCOUNTABILITY

In its assessment of membership and industry trends, CMSA has recently determined that measurable outcomes are paramount to case management accountability in current and future climates. To help case managers meet this challenge, the organization unveiled its Center for Case Management Accountability (CCMA) in September 1996, which appears to be the first profession-at-large collective attempt to provide standardized, conclusive outcomes pertaining to case management intervention.

CCMA is based upon the premise that standards of care can ultimately be achieved through data collection and education. In the first phase of CCMA, dimensions, indicators, protocols, and reporting formats that can demonstrate the value of case management to its customers will be defined.

Dimensions might include cost, client satisfaction, client knowledge, and final outcomes (health status, client empowerment).

In its strategic plan, CCMA is targeted as a driving force to help case management thrive, not merely survive, in an era of health consumerism and managed care. The plan states, "The long-term purpose behind CCMA is improvement. As the voice of leadership in case management, CMSA wants not merely to demonstrate value but to maximize it. Through CCMA, the organization and its members will identify what works best in enhancing client's health status and in achieving net health care cost savings."

Central to CCMA is the creation of a pooled database, which will allow members to pool their processes and outcomes data in a central repository. Pooled outcomes data can then facilitate establishment of norms and trends to measure industry-wide performance and quality improvement. Future consistency across the continuum of care will be pursued through linkages to other organizations defining health care accountability standards, as well as a commitment to define generally accepted accountability standards compatible with state and local legislation across the country.

This demonstration of the value of case management through outcomes and accountability is an aggressive step toward standards of care that is both purposeful and measurable. It can supply case managers with the tools necessary to "watch the store"—to police this exploding profession, and to ensure credibility and advanced practice amidst speculation and claims of substandard care.

The reporting of outcomes is simply a benchmark to accurately reflect the complex nature of case management. It is a validation of an extremely effective recipe for quality driven health care. It is an attempt to improve a system by first measuring the system. It is an answer to the expectations of the payers and the purchasers for suitable report cards. Finally, it is a response to the repetitious claim that case management costs too much.

THE CALL TO POOL RESOURCES

The greatest challenge now facing case managers is that of collaboration and participation to fuel this and other potential outcomes projects. Just as the American Medical Association reaches milestones with physician participation, case managers are being called upon to pool resources to substantiate outcomes and standards of care. The profession is now being driven largely by the will of its own case managers, and whether the curve in the road ahead leads to a ravine or a superhighway depends upon the drivers.

A Framework for Integrated Quality Improvement

Catherine Willoughby, Ginette Budreau, and Debra Livingston

In recent years, quality improvement (QI) activities have grown in scope and importance, as has the challenge of organizing and administering quality programs. This is due, in large part, to changes in internal and external forces driving QI programs. The Joint Commission on Accreditation of Healthcare Organizations, one external driving force, now encourages us to think beyond departmental QI to the entire organization. We are to view improvement more broadly as improving organizational performance.[1] Improving organizational performance includes standards development, staff education, performance appraisal, competency assessment, continuous quality improvement (CQI), research and research utilization, risk management, case management, and more.

In addition, a relatively new market model of health care delivery has made the margin for poor performance and error narrower than ever, and data are required to document quality outcomes clearly. Quality data are being collected in many different forms, to meet a variety of objectives, by clinicians, administrators, regulators, and third party payers.

The complexity and diversity of quality programs create the need for an organizing, integrating framework that acknowledges the contributions of all areas and provides links for enhanced effectiveness and efficiency. Such a

J Nurs Care Qual 1997; 11(3): 44–53
© 1997 Aspen Publishers, Inc.

framework was developed by members of the Division of Psychiatric and Chemical Dependency Nursing at the University of Iowa Hospitals and Clinics (UIHC). The QI framework defines the various components of a quality program and organizes these components into four broad categories: maintenance indicators, CQI activities, time-limited QI activities, and sentinel events (Figure 1).

MAINTENANCE INDICATORS

Maintenance indicators are identified first, not because they are considered the most important but because they are considered the most elemental. They reflect the basic foundation upon which a quality program is built. Maintenance indicators are measured and compared against an absolute threshold. The emphasis is on individual compliance, and the work is rarely multidisciplinary. In the early years of quality work, this was the sole focus of most departments of nursing. In contemporary quality programs, there are two primary types of maintenance indicators: structural indicators and competency indicators.

Maintenance indicator data are usually the clearest and easiest to interpret. A threshold is either met or not met; statistical tools are not necessary to determine whether a problem exists. Maintenance indicators are basic and useful indicators of individual compliance or adequate mechanical function that support the delivery of care, but they do not address the processes of care.

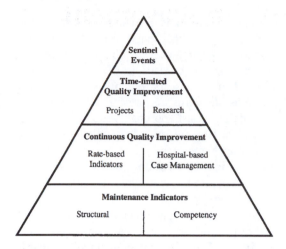

Figure 1. QI framework.

Structural indicators

Structural indicators provide data that indicate that basic structures are in place and running smoothly. At the nursing unit level, this includes such things as equipment and documentation checks. On the psychiatric units at UIHC, structural indicators include checks on crash cart supplies, glucometer calibration, and medication refrigerator temperature as well as chart audits to monitor compliance with documentation standards. In a more technical setting (e.g., an intensive care area) where there is more equipment, the list of structural indicators may be longer.

Competency indicators

Competency indicators are intended to document and monitor the ability of staff to perform safely and effectively in a given setting. They focus clearly on individual performance and compliance. The Joint Commission mandates that staff competence be assessed and maintained on an ongoing basis.[1]

The first step in establishing professional competency is documenting the formal education and licensure that are the conditions of employment. Second, the organization assesses and ensures the ability of individual staff to meet the requirements of specific positions through organizational and unit-specific orientation programs. Finally, ongoing evaluation of employee competence is necessary.

A wide variety of competency assessment methods can be used, including successful completion of written tests, skill demonstration in classrooms, and peer review in the practice setting. The Joint Commission standards do not prescribe any particular methodology as long as objective performance criteria are used.

CQI ACTIVITIES

Improving processes of care is the focus of the second and third categories of the framework, which focus on QI rather than quality maintenance. CQI is based on the philosophy and methodology developed by Deming and Juran and tested in the Japanese industrial setting. The central belief is that quality can be continually improved by using reliable techniques to study and refine processes. This is in contrast to the traditional idea that the best performance can be obtained by searching out and eliminating problems. In 1987, the Joint Commission issued a report on a national demonstration project that verified successful application of CQI principles in health care settings.[2] Soon after, the application of these principles in health care organizations became a basic Joint Commission expectation. Organizations have realized their value in terms of improved care, increased efficiency, and reduced costs. CQI activities, the second category identified in the framework, is subdivided into two types of activities: rate-based indicators and hospital-based case management and variance tracking.

Rate-based indicators

Rate-based QI indicators are the foundation of CQI. The Joint Commission defines an indicator as a "valid and reliable quantitative process or outcome measure related to one or more dimensions of performance such as effectiveness and appropriateness."[3(p.255)] An indicator is a statistical value that gives an indication of quality or performance over time. There is no one particular improvement process prescribed by the Joint Commission. The expectation is that there will be some method used to select functions or processes to assess, measure, evaluate, improve, and reassess for results. This process must be grounded in sound statistical methodology. It is in this aspect of QI work that tools such as flowcharts, cause and effect diagrams, and Pareto charts are used to analyze processes. Run charts and control charts are used to display and analyze trended data.

Variation in indicator data collected over time is studied to determine whether a problem exists or a process has changed. The variation can be of two types. Common cause variation is the result of anticipated variation within the system. For example, it is assumed that some medication errors will occur on a busy medical unit and that the number of reported errors will vary somewhat from month to month. When the variation occurs within statistically determined control limits, it is considered common cause variation. A process under study is considered stable when it varies only within the expected, predictable range. When one or more data points fall outside the statistically determined control limits, it is called special cause variation.[4] If the number of reported medication errors falls above the upper control limit, it is presumed that there is a related special circumstance, such as unusual staff turnover or confusion about a pharmacy system change. The process is considered unstable. System improvements cannot be made until special cause variation is eliminated.

Hospital-based case management and variance tracking

CareMaps™ or clinical pathways are QI tools that allow multidisciplinary teams to provide hospital-based case management by examining the processes and outcomes of care through variance tracking and analysis. Variance data, collected quarterly from population-focused CareMaps™, provide a rich source of data for quality assessment and improvement (QAI).

At UIHC, CareMaps™ are developed by multidisciplinary teams that are usually chaired by a nurse case manager. The maps serve as collaborative guidelines that time and sequence the interventions of the key health care providers for a particular patient case type.[5] By delineating the desired processes and outcomes of care, they serve as standards of care for intended patient populations. Cost and quality are monitored on every shift by review of compliance with the CareMap™ for each patient. As individual patient variances are identified, the health care team discusses the causes and attempts to get the patient back on track.[6]

In addition to this concurrent audit of individual patient variances, aggregate variances are analyzed. These are the cumulative variances that occur among the patients on a particular map that are aggregated and reported quarterly.[6] At UIHC, case managers collect individual patient variances and send these data to the Office of Outcomes and Evaluation for statistical analysis and graphing for ease of interpretation. Compiled variance data are then provided to the multidisciplinary team that developed the CareMap™. The multidisciplinary team members look for patterns in the data and determine whether the variances are related to systems, practitioners, or patients. In this way, QAI activities are returned to the attention of the clinicians most involved in the care of the patient population.

System variance is the most useful for identifying QI opportunities. System variance is deviation from the map that originates from the processes of patient care delineated on the map. Examples are delays in laboratory turnaround times due to inadequate staffing or inability to transfer a patient out of an intensive care unit (ICU) because of a lack of beds.

On one unit, variance data indicated a delay in cardiac rehabilitation contributing to slower progress among patients with myocardial infarction. This was determined to be due to lack of time by physical therapists and nurses on the weekends, when staffing was lower. The result of QI work was that the hospital's cardiac rehabilitation program was extended to include weekends, providing for more continuity of care and faster patient progress.

Practitioner variance results from failures of individual clinicians to order or perform tests or interventions that are specified on the map. When the failure is due to an individual performance problem, it is dealt with through existing managerial lines of communication. An example of practitioner variance of a different sort was found in the cardiovascular ICU. According to variance data, the length of stay of patients undergoing angioplasty was prolonged because physicians were not always available to remove the femoral catheters at the time specified on the CareMap™. In response, the cardiovascular ICU nurses received education and training and began removing the catheters themselves. This change in practice resulted in a 44 percent decrease in the number of hours patients had to lie flat in bed.

Patient-related variances are the result of individual patient characteristics, such as age or comorbidities. They rarely require any action on the part of the CareMap™ team, and they rarely result in modifications of the map. These variances tend to be the least useful for identifying opportunities to improve cost and quality.

After evaluating quarterly variance data, the multidisciplinary team may decide to continue to monitor a variance, change the CareMap™, change practice, or share the data with other departments or programs for further review and action.[7] At UIHC, case managers serve as members of many of the unit-based QAI committees, and variance evaluation provides topics for QI work. QAI and case management share the common goals of promoting more effective, efficient care. The complementary nature of the relationship between their two different approaches is illustrated in some settings where case management represents the majority of the units' QI work.

TIME-LIMITED QI ACTIVITIES

Quality projects

This type of QI activity has as its goal the resolution of an identified problem or implementation of an innovation. In contrast to the ongoing collection of data over time that is characteristic of continuous quality indicators, the use of data for quality projects is time limited. There are often data that support the need for a project. For example, the idea for a project may grow out of ongoing data sources, such as risk management or epidemiology, or continuous quality indicators. Data are also used to verify successful completion of a project. The Joint Commission has established as an improvement process standard that organizations must include follow-up measurement as part of the planned change strategy to ensure that desired outcomes are met.[1]

Members of health care organizations make many improvements as they make changes and solve problems in their day-to-day work. In spite of improvements in care, enhancements of efficiency, and increases in productivity, relatively few of these positive outcomes have been conceptualized as QI. The inclusion of a project category in the framework provides an opportunity to put a QI frame around this significant work. In implementation areas at UIHC, this has resulted in staff viewing more of their work in terms of quality.

Projects can be reported at any level in the organization. Some that are smaller in scope may be reported at the unit or divisional level, and they may or may not be multidisciplinary. The majority of the larger departmentwide or organizationwide projects are multidisciplinary or interdepartmental. Source of project ideas include problems or ideas identified by staff, patients, and visitors.

A UIHC example of a QI project that affected the entire hospital was the work that was done to provide and maintain a supply of wheelchairs at the main entrance. This project resulted from years of futile attempts to keep wheelchairs available for arriving patients. A team of staff from various departments, including Patient and Guest Relations, Housekeeping, Plant Operations and Maintenance, and Nursing, collected data on the problem, identified root causes, and then developed and implemented a plan. A fleet of red wheelchairs was stationed at the main entrance; these red wheelchairs are easily distinguishable from those used elsewhere, so that they are not inadvertently left in other areas. After the implementation of the "Red Fleet," the Housekeeping Department found close to 100 percent compliance with the new system, and the problem was solved.

In the case of a large project such as this, it is necessary to identify a facilitator to coordinate the work of staff who represent all stakeholders. Members of the team are given direction and support as needed from the QAI committee at the appropriate organizational level. At UIHC, a project report form has been developed that gives direction for process and outcome expectations (Figure 2). This report form is attached to the quarterly QAI report and is distributed through the organizational QI reporting structure.

Research

Clinical nursing research is conducted and utilized to improve patient care outcomes and other aspects of quality. Because of their shared goals, nursing research and QAI are closely related. At UIHC, when a practice problem or opportunity to improve care is identified, individuals or groups such as a unit-based QAI committee, divisional research committee, or members of an ad hoc team investigate the problem. Based on our experience with the Iowa Model of Research-Based Practice, QAI data often serve as the problem-focused triggers that lead the nursing staff to evaluate existing research literature to determine whether a change in practice is indicated.[8]

Projects that start out strictly for QAI purposes may become research utilization projects or stimulate the conduct of research as the literature is reviewed and plans evolve. The Iowa Model provides an easy to follow, practical guide to help nurses through the decision-making process to determine whether a quality concern is best addressed as a QAI project, a research project, or a research utilization project. In one case, a pediatric unit-based QAI committee identified an opportunity to improve sedation for children undergoing computed tomography and magnetic resonance imaging. The committee collaborated with the divisional research committee to develop a research-based protocol for the administration of intranasal midazolam. Ongoing evaluation of the practice change indicated that a higher percentage of children were able to complete their examinations within a shorter length of time.[9]

Regardless of which committee or team is chosen to address a quality concern, unit and divisional QAI committees are informed about any resulting plans to change practice. Because of the expertise of QAI staff in identifying and monitoring important processes and outcomes, they serve in a consultative role and often assist in gathering or providing baseline and follow-up data. A departmental research utilization project report form is filled out by any nurse who initiates a research utilization project. This provides built-in reminders for the staff to consult and collaborate with QAI staff during data collection stages. As new research-based protocols and standards of care are implemented, the QAI staff develop and monitor quality indicators. For example, an indicator to evaluate satisfaction with pain control was established after implementation of Agency for Health Care Policy and Research clinical practice guidelines on acute pain management in pediatrics.[10,11]

When it is necessary to continue to evaluate changes associated with a time-limited QAI project, research, or research utilization, one or more indicators are developed for data collection and interpretation over time.

SENTINEL EVENTS

Sentinel events are a critical component of every quality program. According to the Joint Commission's Accreditation Manual for Hospitals, a sentinel event is an occurrence that, when noted, requires intensive assessment.[1] Sentinel events are grave, untoward outcome or process errors of care that had or could have had serious negative effects on the patient or others. Many times when a serious event (e.g., a successful suicide or a serious medication error) occurs, there is more than one contributing factor that must be identified. Identifying and eliminating causal factors will improve care and decrease the likelihood that such an event will occur again.

QAI PROJECT SUMMARY REPORT

Project title _____

Purpose/rationale _____

_____

_____

_____

Important functions addressed _____

Dimensions of performance addressed _____

Project summary (include relevant data)

Improvements in care and/or organizational performance (include relevant data)

Additional comments (including any future work planned related to this project)

Date started: _____ Date completed: _____ Date report filed: _____

Departments involved: _____

Report submitted by: _____ Signed: _____

This material has been prepared for use by a University Hospital Staff committee investigating ways to reduce morbidity and mortality.
Written: 4/95

Figure 2. QAI project report form.

When sentinel events occur, the process of review must include consideration of all the potential direct and indirect circumstances leading up to the event. What were the systems issues at play? Where and how did processes fail? One must ask whether current standards of care were maintained. After a thorough analysis of contributing factors, the review team identifies where improvements are needed and how to implement these changes. In a health care organization, the team assigned to this task often comprises frontline managers, case managers, and practitioners across departments.

Although most health care organizations have a system in place for reporting unusual occurrences through incident reports, the UIHC form and reporting process for sentinel events are more detailed. The use of a sentinel event report form (Figure 3) is helpful because it guides appropriate personnel through the review process. The form provides a mechanism for reporting the sentinel event and the corrective process. Although it emphasizes the seriousness of each event, it minimizes placing blame on specific individuals.

IMPLEMENTATION

The QI framework described in this article was developed by a nurse manager on a child psychiatry unit to guide her in understanding and organizing the unit's QI program. Expert nursing staff and/or appropriate councils across the UIHC Department of Nursing were asked to develop the characteristics and examples for pieces of the framework within their practice domains. For example, the Case Management Council wrote the hospital-based case management section, an education nurse specialist developed the competency indicators subheading, and representatives of the Department of Nursing Reasearch Committee developed the section on research.

Today, the Department of Nursing QAI Committee endorses this framework, and it is widely used throughout the department. It is an outline that is used to conceptualize, describe, organize, and plan for the diverse QI activities that exist in a multifaceted, integrated quality program. Divisional QAI reports and manuals are organized around the QI framework categories.

Although the framework was developed for use in a department of nursing at a university hospital, it is flexible enough to be tailored to any health care setting: inpatient or outpatient, community based or institutional, long-term or acute care. Within an organization, the framework can be adapted depending on unit-based and/or organizationwide conditions and priorities. The tailoring that is done determines the composition of each category.

Consider the problem of patient elopement from a psychiatric unit. On a child psychiatry unit, that would be considered a sentinel event. The legal aspects of caring for minors and typical parental expectations are conditions that make close supervision of patients an extremely high priority. The elopement of a child is a dangerous and rare occurrence. When it happens, it is documented and responded to by a multidisciplinary team, whose members attempt to analyze the event and make recommendations to prevent future occurrences.

In adult psychiatry, where patients are more autonomous, elopement happens more frequently, and it is not always dangerous. Voluntary adult patients who are not on restricted supervision levels may walk away from an activity or fail to return from pass. Because this type of elopement does not usually have the same safety and legal ramifications as the elopement of a child, it may be documented only by an incident report. This example illustrates how one problem can be addressed differently and fit in a different place in the QI framework even within closely related specialty areas.

Should the frequency of adult elopements increase, the unit-based QI committee might decide to initiate a CQI activity or a QI project to

Department of Nursing
QAI
Sentinel Event Follow-Up

Date: _____   Unit: _____

1. Review of the event

    a. Detailed description of event

    b. Other disciplines involved (include these people in the follow-up below)

    c. Impact of event on patient/others

    d. Possible causes or contributing factors

    e. Immediate action taken

    f.   Suggestions for additional actions/corrective measures

                        Signature of individuals involved in this process
                        Name _____ Discipline _____
                        Name _____ Discipline _____
                        Name _____ Discipline _____

2. Corrective measures

    a. Plan for additional corrective measures to be implemented

    b. Implementation of corrective measures

    c. Evidence of resolution

                        Signature of individuals involved in this process
                        Name _____ Discipline _____
                        Name _____ Discipline _____
                        Name _____ Discipline _____
                        Date _____

This material has been prepared for use by a University Hospital Staff committee investigating ways to reduce morbidity and mortality.
Written: 4/95
Revised: 9/95

Figure 3. Sentinel event form.

address the concern. This illustrates the other dimension of flexibility that is possible in implementation of the framework: An issue can be categorized and managed by moving it from one place in the framework to another as deemed appropriate by the clinicians in the area.

• • •

In the Department of Nursing at UIHC, this QI framework has been instrumental in improving the organization and understanding of the QAI program. It has the potential to be a useful tool for staff in all departments as our organization proceeds toward more horizontal integration of services. In the spirit of CQI, this framework will be refined as concepts and methods of health care quality evolve.

REFERENCES

1. Joint Commission on Accreditation of Healthcare Organizations. "Improving Organizational Performance." In *1995 Comprehensive Accreditation Manual for Hospitals*. Oakbrook Terrace, Ill.: Joint Commission, 1994.

2. Berwick, D.M. "Curing Health Care: New Strategies for Quality Improvement, a Report on the National Demonstration Project on Quality Improvement in Health Care." San Francisco, Calif.: Jossey-Bass, 1990.

3. Joint Commission on Accreditation of Healthcare Organizations. "Glossary." In *The Measurement Mandate: On the Road to Performance Improvement in Health Care*. Oakbrook Terrace, Ill.: Joint Commission, 1993.

4. Fields, W., and Siroky, K.A. "Converting Data into Information." *Journal of Nursing Care Quality* 8 (1994): 1–11.

5. Zander, K. "Second Generation Critical Paths." *Definition* 4 (1989): 1–2.

6. Bower, K. "Standards as a Bench Mark of the Case Management Approach to Care Delivery." In *Encyclopedia of Nursing Care Quality*, Vol. 2, edited by P. Schroeder. Gaithersburg, Md.: Aspen, 1991.

7. VanBuskirk, M.C., and Vanderbilt, D. "Evaluating Patient Care by the Use of a Diabetic Ketoacidosis CareMap™ in an Intensive Care Unit Setting." *Journal of Nursing Care Quality* 9 (1995): 59–68.

8. Titler, M.G., et al. "Infusing Research into Practice To Promote Quality Care." Nursing Research 43 (1994): 307–313.

9. Weber, E.R., et al. "New Routes in Pediatric Conscious Sedation: A Research-Based Protocol for Intranasal Midazolam." *Journal of Nursing Care Quality* 10 (1995): 55–60.

10. Acute Pain Management Panel. *Acute Pain Management: Operative or Medical Procedures and Trauma. Clinical Practice Guideline*. DHHS Pub. No. AHCPR 92-0032. Rockville, Md.: Agency for Health Care Policy and Research, 1992.

11. Schmidt, K., et al. "Implementation of the AHCPR Pain Guidelines for Children." *Journal of Nursing Care Quality* 8 (1994): 68–74.

The Integration of Primary Care and Case Management in Chronic Disease

Cheryl Phillips-Harris

System integration, a concept hardly mentioned in the early 1980s, is now the focus of discussion for payers, hospital organizations, and providers alike. Central to integrated health care delivery is an understanding of chronic care and how it differs from an acute care model (Table 1). Chronic care can be defined as "the ongoing provision of medical, functional, psychological, social, environmental and spiritual care services that enable persons with serious and persistent conditions to optimize their functional independence and well being from the time of onset until problem resolution or death."[1] Simply put, chronic diseases are conditions for which there is no specific cure and whose course is one of progressive decline and obstruction of daily activities. Studies have estimated that the number of Americans with chronic illness that limits normal activities for their age group equals roughly 34 million and that 40 percent are under age 65.[2]

In a typical case of chronic disease, no one person or provider assumes complete responsibility for ensuring the delivery of needed services. Patients and families serve as their own care managers and frequently lack the necessary resources to organize the medical, community, and support services needed.[3] The maze of reimbursement regulations adds to the fragmentation of care delivery. For any given level of care,

there are multiple payers, each with their own needs testing and benefits coverage. Case management is often facility specific or, at best, service limited. The same maze of reimbursement rarely compensates providers or case managers for the coordination of care across settings and over periods of time. Changes of levels of care are "hand offs" and often result in "fumbles." As organizations move into risk-sharing arrangements and capitation-based financing, case management has shifted into the world of utilization review and resource allocation. Patients and their families frequently view case managers as advocates of the system, physicians as the advocates of the patients, and the delivery of care as caught in the turbulent waters between.

DEFINITION OF INTEGRATED CARE

Stephen Shortell has defined an organized delivery system as a "network of organizations that provides or arranges to provide a coordinated continuum of services to a defined population and is willing to be held socially and clinically accountable for the health status of the population."[4] Integrated care is client or patient focused. Services are provided to meet specific needs, and access to the services is simple and may be accomplished anywhere along the continuum. Further, services are flexible and not facility limited. Care coordination is longitudinal (it extends over time and across levels of care), and clinical, functional, and demographic data

Quality Management in Health Care 1996; 5(1): 1–6

Table 1 Changing the Focus of Care

Acute care	Chronic care
Episodic	Continuous
Needs reacted to	Needs anticipated
Focus on cure	Focus on function
Reliance on diagnostic tests	Reliance on care management
Diagnosis driven	Whole-patient care

are linked through information systems and available at all levels of care to all providers. Integrating care for a patient with a chronic illness means the patient or the family can get needed assistance with a single phone call. It means that someone (an individual or a team) will coordinate access, care, and information between the hospital, nursing home, primary care office, specialists, physical therapists, or wherever the patient receives services.

The potential is greater for achieving integration of care using a capitated system of reimbursement rather than a traditional fee-for-service system.[5] However, merely having a capitated contract does not guarantee integrated care delivery. In fact, there is considerable concern that the organizational structures of health maintenance organizations might pose barriers to the frail elderly[6] and that the financial incentives may actually reduce the availability of needed services.[7] There are demonstration models, such as the social health maintenance organization (SHMO)[8] and the Program of All-inclusive Care of the Elderly (PACE),[9] that have shown that, with interdisciplinary case management, cost-efficient care can be provided to a frail and chronically ill population within a managed care structure. When health care services are integrated, the fragmentation often surrounding chronic illness can be prevented.

COMPONENTS OF INTEGRATED CASE MANAGEMENT

Prevention

Organizations can set standards in vertical and horizontal integration from an operational,

contractual, and facilities standpoint and yet fail to provide integrated care at the patient service level. See the box entitled "Components of Integrated Case Management" for a list of components necessary to provide integrated care coordination. The foundation of integrated case management is disability prevention and wellness. Prevention programs need to include primary prevention to avoid disease (e.g., influenza vaccines), secondary prevention to detect asymptomatic disease (e.g., mammograms, blood pressure screens), and tertiary prevention aimed at avoiding further functional decline when possible (e.g., screening for incontinence and falls). Barriers to the focus on prevention include the initial costs of screening and services; an enrollee population that often moves from one system to another; the pervasive belief that prevention is relevant only to a younger, healthy population; and the lack of interdisciplinary teams to provide an organized, population-based system of prevention services.

Risk Identification

In order to coordinate needed services, providers require a process to identify patients with potential needs and classify these individuals by relative risk. Risk identification begins at the time of enrollment or at the earliest encounter.

Components of Integrated Case Management

Prevention and wellness programs

Risk screening

Assessments to identify specific needs of members

Services that are flexible and client centered

Interdisciplinary focus

Care coordination that is longitudinal (over time and across settings)

Information processes that link data to all providers

Easy access for members, caregivers, and providers

Outcomes tracking

The first step is for providers to define what "risks" they wish to measure. From the consumer's perspective, the risks include increased illness, decreased function and independence, and increased probability of death. Providers are concerned with the possibility of complications, lengthy and expensive treatments, and missed diagnoses or failed treatments. Lastly, the risks from the health system's and payer's perspective include inappropriate use of services, increased costs, and suboptimal outcomes.[10]

Several organizations, including insurance companies, hospital systems and provider groups, have initiated various risk identification tools.[11–13] These tools range from health risk appraisals for identifying an individual's lifestyle and behaviors to comprehensive geriatric assessments that target small groups of high-risk individuals. Each has a potential role in integrated case management, and the use of any one screening process is largely determined by the resources available to the system. Unless the information is tied to an intervention process (e.g., health promotion, educational programs for persons with specific diseases, specific services that meet individual needs), then there is no benefit to the patient, provider, or health system. Several questions remain to be answered about risk identification.

- Do the tools produce valid measures of risk? Typical predictors of hospitalization include age over 79 and living alone, poor self-perception of health, more than six medications taken on a daily basis, and two or more hospitalizations or emergency department (ED) visits within the past six months.[12,14]
- How is the information shared with providers? Sharing can be accomplished by providing a list to primary care physicians of their "at-risk" patients, providing a summary of risk factors, or having the risk screening tool completed and scored in the physician's office.
- Should systems rescreen, and if so, when? Some systems have taken the approach of

annual rescreening based on age criteria (e.g., all persons over age 75), whereas others track utilization criteria (e.g., number of ED, hospital, and physician visits or the use of ancillary services such as home health) to determine who needs rescreening.

- How will the system determine if the risk identification program is working? Clearly, the link to outcome data, such as admission rates, total cost of care, and functional decline, is essential to measure the success of such a program.
- Who should pay for the risk identification program? Most organizations have found it best to share the cost between the hospital and medical groups since the potential benefits would be seen by both entities.

What Is Primary Care?

When asked to define *primary care,* insurance executives, hospital system administrators, and medical group leaders typically equate primary care with physician care. In fact, considerable energy has been expended by physicians themselves in defining turf (e.g., deciding who has precedence and under what circumstances specialty physicians may serve as primary care providers). Primary care can best be defined as a *function* of care delivery that is comprehensive, accessible, and coordinated. In addition, it is person focused and holistic, and the patient maintains an active and accountable role in the management of his or her disease. Primary care is optimally delivered in an interdisciplinary manner that allows each member of the team to contribute his or her skills and scope of knowledge.

Physicians often feel that such an approach represents a "loss of control" over patients and treatments and that the team process consumes valuable time and is redundant. In fact, a well-organized interdisciplinary team should *increase* control, since the services will not be fragmented, nor will information be "lost" between the levels of care. Needs can be anticipated rather than reacted to. Time management is also improved when each member of the team collects and shares data. Multiple assessments (e.g., of home safety, caregiver resources, medicines, and cognitive and affective disorders) can be done at various sites without requiring the physician to be present. The team can also serve as a problem-solving resource for the physician, patient, and family. Ideally, it does not function in isolation from the physician but also does not require the constant involvement of the physician. The team and the physician should work sharing information and discussing clinical options. Through this process, primary care becomes a team function.

MODELS OF INTEGRATED CARE

Multiple health care delivery systems have taken various components of integrated primary care and developed geriatric assessment and consultation programs.[11,15,16] Many of these provide the initial assessment, make recommendations to the physician, and provide future consultation only as requested. One model integrated case management program is the Geriatric Care Coordination Program (GCCP) in Sacramento, California. This program uses screening, assessment, and care coordination in a longitudinal approach. It works with the physicians and follows the care of the frail, at-risk older patients until problem resolution or disenrollment. The population consists of Medicare HMO enrollees linked to the Sutter Medical Group, under Sutter/CHS. Sutter/CHS is a nonprofit, multiservice health care system with approximately 6,000 affiliated physicians in Northern California. The Sutter Medical Group is a foundation-model multispecialty group based in Sacramento. The GCCP, which services approximately 60 primary care physicians, is a pilot project created for the purpose of evaluating the benefits of this type of program throughout the region. To date, the GCCP has screened over 4,000 enrollees and is actively involved in the care of over 300 seniors.

At the time of enrollment, members are sent a screening questionnaire that requests information about past utilization, number of medications, self-perception of health and disease-group categories, use of durable medical equipment and other services, degree of independence in activities of daily living and instrumental activities of daily living, caregiver needs and resources, and depression. Those patients who do not return their questionnaires are contacted via phone. All data collected are scored and entered into a database that is shared with the after-hours advice center and the social services triage center.

The scores are stratified into four levels of risk (see box entitled "Risk Stratification"). Those at Level II are given disease-specific resources such as educational materials and information regarding self-directed care. Those at Level III are referred to social services in order to coordinate community and caregiver resources. Finally, those at highest risk (Level IV) are referred to the care management team, which consists of a geriatric physician, a geriatric nurse practitioner, and a master's level social worker. For each patient, an assessment is performed in a clinic setting, the home, an acute care hospital, or a nursing home. A care plan is developed with the

---

Risk Stratification

Level I: No identified risk factors; patient may benefit from primary prevention and health promotion.

Level II: Patient has stable chronic disease; may benefit from early detection and primary and secondary prevention and health promotion.

Level III: Patient has chronic disease, with predominantly social needs and need for caregiver; would benefit from care planning and clinical management to prevent further functional decline.

Level IV: Frail elders with multiple medical, social, and functional problems; at high risk for placement, hospital admission, functional decline, or death.

patient and family and communicated to the primary care physician. The team then follows the patient over time, with interventions based on need, and it does not "sign off" the case until problem resolution or disenrollment. Changes in the patient's clinical and functional status are shared by the primary care physician and the team.

Since patients will shift between levels, there must be additional mechanisms for case finding. Patients are also identified by utilization review and physician referral. In addition, several "triggers" were developed to be used by the concurrent review nurse in the acute care setting to identify at-risk patients (see box entitled "Acute Care Triggers for Referral to the Geriatric Care Coordination Program"). The case management team also assists in coordinating placement to other levels of service within the Sacramento area. If the primary care physician is not available to attend a patient in the nursing home, the team, including the geriatric physician, assumes the responsibility for care. If the physician does attend the patient, then the team plays a consulting role. The team also facilitates home health care when the patient is ready to return home. Information is shared by the geriatric physician, the primary care physician, other providers, and the managed care authorization staff. As a consequence, the responsibility for primary care is shared and the contribution of each of the disciplines within the team is strengthened.

PATIENT RESPONSIBILITY AND SELF-DIRECTED CARE

An argument has been made that, in fact, the true primary care provider is the patient. In any case, no model of integrated care coordination is complete without the patient (or health plan member) as an integral part of the team process. In order to function as part of a team, the patient needs to access resources and information, including information on how the health care system works, how it is organized, how decisions are made about the allocation of resources, and how the patient can enter the system.

Patients also need information about health and wellness and how to make basic lifestyle choices that will positively impact their lives. They need preventive services (e.g., screening and immunizations) that are easily accessible. They need resources to assist them in managing their own illness, including disease-specific educational materials and classes, and easy access to advice. Many organizations link "advice lines" to the physician's office through the information system, thus allowing the advice nurse to transmit the patient's concerns and schedule appointments.

As part of a team, patients must also accept certain responsibilities. To avoid being placed in a passive, non–decision-making position, they must share as well as receive information and modify their behavior based on the advice they get. When individuals and families are given the tools to participate in and manage care, they can become a strong and integral component in the process of integrated primary care.

Acute Care Triggers for Referral to the Geriatric Care Coordination Program

New confusion (delirium)
Dementia
Depression
Incontinence
Poor nutritional status, malnutrition, or poor oral intake during hospitalization
Falls (within past year or during hospitalization)
Use of restraints
Polypharmacy (five or more medications taken daily)
Prolonged immobility
Lack of community or social support or resources
Needs expressed by individual, family, or caregivers
Anticipated need for placement or extended home health care
Prolonged hospital course beyond anticipated length of stay

REFERENCES

1. Bringewatt, R. Position paper. Minneapolis, MN: National Chronic Care Consortium, April 1993.

2. LaPlante, M. "The Demographics of Disability." *Milbank Quarterly,* 1991 suppl., pp. 55–77.

3. Schlesinger, M., and Mechanic, D. "Challenges for Managed Competition from Chronic Illness." *Health Affairs,* 1993 suppl., pp. 123–36.

4. Shortell, S., et al. "The Holographic Organization." *Healthcare Forum Journal,* March–April 1993, pp. 20–26.

5. Paone, D. "Care across the Continuum." *Case Review* (Fall 1995): 11–12.

6. Bates, E., and Brown, B. "Geriatric Care Needs and HMO Technology: A Theoretical Analysis and Initial Findings from the National Medicare Competition Evaluation." *Medical Care* 26 (1988): 488–98.

7. Freeborn, D., et al. "Consistently High Users of Medical Care among the Elderly." *Medical Care* 28 (1990): 527–40.

8. Harrington, C., and Newcomer, R. "Social Health Maintenance Organizations' Service Use and Costs, 1985–1989." *Health Care Financing Review* (Spring 1991): 37–52.

9. Shen, J., and Iversen, A. "PACE: A Capitated Model towards Long-term Care." *Henry Ford Hospital Medical Journal* 40 (1992): 41–44.

10. National Chronic Care Consortium. *Final Report on Risk Identification Initiative.* National Chronic Care Consortium, 1995.

11. Kramer, A., Fox, P., and Morgenstern, N. "Geriatric Care Approaches in Health Maintenance Organizations." *Journal of the American Geriatrics Society* 40 (1992): 1055–67.

12. Boult, C., et al. "Screening Elders for Risk of Hospital Admission." *Journal of the American Geriatrics Society* 41 (1993): 811–17.

13. Defriese, G., and Crossland, D. "Health Status and Health Risk Assessment among Older Adults." *Generations* 18, no. 1 (1994): 51–56.

14. Pacala, J.T., Boult, C., and Boult, L.B. "Predictive Validity of a Questionnaire That Identifies Elders at Risk for Hospital Admission." *Journal of the American Geriatrics Society* 43 (1995): 374–77.

15. Naylor, M., et al. "Comprehensive Discharge Planning for the Hospitalized Elderly." *Annals of Internal Medicine* 120 (1994): 999–1006.

16. Evans, K., Yurkow, J., and Siegler, E. "The CARE Program: A Nurse-Managed Collaborative Outpatient Program to Improve Function of Frail Older People." *Journal of the American Geriatrics Society* 43 (1995): 1155–60.

Managing and Redesigning the Continuum of Care: The Value Chain Model

Kathy Fleschut, Chip Caldwell, and B. Eugene Beyt, Jr.

Systems of care that improve the quality of life for the populations served are developed either on a virtual basis, driven in large part by financing mechanisms, or are built around physician- and provider-directed systems of care which bear clinical and financial risk. In either case, the health and well-being of the population has to be managed, measured, and continuously improved through the redesigning of processes. Further, the incentives for all stakeholders need to be aligned in order to produce the partnership between patients, physicians, providers, and payers that is necessary for controlling demand, managing acute and chronic illness, and defining measurable outcomes. In the new health care environment, the integration of clinical medicine, systems thinking, and quality management disciplines provides needed tools and skills and can help identify key leverage points and learning opportunities to improve the quality of the health care services delivered.[1,2] Within this framework, this article presents a conceptual plan and model designed to assist care managers, physicians, and organizations in managing and redesigning the continuum of care.

A SYSTEMS APPROACH

A system dynamic model of care that assumes risk and measures and improves the health of the population served has been previously de-

scribed[3] and may serve as the underpinnings for the clinical management and redesign of the continuum of care. Represented in terms used in system dynamic modeling, the population at risk may be divided into two "stocks," those individuals who are healthy and those who are receiving active intervention for an acute or chronic illness. Management of the continuum of care becomes essential as patients "flow" from one group to the other. This high-level system model is useful for identifying the leverage points of assumption of risk, alignment of incentives, development of a system of care, management of demand, and measurement and redesign of clinical processes. System models can be constructed with specific details and in response to unique considerations; however, a general model serves as a framework to address redesign and management of the continuum of care (Figure 1). The continuum is bascially the system of health-related processes beginning before birth and ending with death. In addition, it is useful to think of the continuum of care as having discreet access points that correlate in a general way with most health delivery systems' organizational groupings. Obviously such groupings, although artificial, may nevertheless assist in uncovering management and redesign options.

CREATING A MODEL OF CARE

The current reality, which includes cost-containment strategies within the insurer–payer

Quality Management in Health Care 1996; 5(1): 42–48
© 1996 Aspen Publishers, Inc.

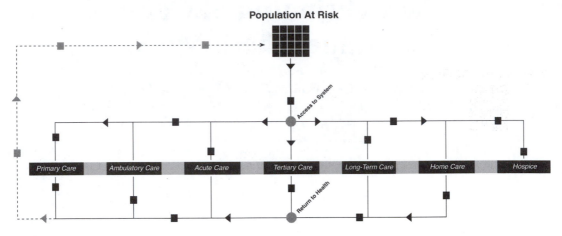

Figure 1. Continuum of care.

community as well as new reimbursement alternatives such as capitation, is forcing many health care systems to develop the core competencies needed for managing care. Pressures on and within an organization can promote quick fixes and tampering, and can obstruct the development of a planning process. It is important that the organization avoid these kinds of pitfalls by involving stakeholders early in the development. Fostering stakeholder participation begins with active dialogue within a "safe container"[4] directed toward creating a shared understanding and vision of the organizational's model of the continuum of care.

A quality planning team should be formed, with representatives from each segment of the continuum, as well as from the case management and quality management departments. Such a team, which will include appropriate clinicians, should be empowered to design and improve the care processes along the continuum. To achieve this mission, the team would need to accomplish two things: (1) develop the necessary resources and structures and (2) develop a model showing how the system would manage and redesign care. The first task would consolidate the necessary care management human resources into one management structure in order to reduce duplication and synergize efforts to manage patients across the continuum, and the

second would generate the organizational linguistics needed to communicate effectively and systematically on management and improvement issues. The management, improvement, and redesign of this core competency for a system of care constitute the central initiative for meeting the challenges of the current reality.

MANAGING THE MODEL OF CARE

As the planning process proceeds, attention turns to designing and articulating the continuum of care model appropriate for the organization. Figure 2 presents one proposed model. The model begins at an access point along the continuum of care through which patients in the population risk pool (stock) could enter (flow) into the system. Since the system must have the ability to prevent episodes of illness and provide coordinated interventions that are cost effective while achieving quality outcomes and satisfied customers, risk assessment at the access point is performed. The key task of this model is to identify the risk and health status of the individuals who make up the population pool and segregate the individuals on the basis of underlying or chronic illnesses. Obviously, efforts at the primary end of the continuum to develop partnerships with employers allow the identification and management of high-risk employees. As-

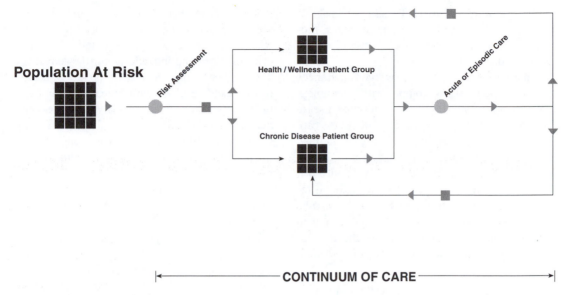

Figure 2. System model of care.

sessment of new members is also performed. Once the initial assessment is completed, patients are placed into two kinds of groups: disease-specific patient groups and wellness and health promotion groups.

Within the disease-specific patient groups (groups of patients with chronic illnesses such as diabetes and congestive heart failure), the risk assessment methodology allows for specific needs to be identified for each patient. Developing a plan or disease-specific clinical pathway of care meeting the patient's needs is the next step. This individual plan or pathway of care is based on the partnership between the physician, the patient, and a community case manager and is focused on achieving mutually shared goals in the most cost-effective way possible. The patient is continuously monitored through the case management program and handoffs are made to appropriate inpatient teams if the need for more intensive treatment arises.

A common occurrence within the disease-specific patient groups is an acute event (as shown in Figure 2) requiring acute or episodic care. When this occurs, the patient care is overseen by a multidisciplinary team of clinicians, including the primary care physician and the community and institutional case managers. Upon admission to the institution, the patient is placed on the appropriate pathway of care, with the primary nurse and physician having the lead role in supporting and directing the management of care and the allocation of resources. Following the institutional intervention, the management of care is handed back to the physician and community case manager, and the patient is placed back into the disease-specific group.

For those patients for whom the initial risk assessment fails to identify any specific disease or condition, the chief goals are to reduce clinical risk, promote healthy behavior, and manage the demand for services. To achieve these goals, health promotion activities in various wellness education programs are developed. They are geared toward educating the patients and the community on how to maintain a healthy lifestyle. Such programs are developed as pathways of care for the particular population in an attempt to increase quality of life and prevent episodes of illness. Community case managers promote the development of organizational relationships with the patients, acting as resource persons and evaluating progress toward set goals. These evolving relationships, which are basically partnerships, promote patient independence and a sense of control over health.

There will always be, however, instances when a patient fails to comply with recommendations or a new onset of a condition or disease occurs. When this happens, episodic illness care may be required, and the same process outlined for the disease-specific patient groups is followed. Management of the patient is handed off, and after the interventional care the patient is reassessed to determine whether he or she can be placed into the wellness group again or is now in need of community case management as a patient in one of the disease-specific groups.

ROLE OF CARE MANAGEMENT AND IMPROVEMENT

The model must be supported by the appropriate deployment of human resources, including community case managers and institutional case managers. From the community perspective, clinicians manage patient care, including specialty referral, risk assessment, and patient education. Institutional case managers manage inpatient utilization as well as the necessary precertification. Precertification requirements of payer groups are intended to reduce demand for services, and guidelines utilized by insurance companies assist the case managers in determining how resources should be deployed. The case managers, both community and institutional, have the primary function of managing the care of patients and acting as process consultants. As clinical redesign occurs and protocols and pathways of care are further developed, case managers perform the ongoing monitoring needed to ensure that the care is optimally provided in the least costly and most appropriate setting.

A second key task is to determine the health care effectiveness of care management programs by applying quality management tools and techniques to a set of operational and clinical goals. The group mainly responsible for this task consists of clinicians, data analysts, statisticians, quality management consultants, and management engineers. The group works in concert with physicians, case managers, and other clinicians in improving and redesigning the delivery of care. The core competencies of the group include research and development of breakthrough ideas, measurement and statistical analysis, process and outcome measurement, and facilitation of redesign and improvement efforts. The group is a central hub or toolbox for operational quality and patient care improvement activities and is responsible for facilitating teams, developing early warning systems based on established monitors, and developing necessary clinical profiling and key indicators linked with financial results. The group also develops the necessary teams, monitors their progress, develops and maintains key databases, and creates the necessary report cards for accrediting agencies.

LEARNING EXPERIMENTS

As the modeling and planning process moves into the implementation phase, a construct for organizational learning may prove to be very useful. In this process, aims are established, the necessary measures to ensure that the aim has been reached are agreed upon, and a cycle of learning is then implemented. Clinical aims that incorporate measures have been previously published.[5] (See box for an example of one of the clinical aims to be achieved.) Such clinical aims are often focused on key patient populations or high-volume procedures that have wide variation and high cost as a result of the way care is delivered. In order for the clinical aims to be accomplished, participation from multidisciplinary groups from each access point along the continuum is crucial.

The process for agreeing on and redesigning the continuum of care will often lead to the convening of a clinical quality council comprising key clinician leaders. The council will be responsible for managing and redesigning the continuum, and its members, often mostly physicians, should have a vested interest in the well-being of the patient population and should

**Clinical Aim Number 1:
Cardiovascular Disease**

Early intervention: Establish a process for early identification of high-risk patients within a defined population, focusing on serum cholesterol and blood pressure screenings, with a resulting 20-percent improvement in treatment, compliance, and follow-up.

Acute management: Redesign the process of care for treatment of heart disease that results in a 20- to 30-percent reduction in cost and variation without compromising the clinical and functional outcome of the patients.

Chronic management: Establish a clinical pathway of care addressing the chronicity of congestive heart failure that improves the patients' perception of personal health and reduces the readmission rate and cost by 40 percent without compromising clinical outcomes.

have an opportunity to become comfortable with the data validity and measurement systems. The redesign efforts should be prioritized on the basis of opportunity, level of aligned incentives, complexity, and time needed to implement proposed changes. Initial meetings with clinician leaders should be devoted to clarifying the goals, the necessary team membership and roles, the time frames for completion, the financial savings to be achieved, and the necessary support needed from the care management and health care effectiveness staff.

THE VALUE CHAIN MODEL

Figure 3 illustrates the value chain model for managing and redesigning the continuum of care. In this model, the continuum of care is detailed for a specific clinical aim, and measures are established utilizing the "value compass" (with the dimensions of process, satisfaction, cost, and outcome). Baseline data are collected to illustrate the current level of performance and the stability of the existing processes and to ensure that the redesign effort achieves its aim. This framework provides a fertile environment for opportunities for innovation and breakthrough thinking, as such concepts are presented as leverage points within a redesigned system as opposed to meddling in a current system of care. In addition, the process of establishing the value chain often produces the opportunity for in-depth conversations about the complexities of current processes and the frustrations and dissatisfactions that lie below the complacent surface of everyday events.

The core competencies of the value chain model provide the specific organizational language for the continuum of care. As previously mentioned, this shared language fosters a level of conversation, shared insight, and public reflection that increases organizational learning and has demonstrable community benefits. The redesigned value chain then becomes the base for another cycle of improvement and innovation as aims are re-examined and redirected toward new performance levels.

THE RESULT: A CULTURE OF LEARNING

Managing and redesigning the continuum of care based on the value chain model is an evolutionary process. It would be naive not to recognize there are several obstacles to successful implementation. Obviously, the current health care delivery system often creates a cost base requiring unrealistic volume demands and capital spending. This approach leads organizations away from the concept of a continuum of care that promotes health and well-being. Thus, there has to be a continued effort to share the vision and, as important, share the power with clinicians, who are the key determinants of resources utilized and delivery of services. That sharing has to be based on aligned incentives and a systemic organizational structure promoting a culture of trust and dialogue, and it also has to be "data driven," which means that management

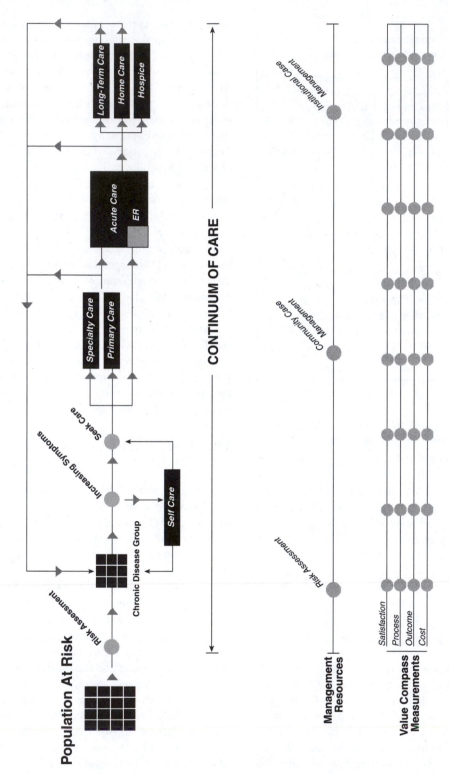

Figure 3. Sample value chain for a clinical aim.

and redesign efforts must be responded to objectively rather than emotionally.

Management of the continuum of care and support of all aspects of the value chain is truly a systemic process and requires many health care workers to undergo a fundamental shift in their view of health care. This shift can only be accomplished through a culture of learning and through understanding system complexity and the likely results of actions taken. Organizational learning, which is essential for redesigning the value chain, will occur if clinical and institutional leaders articulate the aims of systems of care and create learning opportunities to demonstrate redesign and improve the management of the continuum of care.

REFERENCES

1. Caldwell, C. *Mentoring Strategic Change in Health Care: An Action Guide.* Milwaukee, Wis.: Quality Press, 1995.
2. Senge, P.M. *The Fifth Discipline: The Art and Practice of the Learning Organization.* New York, N.Y.: Doubleday, 1990.
3. Bright, S., and Beyt, G. "Lessons in Systems Thinking: A Tale from the Land of Middle Health." *The Systems Thinker* 6 (1995): 1–5.
4. Isaacs, W. "Dialogue: The Power of Collective Thinking." In *Reflections on Creating Learning Organizations,* edited by K.T. Wardman. Cambridge, Mass.: Pegasus Communications, 1994.
5. Berwick, D.M. "Eleven Worthy Aims for Clinical Leadership of Health System Reform." *JAMA* 272 (1994): 797–802.

Managing Critical Pathway Variances

Janice Schriefer

As experience with critical pathways grows, the need for a sophisticated approach to variance management increases. The subject of critical pathway variance management is relatively underdeveloped compared to the literature describing the initial development of pathways. At Fletcher Allen Health Care (Fletcher Allen), we see a similar situation. Over the past seven years, we have developed more than 50 pathways, but many are now abandoned and left in file cabinets for various reasons. Of all the pathways developed, only about 20 currently have active management of variances. Because pathway development is labor intensive, perhaps it is time to contain the development of pathways and emphasize the management of variances for the pathways that are already in use.

Unfortunately, the literature does not provide clear, consensus guidelines on how to document, collect, analyze, and report critical pathway variances. This article reviews the various definitions and approaches that have appeared in the literature, shares the variance management experience at Fletcher Allen, and offers some conclusions and recommendations.

CRITICAL PATHWAY VARIANCE MANAGEMENT: A LITERATURE REVIEW

Defining and classifying variances

Variance is commonly defined as "the state of being variable or variant" or "the state of being in disagreement."[1] Rudisill and associates defined pathway variances as a "discrepancy between expected and actual events in a patient's plan of care."[2(p.30)] At Fletcher Allen, pathway variances are defined as a deviation from the patient care activities outlined on the critical pathway that alters the anticipated discharge date, the expected cost, or the expected length of stay. Although these definitions vary slightly, the concepts are similar.

Many authors have reported standard categories for the causes of variances, such as patient/family, caregiver/clinician, hospital/system, and community. Zander defined each category as follows[3]:

- *Patient/family variance*—anything related to patients or families that causes a variance from the pathway, such as having a complication from a procedure (e.g., an infection).
- *Caregiver/clinician variance*—anything related to the caregiver or clinician caring

The author thanks all the staff of Fletcher Allen dedicated to using critical pathways to improve clinical and financial outcomes. A team approach and a willingness to change are integral to their success.

Quality Management in Health Care 1995; 3(2): 30–42
© 1995 Aspen Publishers, Inc.

for the patient that causes a variance from the pathway, such as a delay in providing a specific treatment needed to move along the expected plan of care.

- *Hospital/system variance*—anything related to the hospital or health care system that causes a variance, such as being unable to schedule a patient for a test due to a backlog of cases.
- *Community variance*—anything related to the care provided outside of the hospital that may cause a variance, such as the lack of respiratory therapists in the community to provide needed home care.

Coffey and colleagues used the same definitions and provide the following examples for each variance category.[4] A patient/family variance occurs when a patient refuses a test that is required prior to discharge. A caregiver/clinician variance occurs when there is a delay in discharge teaching for a parent of an ill child. A hospital/system variance results when the computed tomography scanner breaks down. Last, a community variance happens when the lack of nursing home beds delays a patient's discharge.

While Zander's four-element classification scheme is widely used, it is not universal. For example, Robinson and colleagues saw only two high-level classification elements. They categorized the causes of variance as either system or patient.[5] But these authors expanded the classification detail by using a variance identification decision tree. The variance categories in their decision tree included material resource consumption, human resource consumption, time delays, co-morbid factors, complications, and compliance factors. Such thorough identification of variances is imperative to minimize adverse effects on quality and fiscal outcomes. However, while this work adds detail to our understanding of cause-effect relationships in variance analysis, the authors failed to quantify the effects on outcomes.

Bejciy-Spring, who utilized the classification scheme of Robinson and associates, cited frequent causes of variances for laminectomy patients.[6] The common variances related to patients and families included very young or very old patients, no family or significant other at home, and activity intolerance. The causes for systems variances included bed not being available, appointment times not available, breakdown of equipment, home health care not available, no third party coverage for necessary procedures, and lack of extended care facility placement. Even though the author referred to improved resource utilization, the actual improvements were not quantified.

While Robinson and coworkers and Bejciy-Spring used derivatives of Zander's model, Hoffman took a different approach to classifying variance.[7] Hoffman used the categories often found on the left-hand side of the pathway (evaluations, tests, consults, treatments, medications, activity, diet, elimination, education, discharge, and complications) and tabulated the frequency of variances within each category. The advantage of this method is that staff are already familiar with the standardized pathway categories.

Instead of the rigid categories suggested by Zander and others, Mikulaninec[8] recommended individualizing pathways based on the patient's co-morbidities and socioeconomic factors. Thereafter, any deviations from the pathway are termed variances, and a plan is developed to address them. This approach allows pathways and variance classification to be tailored to fit individual patient conditions. Mikulaninec suggested that one look at each variance individually—in light of unique patient conditions—and develop a specific plan to address each variance. The author reported a two-day length of stay reduction by applying this approach to an amputation pathway.

It should be noted that in all of the classification schemes described above, a variance can be either positive or negative. A positive variance occurs when a patient meets the expected outcomes for a critical pathway *prior to* the timeline established. For example, a patient undergoing a total hip replacement may be ready for discharge on the fourth postoperative day rather than the expected length of stay of five days.

While there is much written on the definition and classification of variances, the active management of variances receives relatively little attention in the critical pathway literature. Most articles only briefly mention variance management. There are only a few articles that focus on variances in particular. But, the experience at Fletcher Allen appears to indicate that careful management of variances from the critical pathway often results in care improvements.

Collecting variance data

Just as there are many schemes for classifying variances, the literature also provides a variety of examples of practical ways to collect data on variances. These approaches tend to fall into one of four categories: notations directly on the critical pathway document itself, retrospective chart review, the use of a separate variance data collection sheet, and the use of computerized systems.

It should be noted that the critical pathway literature provides very little detail on the mechanics of variance documentation directly on the pathway. However, anecdotal reports indicate that many institutions utilize this approach. Most pathways have a section at the bottom labeled "variances," where the appropriate provider is expected to document the variance directly on the pathway.

Another method of collecting variance data is a retrospective chart review. Again, the specifics of such a review are difficult to find in the pathway literature. However, the article by Farley in this issue gives an example of this technique. As noted by Ferguson, if the chart review approach is used, it is helpful to have a standard audit tool to ensure consistency of data collection.[9]

Hoffman outlined a method where nurses write variances on a variance tracking tool attached to the pathway.[7] Nurses follow up on these variances and address them. After patient discharge, the variance tracking tool is sent to the quality management department for analysis and reporting of trends. Hoffman did not describe the frequency or accuracy of these reports, nor how data integrity is assured. The re-ports are used primarily to provide feedback to the interdisciplinary team that is managing the pathway. Utilizing this method, Hoffman cited improvements that included a reduction in complication rate of 11 percent and a reduction in length of stay of three days.

Similarly, Hampton used a tool separate from the pathway to document both the variances that occur and how they are addressed.[10] In this approach, any discipline involved in the care of the patient can document variances. The nursing staff caring for the patient conducts a follow-up evaluation of actions taken. Hampton recommended no documentation for a positive variance such as an early discharge; documentation of variances occurs only when length of stay is longer than expected. Unfortunately, Hampton failed to give any examples of improved quality and cost-effectiveness associated with this approach. Data from variance analysis are used by quality improvement teams, but it is unclear how often these teams meet and exactly what improvements are undertaken. Like Hoffman, Hampton did not address issues of data integrity or accuracy.

Johnson presented an interesting approach to variance management whereby a daily, interdisciplinary variance review meeting is written directly into the critical pathway.[11] In these meetings, caregivers either confirm that the patient is on track, or immediately create a strategy to address variances. Including variance review as a daily step on the pathway itself may remind staff of its importance and improve the accuracy of the data. Often, staff will postpone documentation of pathway variances until after higher priority tasks are completed, such as administration of medication or wound care. As a result, the variance might not be documented or key details might be omitted. Daily review ensures that the facts surrounding important variances are documented while the events are still fresh.

Although paper systems for collecting variances are more common, computer-based systems do exist. DiJerome described a computerized critical pathway and variance system in use at the Summa Health System (Akron, Ohio).[12]

The advantage of such a system is the ability to adapt the pathway to changes in the patient's condition that are normally seen as variances. This flexible, computerized pathway approach avoids the "falling off the path" phenomenon that has a negative connotation. The computer system also removes the manual steps of data collection and trend analysis of variances. It is a challenge, however, to provide additional training to nurse case managers using the system who have little computer experience. No data were presented relative to the efficiency of the system compared with a paper variance tracking system. In addition, there was no mention of mechanisms to ensure data integrity.

It appears that more institutions are heading toward automated pathways and variance data collection. Lumsdon and Hagland found that while many organizations initially track variances manually, automation and links to clinical information systems are often needed as the dataset grows.[13] Of those hospitals surveyed, 21 percent had an in-house, spreadsheet-based system to analyze variances from pathways; 8 percent had automated critical pathways with caregivers directly entering data into computers; and 6 percent were developing automated pathways. When asked about their plans to automate pathways, 34 percent said they would like to automate but have other information service priorities; 32 percent said they have no plans to automate pathways; 23 percent plan to develop automated tools for variance analysis; and 21 percent plan to automate charting based on critical pathways within one year.

Analyzing and reporting variances

After data are collected, the next steps in variance management are analysis and reporting. The literature reports a variety of approaches to these tasks.

On the analysis side, Strong and Sneed performed a controlled trial to evaluate variances from a coronary artery bypass graft (CABG) critical pathway to determine those that significantly influenced postoperative length of stay.[14]

Using correlation between variables, they discovered that the variances of slow activity progression, prolonged telemetry use, and inspirometer use had the greatest impact on length of stay. Interestingly, Fletcher Allen found that prolonged telemetry use and slow activity progression were the two most frequent variances for CABG patients (confirming Strong and Sneed's findings).

Another method of analysis was described by Ferguson.[9] At Johns Hopkins Hospital, nurse case managers code variances as a nursing diagnosis and use the nursing process (i.e., data collection, assessment, planning, and evaluation) to improve care. The pathway includes an activity that reminds case managers to evaluate variances daily (similar to Johnson's daily variance review meetings[11]).

On the reporting side, Bueno and Hwang described quarterly variance management summaries on patients covered by specific nurse case managers throughout the Robert Wood Johnson Hospital (RWJH).[15] According to the authors, analysis of pathway variances is vital to achieving expected patient outcomes, timely discharge of patients, and appropriate utilization of resources. At RWJH, nurse case managers identify variances from a variety of sources including nursing documentation, physician progress notes, and verbal communication with providers and patients. Variances due to support departments, such as radiology or the catheterization laboratory, are compiled and reported to the director of the department for action. The RWJH system uses a computer scanner to compile, analyze, and report variances in an automated fashion. The savings accruing from pathway variance management were not quantified.

Metcalf described the reporting mechanism at the Alliant Health System, where the focus is on identifying trends in pathway variances.[16] Trends include patient characteristics that contribute to variances, as well as variance trends in the use of resources to care for patients on the pathway. If cost variances, adverse quality variances, or noncompliance patterns are seen, statistical monitoring is initiated. Monthly variance reports are disseminated to medical and nursing staff. Notably, nursing directors, head nurses, and utilization review staff share responsibility for analyzing and reporting variances. A length-of-stay reduction of 2.6 days for joint replacement patients was reported after implementation of a pathway and this associated documentation system.

The role of case management

Case managers often pull together the pieces of classification, collection, analysis, and reporting of variances. Many institutions employ case managers, who are often nurses, for particular patient populations. When a pathway is written for such a population (e.g., hip replacement or open heart surgery patients), the case manager manages the variances experienced on the pathway. Variance management and case management need to be thought of as integrated and mutually complementary.

For example, Woodyard and Sheetz looked at whether or not tests and treatments were accomplished as planned on the pathway.[17] They recommended evaluation of variances on a shift-by-shift basis to produce optimal outcomes. Then, nurse case managers can use focus documentation to address variances. Most important, variances provide structure for change-of-shift reporting and for the multidisciplinary discharge planning process. Likewise, the focus on variance management during change-of-shift reporting provides concurrent management, which is more effective than retrospective review. Woodyard and Sheetz reported a 50 percent improvement in patient teaching and retention resulting from a quality improvement project that inaugurated changes in the pathway.

Crummer and Carter reported on the use of nurse case managers to record and track variances, in addition to intervening to address the variance.[18] Under this system, the case manager develops and implements a quality improvement process for any recurrent variances from the pathway. While Crummer and Carter felt that pathway variances provide quantitative data on the correlation between effective resource utilization and patient outcomes, no data were given to support this conclusion.

Romito described a nurse case manager's role in creating a pathway for stroke patients.[19] Whenever a variance from the critical pathway occurs, the discharge date is adjusted accordingly and the plan is continued from there. Moreover, weekly rounds are used to review positive and negative variances. Romito cited numerous anecdotal improvements due to pathways, including length of stay reductions, improved charting, increased communication with insurance companies, and increased patient understanding of the plan of care.

A modified approach to case management employs a team to manage care overall, instead of just for individual patients. Giuliano and Poirier described a multidisciplinary practice group that met regularly to review trends in critical pathway variances.[20] Patients and family members were also invited to the practice group meetings to discuss individual variances from the pathway. Strengthened teamwork between nurses, physicians, and patients was seen to result. Notably, nurse case managers track and analyze the variances, with the goal of continually improving the clinical outcomes.

As noted by Guiliano and Poirier and other case management advocates, involving patients and families with critical pathways is essential. Fletcher Allen recommends that every pathway team develop a patient and family version of the pathway so that patients can be more involved in the management of their own care. Mosher and colleagues found that patients and families appreciate getting a copy of the pathway.[21] Patients know what to expect each day and feel motivated to meet the targets on the pathway. Perhaps simply sharing the pathway with patients and families helps prevent some variances.

It appears that critical pathway documents provide a means for securing higher levels of patient and family involvement. For instance, Latini and Foote created a pathway for the first 72 hours of a trauma patient's stay.[22] They provided copies to patients' families, who reported decreased stress and frustration as a result of being informed. Because the family understood the plan according to the pathway, it gave them a sense of control. At Fletcher Allen, CABG patients receive a copy of the pathway from the case manager either on their preoperative visit day or in the coronary care unit if they are an emergent case. A patient/family videotape accompanies the pathway.

Link between variance management and continuous improvement

Berwick emphasized the connection between critical pathways and continuous quality improvement (CQI).[23] The pathway helps physicians engage the positive challenge of reducing variation as part of the general improvement process. In fact, CQI and pathways work well together.

It is no coincidence that Fletcher Allen's experience with critical pathway variance analysis echoes the literature. The majority of authors support the use of teams to manage pathway variances. Moreover, the teams are best equipped to resolve variances if the CQI approach of focusing on the process and utilizing teamwork is employed. Variances are rarely the result of one professional group. Therefore, all the key players for a particular patient population must meet as a team on a regular basis to uncover opportunities for improvement in the process of care. If the team meets for one year, solves a problem variance, and disbands, the entire thrust of CQI is lost. Variance management requires ongoing perseverance and dedication.

As an example of what can happen when critical paths are not linked to CQI efforts, Falconer and associates performed a controlled study with stroke patients.[24] They found that using a critical pathway failed to provide improvements in the cost of care and clinical outcomes. But, although quality improvement is mentioned as a factor in health care, the study failed to integrate CQI into the research. If the critical pathway team had used a CQI approach to follow up on variances, it might have made incremental improvements in care. Instead, it appears the authors simply ended the study after tracking 53 patients on the pathway.

Coffey and associates explained that timely analysis and management of variances from a critical pathway may bring about improvement in the form of decreased complications and resource consumption.[4] They shared data on significant cost savings at the University of Michigan Hospitals in populations where pathways were initiated, and they stressed the importance of using variance data to update and improve the critical pathway continuously. This practice is especially important in light of the rapid technology changes that can dramatically change a care process. Further, these authors emphasized that methods used for variance analysis and outcome measurements will depend on the original goals for implementing the critical pathway.

Wood and coworkers stressed the importance of focusing on positive variances as a way to bring about improvement stating that "The purpose of identifying variances is to evaluate what works and what needs refinement."[25(p.57)] Often, a positive variance (achieving outcomes earlier than anticipated) provides clues for more cost-effective care. Unfortunately, the authors failed to provide an example. They did, however, provide a copy of the variance tracking tool that is attached to their pathways. It appears to be a useful tool with an area to document the variance, the action taken to correct the variance, and the outcome of that action.

Grudich described the use of a critical pathway to bring about an improvement in operating room efficiency.[26] By tracking variances from the pathway, Grudich discovered that surgeons and anesthesiologists not arriving on time accounted for 43 percent of all operating room variances from the schedule. Using such data helped to increase the staff's understanding of the variances from the critical pathway and led to work toward improvement.

VARIANCE MANAGEMENT AT FLETCHER ALLEN

At Fletcher Allen, the approach to variance management is based on several observations mentioned in the preceding literature review. In particular, a form of case management is used with a number of pathways, and continuous quality improvement techniques are employed in the management of pathway variances. Fletcher Allen's approach also extends the effort in ways not covered in the literature review. These efforts include establishing a plan for staff education on variance management, involving the utilization review staff in collecting variances, and using algorithms to address common variances. The Fletcher Allen critical pathway system uses a four-step model that includes development, use, measurement, and improvement. Variance management is most important during the measurement phase of the model.

This section describes Fletcher Allen's variance management methodology and outlines its approach to staff education, documentation, collection, classification, analysis, and reporting of variances. In addition, a variance case management success story is presented, detailing the creation of algorithms to address variances, the ways to predict variances, and the link to information systems.

Staff education

Clear and consistent staff education on the use of pathways and the plan for variance management is essential. Often, staff lose interest in pathways and neglect to document variances because they never received instructions on the process nor any regular feedback. Formal variance tracking training for staff is therefore important. It can be accomplished in a grand rounds format, through inservices, or at staff meetings. It is important to remember to provide coverage for staff so that they can attend these educational sessions.

Traditional training sessions are not the only way to educate staff. Some teams have posted written instructions for pathway use and variance documentation, with good anecdotal results. Asking staff for their input on the most efficient process for variance documentation builds a sense of ownership. At Fletcher Allen, the staff are surveyed on the best approach to document variances. Because staff are expected to document the

variance, they should have control over the method used. If staff excel in the use of pathways and documentation of variances, it is important to provide positive feedback on their efforts.

Another staff education issue is the classification of variances. It is important to define the variances clearly. For example, if a patient requires oxygen therapy for longer than stated on the pathway, a decision must be made as to when to record the prolonged oxygen as a variance. Once the variance definitions are clarified and agreed on, all staff members should be informed.

Variances documentation

Staff education regarding documentation has become increasingly important at Fletcher Allen. In 1992, the Critical Pathway Steering Committee, a multidisciplinary group, created a manual for teams interested in critical pathways. The manual has a section that pertains specifically to documenting variances. Next to each intervention on the pathway, the caregiver is expected to check a box as to whether the activity was met, unmet, or not applicable (see Figure 1). If an intervention is unmet, there is a variance from the pathway. When a variance occurs, the provider is expected to document the nature of the variance and develop an immediate action plan. If a caregiver (nurse, therapist, dietitian, or pharmacist) needs extra room to explain the variance, he or she can use the patient's chart and simply add a note to the pathway referring to the appropriate sections of the chart.

This approach has met with some resistance. Staff complain that there is insufficient space to document on the pathway when a variance occurs. The unit specialist, who types the pathways, has been asked to provide additional space in the variance section. In addition, staff complain about a lack of time for documenting variances due to other priorities such as administration of medication. A staff-based committee has been established to address this critical pathway documentation issue.

It is difficult to quantify the exact number of variances recorded per day on a pathway. Of

M = Met U = Unmet N = Not Applicable	**USAP WITH CATH Critical Pathway** **Fletcher Allen Health Care** Expected LOS: _3.7_ DRG: _140_			(addressograph)

Date	Pre-CATH		CATH		Post-CATH		Expected	
Shift/Day/Week	Hosp Day 1 2 3 4 5 6 7 8 M U N		Hosp Day 1 2 3 4 5 6 7 8 M U N		Hosp Day	M U N	Outcomes	M U N
Consults	• Nutrition screen						• LOS within DRG	
Tests	• PTT qd if on Heparin ✓ • K if <4.0 on admission ✓ • EKG ✓ • Weight ✓ • If external transfer reassess EKG, CXR, Labs		Post-CATH: • IV Therapy • Evaluate for scheduling of exercise testing		• Possible exercise test			
Measurements/ Treatments	• Saline lock L arm for CATH IV only ✓ • Telemetry prn ✓ • VS q shift ✓ • O2 prn ✓		• Convert saline lock to KVO IV (separate line) • VS q shift—pre CATH • VS per protocol—Post CATH • O2 prn • Pre-CATH check voiding qs q shift • Post-CATH: Evaluate for I&O CATH		• DC post-CATH bandage • DC IV • Check voiding qs q shift		• Voids as usual • VS usual	
Medications	• Ongoing or ✓ • If external transfer identify current meds ✓ Pre-CATH: Eval for: • Diuretics ✓ • Hypoglycemics ✓ • Dye allergies ✓		Post CATH: • DC ASA and NSAIDS If CABG see CABG cp day 1 • Evaluated for Heparin		• Ongoing • Re-evaluate DC meds • Prescriptions		• After hours pharmacy needs will be met • Off ASA and NSAIDS if CABG • States use and precautions of all meds • Has prescriptions • No adverse drug reaction (inpatient)	
Mobility/ Precautions	• Evaluated activity level ✓		• Brachial: bedrest x2 hr • Femoral: bedrest x8 hr • As tolerated p BR		• Ad lib		• No ischemic symptoms with discharge activity	
Diet/Nutrition	• Lo chol; NAS, lo fat ✓ • NPO p MN x meds ✓		• Resume diet after CATH • Encourage fluids		• Ongoing		• Identify resources available for diet evaluation and changes (mgt)	
Discharge Planning (Ed., Psych/Soc. Homecare)	• CATH teaching ✓ • Financial aid needs evaluated ✓		• Test results/plan		• Discharge pharmacy needs • Teaching: Review meds, risk factors, follow-ups, CRII • States action if chest pain		• States two risk factors & identifies resources • States action if chest pain • States return visit with M.D. • States date of testing (ETT) • Able to get prescriptions filled • Transportation arranged • Pt states post-procedural activity restrictions, care of puncture site	
Variance Facts/Analysis	*Unable to do weight*							
Plan	*Get bed scale*							
Signatures & Initials	*Janice Schriefer*							

Change critical path to:_____

Figure 1. Example of a pathway with met, unmet, and not applicable categories. Unmet means a variance has occurred. Staff use the space provided at the bottom of the form to document the variance and the plan to address it.

course, this number is dependent on the patient's condition and individual needs. However, a recent audit revealed that, at Fletcher Allen, there is an average of 1.3 variances per patient stay. The length of written comments for each variance was seen to depend on the severity of the variance and the complexity of the plan needed to address it. Although the amount of time spent documenting variances has not been measured, staff are encouraged to be as concise as possible.

Variance data collection

Because pathways are a formal part of the medical record at Fletcher Allen, the medical record containing the pathway leaves the unit after the patient is discharged. Consequently, the quality management staff person collecting variance data must go to the medical records department to extract the data. This process is a labor-intensive one; however, some options are available. One solution is to place a carbon on the back of the pathway. Then, when the patient is discharged, the secretary can detach the carbon and mail it to the quality management staff for analysis. This approach is being piloted on the coronary artery bypass graft pathway. Unfortunately, it is still a paper system. However, until computerized systems are in place, it appears to be an excellent option. The CABG pathway team at Dartmouth-Hitchcock Medical Center in New Hampshire also uses a carbon copy method.

Another variance collection method being tested at Fletcher Allen incorporates the utilization review (UR) staff. The quality and utilization management department decided that the UR staff could incorporate review of critical pathways into their regular chart review for utilization purposes. So, the UR staff created a data collection tool to aggregate variances. For the most part, UR staff collect the variances of greatest concern including those that impact length of stay, cost per case, patient satisfaction, provider satisfaction, and readmissions. An example of a variance report based on data collected in routine UR reviews from the total hip replacement critical pathway is shown in

Figure 2. A similar reporting format is used for all pathways.

An added benefit of having the UR staff involved with pathways is their knowledge of inappropriate hospital days. The UR department previously tracked a data element called "barrier days" (i.e., patient days spent in the hospital waiting for a treatment or procedure). These data are used to direct pathway teams to some of the key bottlenecks or system variances in a particular critical pathway. The teams review this information on a regular basis and plan strategies to tackle the variances. In order to avoid parallel and duplicative efforts, the UR staff are phasing out barrier day tracking and replacing it with pathway variance tracking.

The UR staff also maintain data on the number of insurance refusals to pay for services and the number of readmissions. The payment issue is an important system variance to measure. Typically, the nursing staff are unaware of such issues, which makes the UR staff vital to the pathway team. More important, UR's tracking of unplanned readmissions within ten days of discharge is crucial as inpatient length of stays are shortened. These data can be fed back to the multidisciplinary pathway team for discussion. Fortunately, readmissions have not been problematic for the pathway teams at Fletcher Allen.

The process of collecting variances can be fatiguing. It is important to recognize this potential for burnout and respond appropriately. For example, at Fletcher Allen, the nurse manager for the cardiac surgery unit was collecting variance data for years and never complained. However, her enthusiasm started to diminish. The team quickly decided that summarizing variances every other month would be adequate. An automated clinical information system, with critical pathway variance collection built in, may be the long-term solution to the problem of fatigue associated with ongoing data collection.

Variance management

At Fletcher Allen, the most successful model for pathway variance management is the use of a

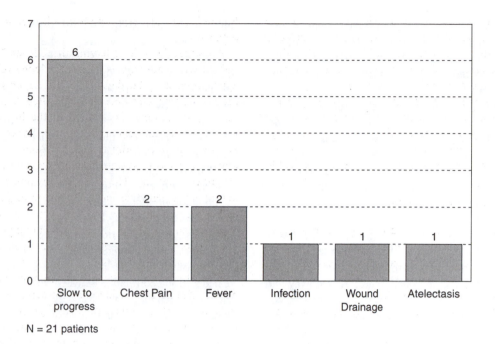

Figure 2. Total hip replacement critical pathway variances (N = 21), illustrating the variances collected and reported by utilization review staff. "Slow to progress" means that the patient is unable to maintain activity level suggested on the pathway.

multidisciplinary team that meets monthly and includes nurses, physicians, therapists, and pharmacists among its members. Without a team to solve the problem of negative variances collectively, all the measurement in the world would have little impact. Currently, approximately ten pathway teams meet regularly to manage variances. These teams have the authority to change practice after getting approval from all providers caring for the population under study.

Teams should share variance data with staff caring for the patient population. Posting the variance information in a common staff area (e.g., the staff lounge) may yield many helpful comments from staff. Involving all staff, not just the pathway team members, in the management of variances prevents a team from working in isolation from the other providers.

An approach to managing variance data involves setting priorities based on the length of stay impact of each variance. This perspective is important because a variance, although frequent, may not prolong stays to a great extent. Conversely, an infrequent variance may account for 50 percent of all days greater than the expected length of stay. An example is shown in Figure 3. The CABG case management team needed to decide where to focus its energy. In this case, because infection impacted length of stay, it became an area of focus. This type of analysis assists the team in choosing the right CQI project—the one that will have maximal impact on outcomes.

After analyzing the variances, the results need to reach the right people. A graph, like the one shown in Figure 2, can be shared monthly with the pathway team. Relative to this example, the nurse case managers on the orthopedic unit, in conjunction with the pathway team that includes surgeons and physical therapists, made plans to address the highest variances. Providers are encouraged to post the variance graphs for all staff to review. A similar process is used by other pathway teams actively meeting to manage pathway variances.

A unique way to manage variances involves combining a clinical algorithm with an existing critical pathway.[27,28] One case management team at Fletcher Allen found such a synergy. The team created an algorithm to address a common variance due to atrial arrhythmias. Implementation of the algorithm, which detailed the best method for treating atrial arrhythmias, has resulted in a statistically significant decrease (p <.05) in atrial arrhythmias (see Figure 4).

Other pathway teams at Fletcher Allen have used the same approach to address pathway variances. A cardiology pathway team recognized a variance at the time of admission for the chest pain pathway. Thrombolytic therapy was being delayed due to system variances in the emergency department and pharmacy. So, the team created an algorithm to improve the efficiency of thrombolytic administration. Another team in renal services added two algorithms to handle variances from the dialysis critical pathway. One algorithm addressed anemia, and the other tackled the management of calcium and phosphorus levels.

While managing variances disclosed by either concurrent or retrospective review is important, the ability to *predict* variances before they happen is also crucial to effective management. Fletcher Allen has developed a model for predicting variances from the total hip replacement pathway. An analysis of 60 total hip replacement patients revealed a strong correlation between certain patient criteria and length of stay. The key predictors included age, obesity, living situation, and insulin-

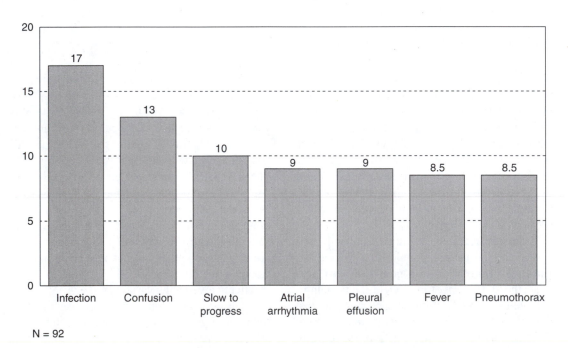

N = 92

Figure 3. Example of the average patient length of stay associated with variances from a coronary artery bypass graft (CABG) surgery pathway (N = 92). All of these variances are patient related. "Slow to progress" means the patient is unable to maintain activity level suggested on the pathway.

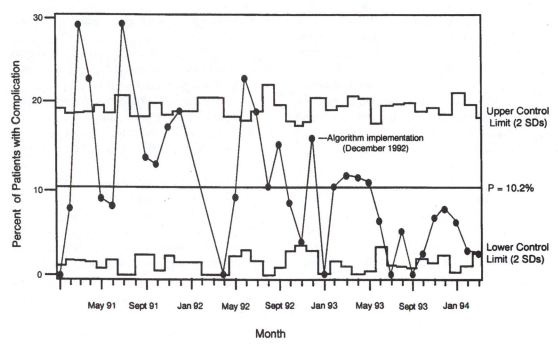

Figure 4. Run chart. Because occurrence of an atrial arrhythmia is such a frequent variance for coronary artery bypass graft (CABG) surgery patients, an algorithm was created to standardize the treatment. The run chart shows improvements after implementation of the algorithm. The chart was created in SAS using a p-chart with upper and lower control limits set at two standard deviations (SDs). Points falling below the lower control limit, and the run of eight to ten points below the centerline, indicate a significant decrease in complications ($p < .05$).

dependent diabetes. The total hip case management team uses these predictors as part of a preoperative screening protocol to identify potential variances before they occur. In addition, patients with certain preoperative factors receive additional support and are not expected to follow the same critical pathway as a patient without high risk factors. The prediction factors can assist nurse case managers in discharge planning, even before the patient is admitted.

Linking pathways and information systems

Because critical pathways often use a paper system, it is important to evaluate the benefits of automation. Currently, the Critical Pathway Steering Committee at Fletcher Allen is working closely with the information services department to link pathways with the clinical and financial informa-

tion system. A software package named Metaphor that links multiple information systems and produces executive decision support capabilities is being used. Under the current implementation, the UR staff collect data on the completeness of documentation and specific variances of interest and enter this information into the UR database for downloading to Metaphor.

The automation of variance data is a big step. While the Fletcher Allen system is in its early stages at this time, the early reports have generated much enthusiasm. Such an advance would not be possible without the UR and information services departments dedicating time to this project.

The long-range plan is to make the information available to both the nurse managers in charge of pathways and the administrators responsible for the patient populations on pathways via a personal computer (PC) network. In the meantime, the quality management, utilization review, and information services departments will have access to the system via PC. Because the Metaphor system links multiple databases for patients on pathways, a relatively powerful machine is needed (i.e., 486 processor, 66 MHz) to run the software. Consequently, acquisition cost may limit the number of machines that can be purchased each year.

CONCLUSIONS

Fletcher Allen's experience has highlighted seven themes that are felt to be common to any health care organization interested in critical pathway variance management:

1. Staff education on variance management is critical to success.
2. Organizations need to establish a system for documenting, collecting, classifying, analyzing, and reporting variances that ensures communication to key clinicians and managers. Posting variance reports for staff review and comments is recommended.
3. Variance management success stories should be publicized and used as models for other pathway teams.
4. The creation of algorithms to address variances should be considered.
5. A method for predicting variances may be useful for planning a variance management strategy.
6. The link between variance management and information systems should be developed in order to simplify and expedite the process.
7. It is critical to recognize and reward teams that eliminate variances and continuously improve care.

The future of the pathway efforts at Fletcher Allen includes further expansion of pathways into the outpatient setting including physician offices, home care, and community partners. In addition, Fletcher Allen hopes to expand the concept of health promotion and disease prevention into pathways.

REFERENCES

1. *Webster's Ninth New Collegiate Dictionary,* S.V. "variance."
2. Rudisill, P.T., Phillips, M., and Payne, C.M. "Clinical Paths for Cardiac Surgery Patients: A Multidisciplinary Approach to Quality Improvement Outcomes." *Journal of Nursing Care Quality* 8, no. 3 (1994): 27–33.
3. Zander, K. "What's New in Managed Care and Case Management." *The New Definition* 6, no. 2 (1991): 1–2.
4. Coffey, R.J., et al. "An Introduction to Critical Paths." *Quality Management in Health Care* 1, no. 1 (1992): 45–54.
5. Robinson, J.A., Robinson, K.J., and Lewis, D.J. "Balancing Quality of Care and Cost-Effectiveness through Case Management." *ANNA Journal* 19, no. 2 (1992): 182–88.
6. Bejciy-Spring, S.M. "Nursing Case Management: Application to Neuroscience Nursing." *Journal of Neuroscience Nursing* 23, no. 6 (1991): 390–97.
7. Hoffman, P.A. "Critical Path Method: An Important Tool for Coordinating Clinical Care." *Joint Commission Journal on Quality Improvement* 19, no. 7 (1993): 235–46.

8. Mikulaninec, C.E. "An Amputee Critical Path." *Journal of Vascular Nursing* 10, no. 2 (1992): 6–9.
9. Ferguson, L.E. "Steps to Developing a Critical Pathway." *Nursing Administration Quarterly* 17, no. 3 (1993): 58–62.
10. Hampton, D.C. "Implementing a Managed Care Framework through Care Maps." *Journal of Nursing Administration* 23, no. 5 (1993): 21–27.
11. Johnson, R.J. "Total Shoulder Arthroplasty." *Orthopedic Nursing* 12, no. 1 (1993): 14–20.
12. DiJerome, L. "The Nursing Case Management Computerized System: Meeting the Challenges of Health Care Delivery through Technology." *Computers in Nursing* 10, no. 6 (1992): 250–58.
13. Lumsdon, K., and Hagland, M. "Mapping Care." *Hospitals and Health Networks* (October 1993): 34–40.
14. Strong, A.G., and Sneed, N.V. "Clinical Evaluation of a Critical Path for Coronary Artery Bypass Surgery Patients." *Progress in Cardiovascular Nursing* 6, no. 1 (1991): 29–37.
15. Bueno, M.M., and Hwang, R.F. "Understanding Vari-

ances in Hospital Stay." *Nursing Management* 24, no. 11 (1993): 51–57.

16. Metcalf, E.M. "The Orthopaedic Critical Path." *Orthopedic Nursing* 10, no. 6 (1991): 25–31.

17. Woodyard, L.W., and Sheetz, J.E. "Critical Pathway Patient Outcomes: The Missing Standard." *Journal of Nursing Care Quality* 8, no. 1 (1993): 51–57.

18. Crummer, M.B., and Carter, V. "Critical Pathways—The Pivotal Tool." *Journal of Cardiovascular Nursing* 7, no. 4 (1993): 30–37.

19. Romito, D. "A Critical Path for CVA Patients." *Rehabilitation Nursing* 15, no. 3 (1990): 153–56.

20. Giuliano, K.K., and Poirier, C.E. "Nursing Case Management: Critical Pathways to Desirable Outcomes." *Nursing Management* 22, no. 3 (1991): 52–55.

21. Mosher, C., et al. "Upgrading Practice with Critical Pathways." *American Journal of Nursing* 92, no. 1 (1992): 41–44.

22. Latini, E.E., and Foote, W. "Obtaining Consistent Quality Patient Care for the Trauma Patient by Using a Critical Pathway." *Critical Care Nursing Quarterly* 15, no. 3 (1992): 51–55.

23. Berwick, D.M. "The Clinical Process and the Quality Process." *Quality Management in Health Care* 1, no. 1 (1992): 1–8.

24. Falconer, J.A., et al. "The Critical Path Method in Stroke Rehabilitation: Lessons from an Experiment in Cost Containment and Outcome Improvement." *Quality Review Bulletin* 19, no. 3 (1993): 8–16.

25. Wood, R.G., Bailey, N.O., and Tilkemeier, D. "Managed Care: The Missing Link in Quality Improvement." *Journal of Nursing Care Quality* 6, no. 4 (1992): 55–65.

26. Grudich, G. "The Critical Path System—The Road Toward an Efficient OR." *AORN Journal* 53, no. 3 (1991): 705–14.

27. Schriefer, J.A. "Reducing the Length of Stay for Post-Operative Open Heart Patients." *Quality Connection* 2, no. 3 (1993): 8–9.

28. Schriefer, J.A. "The Synergy of Pathways and Algorithms—Two Tools Work Better Than One." *Joint Commission Journal on Quality Improvement* 20, no. 9 (1994): 485–99.

Using Computer Systems To Enhance Case Management

Joy L. Luque, Michael J. Pereira, and James D. Brown

It has been estimated that 70 percent of medical costs are attributable to preventable illness.[1] As the population continues to shift toward managed care, providers of health care must develop strategies to manage the care of their members effectively. The initial challenge for a health plan is to identify those members who are or have the potential to be high utilizers of medical services.

Early identification and referral to case management of these members is one strategy that PacifiCare's case management department has implemented in an effort to provide effective medical care to high-risk members and ensure appropriate utilization of resources. In this article, we discuss the development of an on-line triage process to identify actual or potential high utilizers.

PacifiCare of California is one of California's leading managed health care services companies. It serves more than 1.3 million members in its commercial, Medicare, and medical health plans. The company offers a diversified range of health care products, including HMO, PPO, and point-of-service health plans for large, mid-size, and small groups and individual members.

PACIFICARE'S CASE MANAGEMENT DEPARTMENT

The case management department has been in existence for over eight years. Although cen-trally managed, it combines telephonic and on-site case management to handle cases across the state. The PacifiCare case managers are registered nurses. They serve as consultants and resources for the members and help them coordinate services and facilitate the achievement of treatment goals. Staffing is based on a population ratio of 1 nurse per 100,000 members for the HMO membership and 1 nurse per 45,000 members for the PPO membership. Caseloads average approximately 35 cases.

PacifiCare's case management department has historically managed individuals with catastrophic injuries and illnesses. Over the past two years, the department's focus has expanded to include individuals with chronic diseases as well as individuals at risk for illness, disability or death. The management of these cases is proactive rather than reactive; it involves early intervention prior to the acute event, coordination of services, and elimination of any fragmentation of care.

Expansion of the case management program was directed by senior management in an effort to provide needed services to our growing senior population. Health care reform and the growing number of Medicare recipients shifting into managed care were the forces that pushed development of a case management model capable of

Quality Management in Health Care 1996; 5(1): 17–24
© 1996 Aspen Publishers, Inc.

The authors would like to thank Theresa Dobilas, Patti Derouin, Ellen Aliberti, Cindy Natalie, Christina LeGate, Carol Turpen, and Sue Jones for their help.

supporting the care of members with chronic illness. Participants in the development included the case management and the information systems departments as well as many others.

Chronic disease patients account for over half of all high-cost patients and about 60 percent of all hospital admissions.[1] Identification of those members at risk enables health providers and payers to manage risk, not avoid it. The goal is to target interventions that can reduce risk factors that may exacerbate the disease and speed functional decline. Case management intervention needs to be implemented prior to the acute event in order to prevent additional hospitalization and further decline.

COMPUTER SYSTEM REQUISITES

The initial challenge was to find a computer system to assist in the identification of members for case management. The system needed functional capabilities for assessing the appropriateness and potential effectiveness of case management. Essential capabilities also included categorizing cases by criteria, gathering and documenting additional clinical data, and assigning cases to case managers.

In the prior triage system, cases were identified through a custom-built utilization system or by direct communication with a case manager (manual referral). The prior system allowed automated scheduling of referrals. Medical intake coordinators created an authorization (case) number for each episode of care. The system was able to capture diagnosis codes, acuity of care, and location of service as well as authorizations history and claims processing. Those referrals with selected ICD-9 (International Classification of Diseases, 9th Revision) codes were screened nightly and forwarded on-line to the

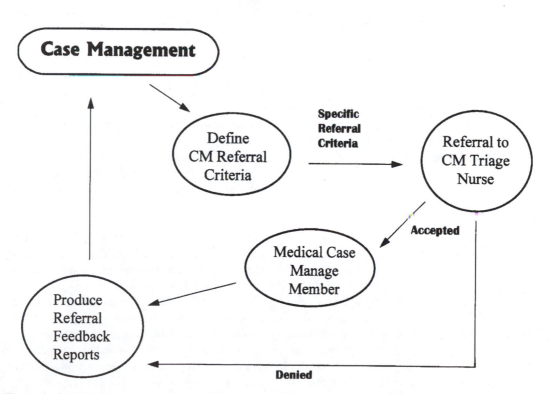

Figure 1. Case management leveling criteria.

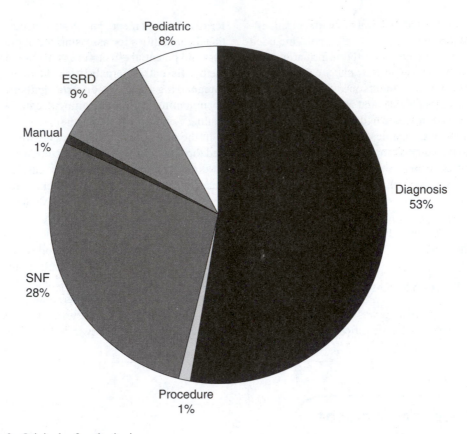

Figure 2. Original referral criteria.

case management supervisor. After an initial review, the cases would be forwarded to case managers for acceptance or denial.

Review of the existing triage system indicated multiple mistakes in the referrals identified and deficiencies in reporting capabilities. A high volume of inappropriate referrals took a large percentage of the case manager's time, reducing the amount of time and resources the case managers spent on appropriate referrals. The system referred a large number of diagnosis codes that did not correlate with high-dollar claims or multiple episodes of care. Also, the reporting capabilities were limited and feedback reporting was not available. Thus, it was difficult to ascertain what changes, if any, needed to be made to the referral criteria. And even if

changes needed to be made, incorporating changes into the utilization system was costly and time consuming.

The utilization system did not facilitate communication between the case management department and other internal departments within PacifiCare. For example, the member services department, whose linkage with the case management department was critical, did not need to use this system and therefore did not have online access to the system.

Customer service was impacted by the lack of coordination between internal departments. Members being case managed were unknown by most internal departments, and at times this obstructed service integration and was identified as an area for process improvement.

STEPS IN THE IMPROVEMENT PROCESS

The case management department evaluated the need for a new automated system and concluded that a new system was required to support the case management process. The next step was to evaluate existing software systems. Most of the case management software programs available focused on hospital-based case man-

agement rather than plan-based case management and were not appropriate for case management within a managed care organization. In addition, they were very expensive, with prices ranging up to half a million dollars. Therefore, the decision was made to develop a customized, fully functional, industry-leading case management computer system in-house.

The information systems department developed a desktop computer program in 1995 to re-

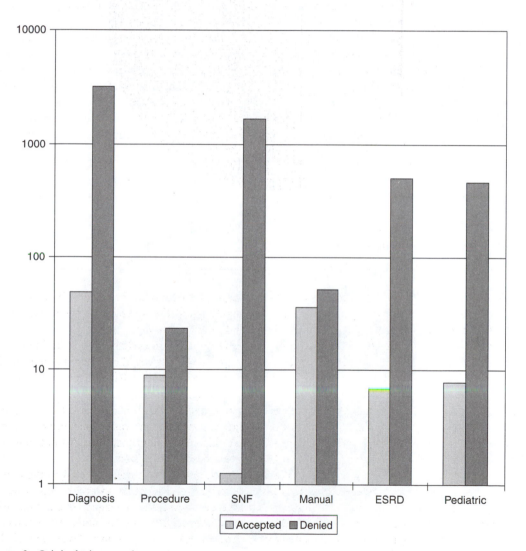

Figure 3. Original triage results.

place the existing system for filtering through preauthorization and concurrent review data. The program incorporated criteria developed by PacifiCare's case management department to identify potential members for catastrophic and chronic medical case management. The initial referral criteria were based on internal data that included ICD-9 diagnosis codes associated with high-dollar claims.

Case management identified members with chronic conditions (e.g., chronic obstructive pulmonary disease) and with end-stage renal disease (ESRD) who were receiving some form of dialysis. Multiple hospitalizations or admission to a skilled nursing facility were among the referral criteria. In addition, procedures associated with high cost, such as transplants, were included. The system was also designed to provide referral feedback reporting, increased software flexibility, and reduced computer-related costs.

Client-server tools were utilized in developing the new triage system. These tools provided increased flexibility and rapid software programming at a lower cost than traditional mainframe software development. This flexibility enabled PacifiCare to quickly and easily fine-tune criteria and improve the appropriateness of case management referrals. Feedback reports on accepted and denied cases for case management have been the basis for refinement of the referral criteria. They have also been used as a performance measure to determine which cases case managers have accepted and which have been denied.

Under the new system, a designated triage staff has been assigned to review referrals to case management and forward cases to the case management staff. The triage staff utilizes on-line triage screens developed specifically for cases identified as catastrophic or chronic. The system links back to PacifiCare's utilization system and therefore

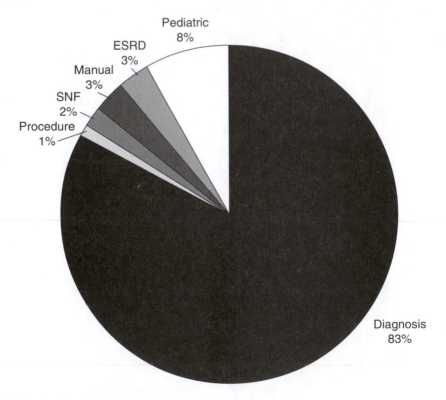

Figure 4. Refined referral criteria (estimated).

provides automatic review of utilization history and claims history. After completion of the on-line triage form, the system utilizes established leveling criteria to determine whether the case should be accepted or denied by case management. These criteria, which provide a more objective approach to the screening of cases, fall into such areas as pharmacy usage, social isolation, and self-health perception (Figure 1).

Reporting systems were designed to monitor the appropriateness of referrals. Standard and ad hoc reporting capabilities allow management to identify trends related to the triage of potential case management cases. Information provided by feedback reporting allows PacifiCare to refine its referral criteria.

Additionally, PacifiCare has been able to add to its diagnosis criteria. By looking at the diagnoses of all cases accepted by case management, it has updated its criteria to include other high-risk diagnoses, such as congestive heart failure and diabetes. Many of these new diagnoses have very specific ICD-9 codes, unlike the broad categories captured earlier (e.g., 250.00 instead of 250).

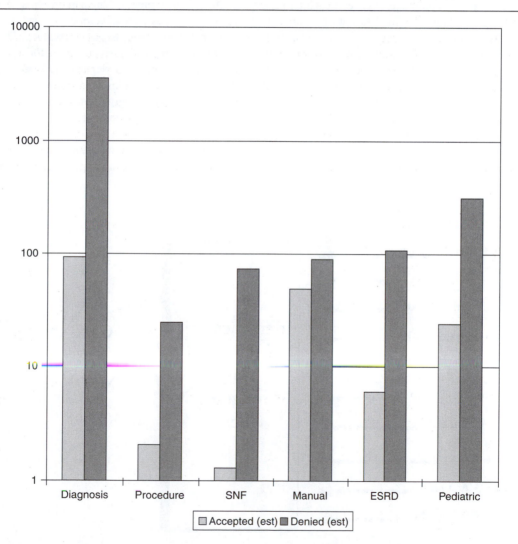

Figure 5. Refined triage results (estimated).

Eliminating codes that have not generated referrals to case management has streamlined the triage process, and case managers are now able to use more of their time performing case management functions rather than reviewing referrals.

PacifiCare has also been able to refine its skilled nursing facility (SNF) criteria. Previous criteria referred any member admitted to an SNF. The intent, once again, was to proactively case manage members who were "at risk." The new SNF criteria identify only those members with three or more admissions to an SNF, increasing the percentage of cases in which case management intervention has a positive impact.

Our ESRD criteria have been redefined. Previously, all ESRD members were referred to case management, whether the member was admitted to a hospital or was having an outpatient procedure, such as dialysis. The utilization system, which tracks outpatient dialysis treatments for documentation for claims payment, was generating referrals monthly on the same patients. Our refined criteria now refer for re-evaluation only those members who have had an acute event (Figures 2 and 3).

Enhancements made to the CSS system allowed electronic referrals to be sent by other departments to the case management department and provided current information about the status of members. On-line information for each case included the case manager's name, phone extension, and notes, facilitating coordination of services within PacifiCare (Figure 4).

The case management department identified internal departments that interface with the health plan members. Department-specific referral guidelines were developed and an interdepartmental flow process was established. The internal departments received education on case management and their department-specific referral criteria. Examples of department-specific criteria included caregiver burnout, severe functional limitations, placement requests, and hospice inquiries.

The customer service system provides two types of feedback on the appropriateness of re-

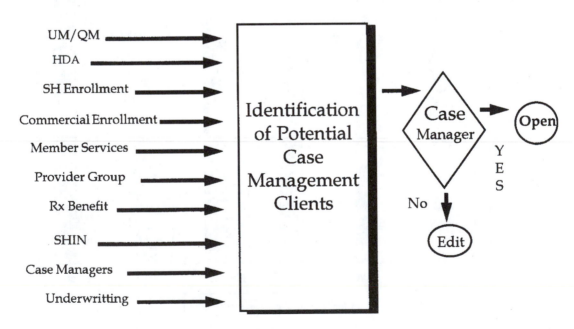

Figure 6. PacifiCare case management interdepartmental process flow.

ferrals: on-line feedback reported to those initiating the referrals and summary feedback reported to management. The first type of feedback employs denial reason codes and textual explanations by the case managers as a way of providing quick and easy-to-understand information to referrers. The second type, which consists of summary reports, is used for refining referral guidelines, monitoring the appropriateness of referrals, and indicating the need for additional departmental training.

PacifiCare's refined criteria have allowed fewer cases to make it through the triage process, and those that do are more likely to be case managed (Figures 5 and 6). However, improvement efforts are not at an end. Continued feedback reporting will allow future revisions to be made to the referral criteria.

One of the future challenges for the case management department is to identify other sources of referrals for early identification for case management. For example, pharmacy data reports can be used to identify members who have been prescribed multiple or specific medications, which would allow PacifiCare to take a proactive approach in managing members who are high utilizers of pharmacy benefits.

●   ●   ●

There is no doubt that an on-line computer system can provide substantial benefits for case management. PacifiCare's system has added consistency and objectivity to the referral process. In addition, reporting systems have facilitated the monitoring and refinement of referral criteria, and on-line systems have improved communication between internal departments. These improvements have supported the case management department's efforts to provide members with cost-effective medical care while striving to improve their overall satisfaction with the health plan.

REFERENCE

1. Lashley, M. "CM and DM Team up for Effective Management of High-Cost Care." *TCM,* no. 3 (1995): 71–76.

PART III

Case Management Administration and Financial Considerations

Activity-Based Costing for Hospitals

Suneel Udpa

The challenges posed by managed care, capitated payments, and other restrictive hospital reimbursement mechanisms such as diagnosis-related groups (DRGs) provide an ideal setting for the implementation of activity-based costing (ABC) in hospitals. Current health care practices and procedures such as DRGs, patient-acuity systems, case management, critical path analysis, utilization review, and others can be used in the implementation of the ABC system.

ABC in the manufacturing sector has remained a focal point of interest for practitioners and academics for a number of years. Studies applying the basic principles of ABC used in manufacturing firms to health care organizations have appeared in health care journals only recently. However, a majority of the studies of ABC in health care settings focus on a narrow application of ABC to a department within the health care organization. For instance, Chan[1] examines the application of ABC to the costing of laboratory tests, Ramsey[2] examines the application of ABC to the hospital's radiology department and a nursing station and finally, Canby[3] applies ABC to the X-ray department of the hospital. In this article, I provide a framework for the implementation of ABC for a health care organization's total operations and its specialized services.

The study described in this article examines the application of ABC to the hospital's inpatient services. Application of ABC to a hospital's outpatient care service requires additional considerations. Outpatient care generally involves a much larger number of units of service with relatively small cost per unit. Also, databases on outpatient services and related costs are often poorly developed and bills are often generated at multiple sites. ABC can nonetheless still be applied to a few selected high-volume and high-cost–low-profit margin outpatient services using the principles and techniques described in this article.

NEED FOR A NEW COST SYSTEM

In conventional cost accounting systems, direct costs such as costs of specific services (e.g., use of the operating room, diagnostic procedures, laboratory tests, pharmacy, and physical therapy) are billed directly to patients. However, indirect costs or overhead for the entire hospital operation (including individual departments) are typically accumulated and divided by the total number of patient days to determine the per diem cost. In this system, hospitals assume overhead cost per patient day is the same irrespective of the patient type, level of care, procedure being performed, or length of stay.

However, not all overhead costs vary on a patient-day basis. For instance, overhead costs relating to admissions and registration do not vary

Health Care Manage Rev 1996; 21(3): 83–96

with the number of patient days but vary with the number of patients admitted, that is, the cost associated with admitting patients is independent of length of stay. Also, the cost per patient day is not the same across all patients. Patients with short stays but who require extensive nursing support have a higher cost per patient day compared to patients who require long stays with minimal nursing attention. Therefore, conventional hospital cost systems can report seriously distorted cost per patient when patient care is diverse in terms of either level of care (acuity) or amount of care (patient days).

Pricing, which historically has not been a key factor in hospital marketing, is now an important criterion through which hospitals compete for business from large organizational buyers such as managed care organizations (e.g., health maintenance organizations [HMOs] and preferred provider organizations [PPOs]), third party insurers, and employers. This price competition and the resulting importance of accurate cost information make the need for a new cost system urgent in most hospitals.

ACTIVITY-BASED COSTING

ABC is an information system that maintains and processes data on a firm's activities and products/services. It identifies the activities performed, traces costs to these activities, and then uses various cost drivers to trace the cost of activities to the final products/services. Cost drivers are factors that create or influence cost and reflect the consumption of activities by the products/services. An ABC system can be used by management for a variety of purposes relating to both activities and products/services.[4]

ABC involves a two-stage allocation process. In the first stage, we assign hospital costs to activity pools such as "admit patients," "cardiac catheterization," "administer ECG tests," and so on. In the second stage, costs are assigned from these activity pools to individual patients, or units of episodic care, using appropriate cost drivers that measure the patients' consumption of these "activity resources."

DEVELOPING THE ABC MODEL

This section details the development and implementation of ABC on a hospitalwide basis, weaving together the principles and techniques of ABC with current health care practices such as case management, critical path analysis, acuity levels, and total quality management (TQM). The steps in developing and implementing the ABC model are outlined below.

Step 1: Form a cross-functional steering committee

In order to establish a process for implementing ABC, first form a committee that will ultimately be responsible for the implementation and evaluation of the ABC system. A cross-functional steering committee could consist of the following members:

1. RN case coordinators/case management specialists
2. physicians
3. accountant
4. information systems manager
5. medical records personnel
6. outside consultant (if necessary).

The committee and its members should meet regularly with physicians, hospital staff, and management to identify issues that could affect the implementation of the ABC system, such as utilization of resources, quality patient care, communication between the nursing staff and physicians, information systems, and process improvements. It is very important to gain staff and physician support for the ABC system. Personnel will more readily accept the new system if they are educated about the nature of the system and are concurrently involved in the development and implementation phases.

Step 2: Identify case types/DRGs for analysis

Case types for analysis are typically selected based on case volume (high volume), financial impact (high cost, low profitability), variance measure (high variance from DRG estimate), quality assurance issues (high risk), or special interest (new service). Also, for initial analysis, case types with predictable hospital delivery paths are selected. When a high-volume or high-cost case type is selected, a decrease in length of stay (LOS) of even 1 day has a very significant impact on costs.

Figure 1 shows a sample graph based on case volume and contribution margin (Price – Variable Cost) per case for each DRG. DRGs in the top left quadrant have the highest case volume and low margin. The hospital is likely to gain the greatest benefit from activity analysis and ABC analyzes these DRGs.

DRGs should not be the only classification system used to develop and implement critical paths and the ABC system. Cost distortions can result when DRGs are broad based and include case types that are nonhomogeneous. In some

cases, it might be more accurate to use the *International Classification of Diseases—Ninth Edition—Clinical Modifications* (ICD-9-CM diagnosis codes) instead of DRGs to analyze particular case types.

Step 3: Profile the health care delivery system

Using case management and critical path analysis, perform activity analysis across all operations and processes that are required to move the patient from preadmission to discharge.

Case management is both a model and a technology for restructuring the clinical production process to ensure that a patient receives needed services in a supportive, efficient, and cost-effective manner. When integrating case management with the hospital cost accounting system, two perspectives of case management should be considered: the hospitalwide systems/processes

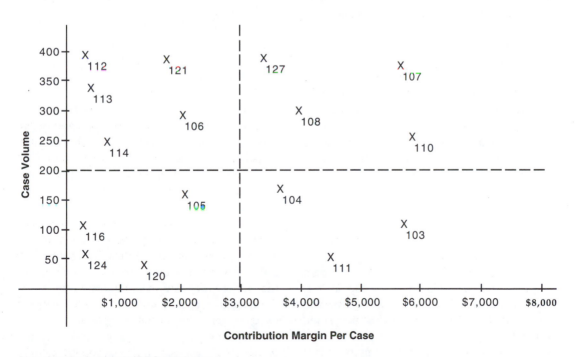

Note: Numbers relate to DRG categories.

Figure 1 Sample DRG Volume—Profitability Matrix.

and the direct patient care delivery system or critical path. Analyzing the hospitalwide processes involves examining in detail the activities involved in the preadmission process, the hospital stay process, and the patient discharge process. For instance, in performing an activity analysis of the hospital stay process, the hospital should review the following activities: ordering and receiving drugs from the pharmacy, ordering and providing therapeutic and diagnostic services, utilizing specialty services, and using all the auxiliary services such as laundry, dietary, administrative, and janitorial.

The direct patient care delivery system or critical path analysis is an abbreviated report that shows the critical or key incidents that must occur in a predictable and timely order to achieve the hospital's medical and financial goals. Critical paths are tools that, once individualized by the primary nurse and physician for a particular patient within the first 24 hours of admission, are used on every shift on each consecutive unit to plan and monitor the flow of care.[5] Table 1 presents a sample critical pathway for acute myocardial infarction for days 0–6.

Case management and critical path analysis are developed and implemented typically by a multidisciplinary group of staff consisting of physicians, nurses, physical therapists, diagnostic specialists, quality and utilization review specialists, and other support personnel. RN case coordinators/case management specialists act as liaisons between this group and the steering committee formed for the implementation of ABC (see Step 1). This linkage is crucial to ensure that clinical information is available to the ABC team for activity analysis and cost information is available to the group developing the critical path.

Case management along with critical path analysis proves a useful framework to analyze activities and to collect data on the type and amount of resources needed and actually used for the delivery of patient care. The data can be used to determine where process improvements can be made and where non–value added activities can be eliminated.

Step 4: Aggregate activities

The number of different actions performed in a typical hospital facility is so large that it is economically unfeasible to create an activity pool for each separate action. Therefore, many individual actions have to be aggregated to form a few separate distinct activity pools. A single cost driver is then used to trace the cost of these activities to different procedures/patients. For instance, the different actions associated with the admissions/registration process such as reservations/scheduling, inpatient registration, admissions testing, and patient placement are aggregated into one activity pool—"admit patients." One must note that as more and more actions are aggregated into an activity, the ability of a cost driver to accurately trace the resources consumed by patients decreases. On the other hand, creating separate activity centers for actions that are either similar or inseparable just adds complexity to the ABC system without providing any new insights into how resources are consumed.

Step 5: Analyze cost flow using cost drivers

The hospital cost management system is used to develop cost information on different activities along the critical path from preadmission to discharge. The procedure involves a detailed analysis of the company's general ledger accounts. In collecting cost information it is necessary to combine certain ledger accounts that are associated with use of similar resources. For instance, salaries and fringe benefit costs that are recorded in two separate accounts are combined for the purposes of allocation. On the other hand, it is sometimes necessary to examine individual bills and vouchers relating to a particular ledger account when similar resources are consumed differently by different activities. For instance, the ledger account Maintenance—Medical Equipment is examined to obtain maintenance expenses relating to medical equipment in radiology, operating room, laboratory, and other departments. Analysis of ledger accounts is not a trivial task because there are over 300 different expense categories at a typical hospital and the

Activity-Based Costing for Hospitals   157

Table 1 Critical Pathway: Acute Myocardial Infarction

Activities	Day 0 (Preadmission)	Day 1	Day 2	Day 3	Day 4	Day 5	Day 6
Admit patients	Patient reservation Insurance verification Routine admission testing						
Provide nursing care		Complete blood chemistry	Complete blood chemistry	Complete blood chemistry	Complete blood chemistry	Complete blood chemistry	Complete blood chemistry
Perform diagnostics		CBC with differential Cardiac isoenzymes q 8 hr PT, PTT, ACT initially and PTT q 6 hr Beta hCG 12-lead ECG daily Chest X-ray	CBC PTT (if on heparin) Cardiac isoenzymes if not at baseline 12-lead ECG daily and per protocol MUGA scan or echocardiogram, if indicated	CBC PTT (of on heparin) Cardiac isoenzymes if not at baseline 12-lead ECG daily and per protocol	CBC PTT (if on heparin) Cardiac isoenzymes if not at baseline 12-lead ECG daily and per protocol	CBC 12-lead ECG daily and per protocol	CBC 12-lead ECG
Provide nursing care		ECG monitoring	ECG monitoring	ECG monitoring	ECG monitoring	ECG monitoring	ECG monitoring
Administer ECG & other tests		HR, RR, BP q 1 hr Rhythm strip q shift and p.r.n. Continuous oximetry Heart sounds, breath sounds q 1–2 hr	HR, RR, BP q 2 hr Rhythm strip q shift and p.r.n. Continuous oximetry Heart sounds and breath sounds q 2 hr	HR, RR, BP q 2 hr Rhythm strip q shift and p.r.n. D/C oximetry Assess other body systems as needed	HR, RR, BP q 4 hr Rhythm strip q shift and p.r.n.	HR, RR, BP q 4 hr Rhythm strip shift and p.r.n. Assess other body systems as needed	HR, RR, BP q 4 hr Assess other body systems as needed

continues

Table 1 Continued

Activities	Day 0 (Preadmission)	Day 1	Day 2	Day 3	Day 4	Day 5	Day 6
Provide nursing care Cardiac catheterization Dispense medications		Heparin IV NTG continuous IV infusion Beta blocker Calcium channel blocker ACE inhibitor ASA Morphine IV, analgesics Stool softener Sedative Antiemetic	Heparin IV Titrate and D/C NTG infusion NTG SL, transdermal Beta blocker Calcium channel blocker ACE inhibitor ASA Analgesics Stool softener Sedative	Heparin IV NTG SL, transdermal or spray Beta blocker Calcium channel blocker ACE inhibitor ASA Analgesics Stool softener Sedative	D/C heparin NTG SL, transdermal, or spray Beta blocker Calcium channel blocker ACE inhibitor ASA Analgesics Stool softener Sedative	NTG SL, transdermal, or spray Beta blocker Calcium channel blocker ACE inhibitor ASA Analgesics Stool softener Sedative	NTG SL, transdermal or spray Beta blocker Calcium channel blocker ACE inhibitor ASA Analgesics Stool softener
Provide meals		Low-salt, low-fat, low-cholesterol, of ADA diet	Low-salt, low-fat, low-cholesterol, or ADA diet	Low-salt, low-fat, low cholesterol, or ADA diet	Low-salt, low-fat, low cholesterol, or ADA diet	Low-salt, -fat, cholesterol, or ADA diet, NPO after 2400 for stress test	Low-salt, low-fat, low-cholesterol, or ADA diet
Provide nursing care		Bed rest (semi-Fowler's) assistance with ADLs	OOB to chair Assistance with ADLs	OOB to chair Assistance with ADLs	Ambulation, ADLs with assistance	Ambulation with supervision	Ambulation with supervision
Provide therapy		IV access Antiembolism stockings Intake and output Oxygen 2 liters/min	IV access Antiembolism stockings Intake and output Oxygen 2 liters/min	IV access Antiembolism stockings Intake and output Possibly D/C O₂	IV access Transfer to telemetry unit Antiembolism stockings D/C intake and output	IV access Antiembolism stockings	Stress test D/C IV access after

continues

Table 1 Continued

Activities	Day 0 (Preadmission)	Day 1	Day 2	Day 3	Day 4	Day 5	Day 6
Provide nursing services—teaching		Orientation to CCU and hospital routines Review of C.P. Cardiac teaching begins	Instruction on diet Cardiac teaching	Orientation to the difference between CCU and telemetry unit Cardiac teaching	Cardiac teaching	Explanation of stress test Complete cardiac teaching	Written instructions: medications, what to report, activity limits, and next appointment
Discharge planning		Social services Discharge teaching	Dietary and cardiac rehabilitation Plan for family teaching	Discharge teaching	Discharge teaching	Discharge teaching Plan discharge	Discharge to home

only information available for each account is the account name and concise explanations of different transactions.

First-stage cost drivers are used to trace the cost of inputs into cost pools for each activity center (see Figure 2). Direct costs are directly assigned to activity centers. For instance, salaries of employees working entirely within an activity center (department) can be directly assigned to that activity center. Common and indirect costs are assigned to different activities centers using different first-stage cost drivers. Table 2 lists different first-stage cost drivers (allocation bases) used to allocate hospital overhead costs to activity centers.

Second-stage cost drivers are used to measure the amount of activity resources consumed by different procedures (DRGs) or patients (see Figure 2). Table 3 lists second-stage cost drivers used for the different activity centers.

Step 6: Educate hospital staff about the ABC system

On-site training seminars are held throughout the design and implementation stage to introduce and educate hospital administrators, nurses, and physicians to the concepts and benefits of ABC, case management, and critical path analysis. Hospital staff meetings are used to report progress and to discuss any problems that the steering committee has encountered. These seminars and periodic meetings have two main objectives: to ensure that the design and implementation are appropriate and to build commitment to the ABC and case management system among the hospital staff.

Step 7: Evaluate and analyze data and results

ABC systems in combination with case management and critical path analysis provide crucial financial and clinical measures to conduct variance analysis and evaluate the efficiency of the health care delivery system in terms of achieving expected patient outcomes, timely

discharge of patients, appropriate utilization of resources, and cost control.

Variances can be categorized into the following:

1. *Patient variances*: These are due to complications or changes in the patient's health, for instance, conditions such as allergic reactions, infections, diarrhea, and hemorrhages that affect LOS and costs.
2. *Caregiver variances*: These can be due to physician variances or nursing variances. Examples include inappropriate use of equipment, untimely tests, insufficient protection, inadequate discharge planning, failure to promptly notify appropriate personnel, and inadequate patient education.
3. *Environmental variances*: Causes for these variances include equipment breakdown, unavailable beds, scheduling problems, lab delays, and power outages.
4. *Price variances*: These are variances caused by paying higher than budgeted prices for supplies, drugs, instruments, and labor.
5. *Efficiency variances*: These usually include duplicated tests or labwork due to faulty procedures, wastage, patient delay, inadequate credit and insurance screening, staffing schedules, inefficient records location and retrieval systems, absenteeism, and medication dispensing errors.

A variance analysis report for each activity center is completed during a patient's stay at the hospital. The report, in addition to providing patient identification and medical information, lists the different categories of variances, possible reasons for the variances, and resources lost or consumed as a result of the negative variances. Resources consumed are measured in units of cost drivers used specific to each activity center, for instance, for nursing care activity pool, resources consumed is measured in number of relative value units (RVUs).

Figure 3 illustrates the application of variance analysis under an ABC system using a hypothetical example based on costs associated with

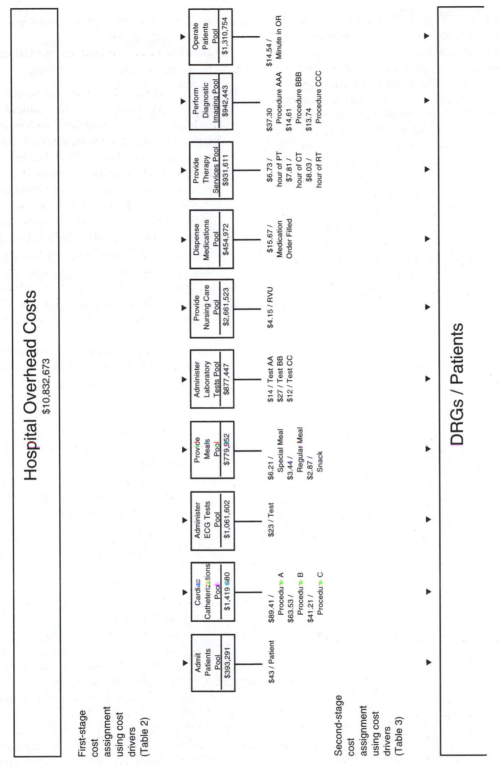

Figure 2 Graphic Example of Activity-Based Costing

Table 2 First-Stage Cost Drivers

	Hospital overhead costs	First-stage cost drivers
Labor-related	Supervision	Number of employees/payroll dollars
	Personnel services	Number of employees
Equipment-related	Insurance on equipment	Value of equipment
	Taxes on equipment	Value of equipment
	Medical equipment depreciation	Value of equipment/equipment hours used
	Medical equipment maintenance	Number of maintenance hours
Space-related	Building rental	Space occupied
	Building insurance	Space occupied
	Power costs	Space occupied, volume occupied
	Building maintenance	Space occupied
Service-related	Central administration*	Number of employees/patient volume
	Central service†	Quantity/value of supplies
	Medical records, and billing/accounting	Number of documents generated/patient volume
	Cafeteria	
	Information system	Number of meals/number of employees
		Value of computer equipment/number of programming hours
	Laundry	Weight of laundry washed
	Marketing	Patient volume

*Central administration costs include salaries of the president, vice president, and other central administrative staff.
†Central service costs include supplying, reclaiming, and sterilizing supplies such as gloves, needles, glassware, syringes, linens, surgical packs, and instruments.

the nursing care activity pool. Although the variance analysis proposed under the ABC system is similar in structure to a traditional variance analysis, there are two significant differences. First, since under the ABC system variance analysis is applied to each activity pool rather than the entire hospital's operation, more homogeneous cost pools and more causal cost drivers are used in the analysis. Second, with the use of a detailed variance analysis report and the emphasis on "activity analysis" under the ABC system, hospital administrators are better able to pinpoint weaknesses in the health care delivery system and focus their improvement efforts.

NUMERICAL EXAMPLE OF ABC IN HOSPITALS

To provide a numerical example of ABC in hospitals, assume the following information:

St. Joseph Hospital offers two services/procedures, DRG 1X1 and DRG 1X2. DRG 1X1 is a procedure requiring high-acuity care with a 5-day stay (LOS = 5 days) in the hospital, after which the patient is moved to a nursing home. DRG 1X2 is a procedure requiring low-acuity care with a LOS in the hospital also of 5 days.

Table 3 Second-Stage Cost Drivers

Activity center	Activities	Cost drivers
1. Admit patients	Reservation/scheduling, inpatient registration, billing and insurance verification, admission testing, room/bed/medical assignment	Number of patients admitted
2. Cardiac catheterization	Scheduling, prepare patient, administer medication, cardiac catheterization, film processing, interpret results, patient education	Number of procedures by type*
3. Administer ECG tests	Scheduling, prepare patient, perform ECG procedure, interpret results	Number of tests
4. Provide meals/ nutritional service	Plan meals, purchase supplies, prepare food, deliver food, clean and sanitize	Number of meals by type†
5. Administer laboratory tests	Obtain specimens, perform tests, report results	Number of tests by type‡
6. Provide nursing care	Transport patients, update medical records, provide patient care, patient education, discharge planning, inservice training	Number of Relative Value Units
7. Dispense medications	Purchase drugs and medical supplies, maintain records, fill medication orders, maintain inventory	Number of medication orders filled
8. Provide therapy	Schedule patients, evaluate patients, provide treatment, educate patients, maintain records	Number of hours by type
9. Perform diagnostic imaging	Schedule patients, perform procedures, develop film, interpret results, transport patient	Number of procedures by type§
10. Operate patient	Schedule patients, order supplies, maintain supplies, instruments & equipment, provide nursing care, transport patient	Number of hours of surgery by surgical suite type

*Cardiac catheterization procedures include therapeutic procedures such as angioplasty, thrombolysis; and diagnostic procedures such as left heart catheterizations, ventriculography, and coronary angiograms.

†Different meal types include special meals, regular meals, and snacks.

‡Laboratory tests include pathological tests, chemical tests, blood tests, immunological tests, and nuclear medicine.

§Diagnostic imaging procedures include routine radiographs of spine, neck, chest, and extremities; mammography; and fluoroscopic procedures such as gastrointestinal series, barium enema, and gallbladder examinations.

Conventional cost system:

The cost of the two procedures under the conventional cost accounting system is computed in Table 4. Note that direct costs are all costs that can be directly assigned to the patient or DRG including physician fees, direct nursing costs, room costs, medications, laboratory tests, and therapy services. Hospital overhead allocated includes hospital and departmental overhead that is not directly assigned to the patient or DRG. In a conventional cost accounting system, overhead is allocated on a patient-day basis, as follows:

Hospital overhead allocated / patient-day = Hospital overhead costs / Number of patient days = $10,832,673 / 54,838 patient days = $197.54/patient day

Activity-based cost system:

Let us next assume that St. Joseph Hospital has analyzed its operations using case manage-

Assume the following information for the nursing activity center of St. Joseph Hospital for the month of September:

Nursing Activity Center
Cost Driver = Number of Relative Value Units (RVUs)

Budget	**Actual**
Activity Level = 600,000 RVUs	Activity Level = 641,331 RVUs
Overhead Costs = $2,700,000	Overhead Costs = $2,661,523
Budgeted Cost per RVU = $4.50	Actual Cost per RVU = $4.15

Information obtained from the Variance Analysis Reports of all patients for the month of September.
Patient Variance = 8,231 RVUs
Caregiver Variance = 11,624 RVUs
Environmental Variance = 14,275 RVUs
Efficiency Variance = 7,201 RVUs

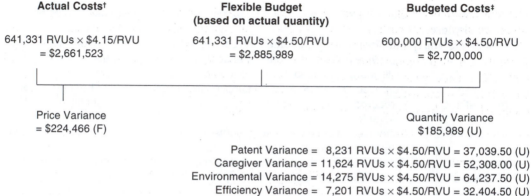

Summary Variance Report for Nursing Activity Center*

Actual Costs†	**Flexible Budget** **(based on actual quantity)**	**Budgeted Costs‡**
641,331 RVUs × $4.15/RVU	641,331 RVUs × $4.50/RVU	600,000 RVUs × $4.50/RVU
= $2,661,523	= $2,885,989	= $2,700,000

Price Variance = $224,466 (F)

Quantity Variance $185,989 (U)

Patent Variance = 8,231 RVUs × $4.50/RVU = 37,039.50 (U)
Caregiver Variance = 11,624 RVUs × $4.50/RVU = 52,308.00 (U)
Environmental Variance = 14,275 RVUs × $4.50/RVU = 64,237.50 (U)
Efficiency Variance = 7,201 RVUs × $4.50/RVU = 32,404.50 (U)

*It is recommended that individual cost drivers be used for different activity pools in analyzing price and quantity variances. In this example, it is assumed that a single cost driver—number of RVUs—adequately captures the consumption of resources in this activity center.

†Here overhead costs for the Nursing Care Activity Center are assumed to be essentially variable in relation to the cost driver used (number of RVUs). For fixed costs, variances can be further divided into strategic and operational capacity variances.

‡For simplicity, budgeted activity level is assumed equal to standard activity level.

Figure 3 Illustrative Example of Variance Analysis under an ABC System

ment and critical path analysis and has identified 10 activity centers (Figure 2) and its first- and second-stage cost drivers (Tables 2 and 3, respectively). It has also analyzed the activities involved within each of the activity centers. Figure 4 presents the analysis of 1 of the 10 activity centers, Perform Diagnostic Imaging Pool, as an illustration.

As shown in Figures 2 and 4, the hospital has determined the amount of overhead cost traceable to each of the 10 activity centers and has computed the overhead rate for each activity center using first- and second-stage cost drivers respectively. In Table 5 these rates have in turn been used to assign the hospital overhead costs to the individual patients/DRGs based on the actual number of activity transactions. Note from Table 5 that the use of ABC has resulted in $3,079.78 in overhead cost being assigned to DRG 1X1 and $835.11 in overhead cost being assigned to DRG 1X2. These amounts are used in Table 6 to determine the total cost of DRG

Table 4 Cost under Conventional Cost Accounting System

	DRG 1X1	DRG 1X2
Patient days	5	5
Direct cost	$8,451.00	$2,421.00
Hospital cost allocated	987.70	987.70
(5 patient days x 197.54)		
Total Costs	$9,438.70	$3,408.70

1X1 and 1X2 under ABC. For comparison purposes, we also present costs for DRG 1X1 and 1X2 under the conventional cost system (see Table 4). Under the conventional cost system, DRG 1X1 is undercosted by over 22 percent and DRG 1X2 is overcosted by almost 5 percent. Using ABC, we have been able to identify the

overhead costs that are traceable to each DRG/patient based on consumption of activity resources and thus obtain more accurate cost data.

Accurate costs reported by the ABC systems reduce the risk that poor case-mix decisions, faulty pricing decisions, and suboptimal capital budgeting decisions will be made because of inaccurate costs. This risk can be particularly high when competitor hospitals can take advantage of a hospital's poor decisions that can occur as a result of inaccurate costs.

• • •

ABC is a relatively new concept for hospitals. Integrating ABC with case management, critical path analysis, and other hospital control processes represents an exciting new development. It provides a structured approach to analyzing activities, costing services, reducing costs, and improving quality. In addition, it brings to bear

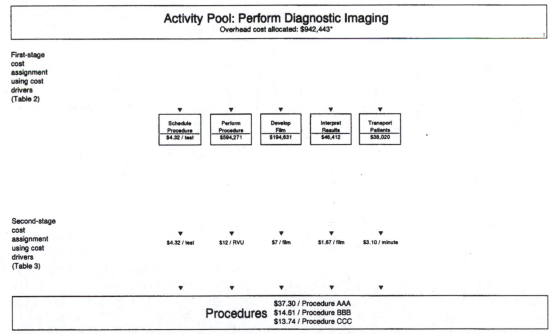

*These are overhead costs relating to the activity center. Direct costs such as salaries of the radiologists, technologists, technicians and staff, cost of supplies and depreciation and maintenance of screening equipment etc. are directly assigned to the activity pools.

Figure 4 Graphic Example of ABC Activity Center: Perform Diagnostic Imaging Pool

Table 5 Overhead Cost per DRG

Activity center	DRG 1X1			DRG 1X2		
	Number of transactions	Rate per transaction	Overhead cost	Number of transactions	Rate per transaction	Overhead cost
Admit patients pool	1 patient	$43/patient	$43.00	1 patient	$43/patient	$43.00
Cardiac catheterizations pool	2 Procedure A	89.41/Procedure A	178.82	1 Procedure C	$41.21/Procedure C	41.21
Administer ECG tests pool	7 tests	$23/test	161.00	4 tests	$23/test	92.00
Provide meals pool	9 special meals	$6.21/special meal	55.89	9 regular meals	$3.44/regular meal	30.96
	6 snacks	$2.87/snack	17.22	6 snacks	$2.87/snack	17.22
Administer laboratory tests pool	4 tests BB	$27/test BB	108.00	3 tests AA	$14/test AA	42.00
Provide nursing care pool	312 RVUs	$4.15/RVU	1,294.80	104 RVUs	$4.15/RVU	431.60
Dispense medications pool	14 medication orders	$15.67/medication order filled	219.38	6 medication orders	$15.67/medication order filled	94.02
Provide therapy sessions pool	7 hrs CT	$7.81/hour of CT	54.67	2 hrs CT	$7.81/hour of CT	15.62
Perform diagnostic imaging pool	2 procedures AAA	$37.30/procedure AAA	74.60	2 procedures CCC	$13.74/procedure CCC	27.48
Operate patients pool	1 hr in OR	$14.54/minute in OR	872.40			
			$3,079.78			$835.11

Table 6 Cost per DRG under ABC and Conventional Cost System

	Activity-based costing		Conventional cost system	
	DRG 1X1	*DRG 1X2*	*DRG 1X1*	*DRG 1X2*
Direct costs	8,451.00	2,421.00	8,451.00	2,421.00
Hospital overhead allocated	3,079.78	835.11	987.70	987.70
Total costs	11,530.78	3,256.11	9,438.70	3,408.70
			Undercosted by 22.16%	Overcosted by 4.47%

the skills of employers from different functional areas of the hospital and helps generate ideas and innovative solutions to the problems at hand.

There are numerous challenges in implementing an ABC system in hospitals. First, collecting the data needed to establish an ABC system is time consuming and expensive. An ABC system is much more complex and detailed than a traditional cost system because costs are allocated to different activity pools and each of these pools is further broken down into several separate activities. This requires detailed analysis of financial accounting records as well as inquiries and interviews to identify and gather costs and other information on specific activities. In some cases, information required for an ABC system is almost impossible to obtain. Also, the statistical analysis required to allocate costs is much more complex for an ABC system. Another barrier to successfully implementing the ABC system is

that many organizations view it as a quick fix and purely an exercise in accounting concerned only with developing better cost data. A successful implementation of an ABC system requires a comprehensive paradigm shift in management—a move from a functional departmental view of the hospital management structure to a more cross-functional view of hospital activities and processes. This requires reeducation of the entire organization from physicians to nurses to administrative staff. For this to happen, the initiative and impetus for change should come from senior management. Very often, changing management's perspective is far more complex and challenging than designing the system.

This article introduces the application of ABC to the management of hospitals. As more and more hospitals gain experience with ABC, their shared experiences will provide further insights into the integration and implementation of ABC in hospitals.

REFERENCES

1. Chan, Y.C. "Improving Hospital Cost Accounting with Activity-Based Costing." *Health Care Management Review* 18, no. 1 (1993): 71–77.

2. Ramsey IV, R. "Activity-Based Costing for Hospitals." *Hospital and Health Services Administration* 39, no. 3 (1994): 385–96.

3. Canby IV, J. "Applying Activity-Based Costing to Healthcare Settings." *Healthcare Financial Management* 49, no. 2 (1995): 50–56.

4. Turney, P.B.B. "What Is the Scope of Activity-Based Costing?" *Journal of Cost Management* 3, no. 4 (1990): 40–42.

5. Zander, K. "Nursing Case Management: Strategic Management of Cost and Quality Outcomes." *Journal of Nursing Administration* 18, no. 5 (1988): 23–30.

Monitoring Case Management Cost Savings

Victoria Hekkers

Many insurance case managers are intimidated and embarrassed by the thought of documenting cost savings. They somehow feel as though they are better nurses, more honest, or more fair by underestimating themselves and the effect their presence has had on the outcome of the case they are managing.

However, these feelings must be overcome; keeping track of case management cost savings is crucial to the continued existence of every case management department.

Determining cost savings is not as perplexing as it might seem. The case manager must ask him or herself, "If I were not involved in this case, in which direction would it gravitate?" The response should result in one of three types of cost savings: Hard, Soft, or Benefit Investigation.

Hard cost savings are, of course, those savings that are reflected by negotiations. Examples of "hard" cost savings are as follows:

The cost of renting a wheelchair is $175 per month and the case manager negotiates a price of $125.

- A lymphoma patient is referred to a local center for a bone marrow transplant. The cost at the center is approximately 30 percent to 40 percent higher than at another distant "Center of Excellence." The case manager is able to either facilitate transfer to the Center of Excellence or negotiate for similar rates at the local facility.

- A patient remains hospitalized and continues to meet utilization review criteria. The case manager suggests to the family that the services might be able to be performed at home (*i.e.,* home care or IV infusion) and then contacts the physician or discharge planner. A discharge is facilitated in this manner.

- An occupational therapist recommends a $1,000 shower chair for a patient in a halo. She also refers it to a non-PPO (70/30) provider who has ordered the specialty item. The case manager learns about the referral and order, then contacts the patient and family, suggesting a less expensive chair for the short duration of need (four weeks until removal of the halo). The patient agrees and the case manager discusses it with the occupational therapist and refers the patient to a PPO provider (80/20). The resulting cost for the commode chair is $199, saving the insurance company $540.80 and the patient $260.20. This is an example of a hard cost saving, as the referral had been made and the item ordered, and without case management intervention, would have been placed in the patient's home at the higher cost.

Case managers, by definition, steer cases to quality, cost-conscious providers and services. For example, the family of a traumatic brain-injured individual plans to place their loved one in

Inside Case Management 1996; 3(4): 2–3

a brain injury program that encourages dependence, is notoriously expensive and has a history of long-term stays. The case manager steers the family toward local, effective, quality-conscious providers who move the patient down the continuum of care while encouraging independence and family involvement.

Although some might consider this a "soft" cost saving, without the intervention of a case manager, the patient would have been referred to a costly long term program. Therefore, the case represents a hard cost savings.

An astute case manager must look at the patient's history to determine cost savings. A terminal oncology patient has numerous hospitalizations, in a short period of time, for pain control. A nurse case manager receives a referral, sets up and coordinates with home infusion, physician-approved hospice, and other interventions, and the patient expires peacefully at home. The hard cost savings should reflect those interventions and include the lack of rehospitalization.

Soft cost savings are sometimes less obvious and sometimes difficult to distinguish. Often, these savings are represented by preventive measures that case managers take to help patients facing potential risks. An example of soft cost savings is a high risk pregnancy patient, with no previous history of premature delivery, who carries the child to term as a result of case management intervention.

In this scenario, if the physician indicates that without case management intervention and assistance, a premature infant would have been delivered, it would be reflected as hard cost savings.

The third type of cost savings is "benefit investigation." These savings come as a result of a case manager's investigation in a patient's insurance coverage. Although insurance companies attempt to determine eligibility, they frequently do so by sending letters to the enrollees or families, asking them to report alternative insurance companies, full-time student status, or COBRA information. Unfortunately, families often misunderstand and report information that is incorrect or misleading, or in some cases, fraudulent.

The case managers frequently obtain and report information that shows that the patient has other primary coverage. This, of course, saves money for the insurance company by identifying another payer for the patient's claim. These savings are classified as Benefit Investigation savings.

This type of insurance case management offers nurses a whole new field of opportunity. It blends nursing, socioeconomics, psychology, and business into a collage of fascinating possibilities.

As nurses begin to value themselves and the impact of their interventions, the true value of cost savings will be recognized and appreciated by the insurance community.

Pricing Specialty Carve-Outs and Disease Management Programs Under Managed Care

Kenneth T. LaPensee

EVOLUTION TOWARD COORDINATED SPECIALIST SERVICES

There is a driving force behind the evolution of managed care: the search for more efficient ways to achieve positive health outcomes for insured populations. Some health policy experts maintain that health services will be structured increasingly around the treatment of particular diseases, both acute and chronic. The rationale for this prediction is that services focused on specific diseases can be the most cost-effective way to deliver care to certain groups of patients. Why? Because services can be coordinated by providers with the greatest expertise in treating these diseases.

Supporting evidence shows that uncontrolled self-referral of patients to specialists under an indemnity health insurance system can be inefficient. However, managed care organizations (MCOs) are working more and more with specialist groups or specialty programs that coordinate disease-specific care and assume at least some of the risk for particular illnesses.

This article focuses on why MCOs contract with specialist groups for disease-specific services, and how they can determine the value of these services, particularly for "specialty carve-out" or "disease management" agreements. This information pertains to MCOs seeking to share

Managed Care Quarterly 1997; 5(2): 10–19
© 1997 Aspen Publishers, Inc.

risk with specialist groups, and the specialist groups trying to assess per member per month (PMPM) or case rates that MCOs offer.

Limitations of primary care coordination

While managed care has prompted a resurgence of interest in primary care, specialist providers are finding ways to participate in spreading the integration and coordination of medical services.

Coordinated medical care requires that someone, mainly the primary care physician (PCP) in current MCOs, has an overview of a patient's medical care. Ideally, the PCP attempts to understand patients in terms of demographic and socioeconomic backgrounds, personal and family medical history, and unique personalities and preferences. Using this information, the PCP tries to manage critical medical conditions that require continuity of care over time. The PCP's mission is to treat these conditions as much as possible, preventing unnecessary use of specialist providers, and coordinate the use of specialists as needed. The PCP becomes a gatekeeper for specialist services.

Coordinating specialty care presents a medical management challenge to PCPs because it requires intensive communication with both the patient and the specialists being used. Added to the PCP's own treatment burden, this responsibility can be onerous. Furthermore, the PCP may not be the most efficient coordinator of the patient's care once the patient has been diagnosed with a certain disease. Having said that, the PCP's role in keeping important patient information and authorizing specialist courses of treatment (rather than each specialist visit) is likely to remain meaningful to ensure continuity of care.

Disability and crisis prevention

The key to reducing costs through medical management is preventing crises that require hospital admissions or preventing onset of disabilities that require long-term expensive services. There are three levels of prevention.

1. *Primary prevention* is the avoidance of increased disease risk through the improvement of health habits, such as the prevention of high blood pressure through weight control.
2. *Secondary prevention* is the avoidance of the occurrence of the acute phase of a disease once a patient has been diagnosed with it, as when the control of blood sugar prevents hospitalization for diabetic complications.
3. *Tertiary prevention* is the avoidance of patient decline or a worsening of a serious patient condition, as when a patient undergoes rehabilitation to counteract the effects of a crisis such as a stroke.

The primary care physician and other managed care organization staff such as patient educators and nutritionists are responsible for promoting primary prevention. However, secondary and tertiary prevention often require guidance from specialists.

Disease management programs

Any discussion of pricing specialist services under managed care should include information on increasingly prevalent disease management programs. There is a growing recognition among MCOs that specialists can be helpful when they participate in coordinating care for certain targeted chronic diseases. These diseases are characterized by:

- long duration after onset
- need for coordinated treatment across a continuum of treatment settings ranging from hospital inpatient facilities to the patient's home
- high cost per episode of care
- a high level of technology or special expertise required for treatment.

The conditions giving rise to disease management programs are cancer, heart disease, musculoskeletal conditions, hypertension, depression, asthma and emphysema, diabetes, trauma, and autoimmune disease.

Initiatives within MCOs to coordinate care for such diseases are called *disease management* (also *chronic disease management* or *disease state management*) programs. The *disease management* term is widely used and applied to a variety of different approaches. In some cases it is seen as a euphemism to mask an effort by medical specialists to gain control of patients in a managed care environment that increasingly favors primary care. Others view disease management as an attempt by pharmaceutical firms to package drug sales to MCOs. Programs that do not promote medical efficacy and efficiency, however, are doomed to failure. Plainly any new system not promoting cost-effective care in the current health care environment cannot succeed.

Although it is unlikely that specialists will beat back the movement toward increased power for primary care providers, specialists and disease management have a legitimate role in managed care. For certain complicated long-term conditions, it simply makes sense to let a specialist coordinate a patient's care related to the condition with minimal interference or delay, while applying incentives to specialist practice to encourage adherence to guidelines.

Disease management programs parallel familiar case management operations in some ways, especially because disease management focuses on a patient with a targeted condition and tries to coordinate the care the individual receives for that condition. In fact, some professionals consider disease management to be a form of case management.[1] While there are important similarities, disease management is a much more powerful concept because it encompasses both secondary and tertiary disability prevention activities. One can think of disease management as being "proactive case management." Table 1 contrasts disease management and traditional large case management programs.

Traditional case management was developed in an indemnity health insurance environment to limit the effects and cost of a medical crisis. Disease management is a "creature" of managed care, and is dedicated to preventing medical crises.

Disease management attempts to manage the health of a group of patients using the techniques of secondary and tertiary prevention. The management effort should result in high-quality care that produces the best outcomes for patients and is cost-effective for the payer. Common features of disease management programs that further these objectives are:

- guidelines for physicians and other professionals for the optimal treatment of targeted conditions;
- risk sharing or case management agreements between payers and specialist groups;
- programs for monitoring the use of particular drug and other treatment interventions to assess patient outcomes and cost;
- educational initiatives to increase patients' knowledge of their conditions and doctors' understanding of the most cost-effective treatments; and
- interventions to modify both patients' behavior so they comply with drug and other treatments, as well as physicians' behavior so they comply with efficacious practice guidelines.

In this author's opinion, the disease management model is effective to use in a carve-out agreement between specialists and an MCO because it can reduce cost for the payer and risk for the providers.

Table 1 Disease management versus traditional case management

Program feature	Case management	Disease management
Strategy	Reactive—initiated in response to a grave crisis	Preventive—initiated before a crisis can occur
Initiating event	Hospital stay for certain condition, or occurrence of a large insurance claim	Diagnosis of certain condition
Oversight and coordination of patient care	Case management nurse	Primary care or specialist physician and managed care organization staff
Financial basis	Discounted fee-for-service	Risk sharing, carve-out, or subcapitation
Level of preventive care	Tertiary only (prevention of patient decline and worsening of condition)	Secondary (prevention of recurrence of illness) and tertiary
Type of illness addressed	Acute illness, or the acute phase of a chronic illness	All phases of a chronic illness
Health care quality improvement emphasis	Ad hoc, for the individual patient being managed	Systematic, for all patients with targeted conditions

PRICING SPECIALIST SERVICES UNDER MANAGED CARE

Current difficulties in pricing disease

Once a managed care organization has identified a need for coordinated specialty care or disease management, the question of how to value these services immediately arises. In today's managed care environment, getting an answer to "What is the cost of this disease on a per case or a per member per month basis?" is rather difficult for a variety of reasons—mostly related to the availability of data.

1. Insurers have set reimbursement rates and tracked costs for medical procedures and products, but not for diagnoses. In fact, capturing the diagnosis code for ambulatory patient claims was not a widespread practice until the late 1980s. Even though diagnosis is now usually captured, until recently insurers have had little reason to track and analyze costs by diagnosis. Almost no "canned" references exist that show the incurred costs of particular diseases across all health care settings.

2. Health maintenance organizations (HMOs) have generally captured little or no information about individual patient encounters that do not involve financial transactions, such as PCP visits or visits to a primary care clinic. When the information is available, the diagnosis is often not recorded.

3. Assessing the cost of a disease or condition is inherently not an easy task. There are pitfalls in the ICD-9-CM diagnosis coding system and the way it has been used that necessitate compensatory analytical strategies in determining disease cost.

4. Even when data on disease cost are available, they are usually in an unprocessed state. Processing raw claims, medical charts, or administrative data can be expensive, especially given the need to compensate for diagnosis data inaccuracies or inadequacies.

Calculating the baseline cost of care from historical encounter data

The above problems can be overcome to some extent, although all of the available data sources are imperfect. Potential data sources are discussed below. A disease-specific database can be constructed that will support pricing of a specialty services or carve-out agreement. Disease-specific claims, encounter, and medical chart data have to be processed to provide an estimate of the *baseline cost of care* rate for the continuum of services covered by the agreement. It's called a *baseline* rate because cost estimates derived from historical claims and encounter data reflect medical practice prior to the specialist service agreement, with its practice guidelines, protocols, and financial incentives for specialists. It is a starting point for managed care pricing.

This baseline rate can be calculated on a case-by-case basis (case rate) or a PMPM (capitation) basis. A specialist carve-out agreement can be rated on either basis. The scope of services covered under the specialty care or disease management agreement determines the proportion of the total disease-specific cost that constitutes the specialist organization's liability. For example, a specialist group may contract with an MCO to provide only inpatient, or only outpatient services, or only services related to a particular subspecialty (e.g., medical oncology but not radiation oncology or cancer surgery).

Data processing to support disease-specific rating follows a pattern such as depicted in the flow diagram of Figure 1.

DISEASE-SPECIFIC RATING OVERVIEW

Data are subsetted by diagnosis

Claims and encounter level data are subsetted according to the set of diagnoses being covered under the specialty carve-out or disease management program. Data on *all* related conditions should be analyzed. For example, if the carve-

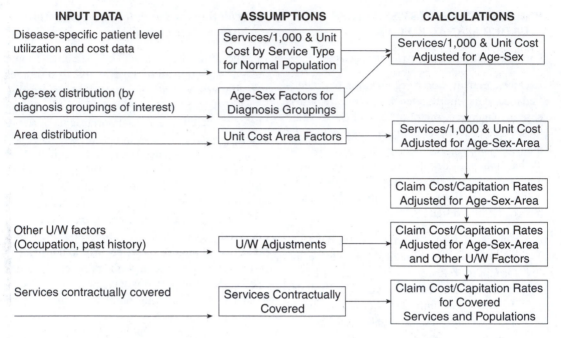

INPUT DATA	ASSUMPTIONS	CALCULATIONS

Disease-specific patient level utilization and cost data → Services/1,000 & Unit Cost by Service Type for Normal Population → Services/1,000 & Unit Cost Adjusted for Age-Sex

Age-sex distribution (by diagnosis groupings of interest) → Age-Sex Factors for Diagnosis Groupings

Area distribution → Unit Cost Area Factors → Services/1,000 & Unit Cost Adjusted for Age-Sex-Area

Claim Cost/Capitation Rates Adjusted for Age-Sex-Area

Other U/W factors (Occupation, past history) → U/W Adjustments → Claim Cost/Capitation Rates Adjusted for Age-Sex-Area and Other U/W Factors

Services contractually covered → Services Contractually Covered → Claim Cost/Capitation Rates for Covered Services and Populations

Figure 1. Disease-specific rating procedure.

out program is for coronary heart disease, data on antecedent conditions such as hypertension or diabetes should also be analyzed.

Membership ("exposure") data are analyzed

The MCO's entire enrollment (membership) file is downloaded. Members in each relevant age, sex, and risk pool category are counted. A frequency distribution of members by all underwriting categories to be used in the model is calculated. This will facilitate the calculation of age-sex factors, disease incidence and prevalence rates, and per capita utilization and cost.

Identification of patients and providers

All unique patients with targeted diagnoses are identified and counted to provide a numerator for cardiovascular (CV) disease prevalence and utilization rates, and a denominator for CV disease case rates.

Identification of all relevant services

All services provided to this set of patients are identified and linked to each patient and also to the providers delivering the services. This is done to create episodes of care at the patient level, and to perform specialty profiling and cost at the provider level, if desired. For example, a PMPM rate for outpatient oncology services may need to be divided between medical oncologists, radiation oncologists, and surgeons.

Calculation of cost components

Services are divided into two categories:

1. services provided to patients that are not related to patients' disease-specific encounters (e.g., a diabetes patient has an admission for an automobile injury), and
2. services provided to patients that are related to conditions covered by the contract.

For those services that are related to patients' covered conditions, the basic health care cost components are calculated:

- average cost per service, by type of service ("average unit cost")
- service utilization rate, by type of service (services per 1,000 members)
- average cost per unique patient or claimant, by diagnosis or predefined set of services (related to "case rate").

Calculation of age-sex factors

Age and sex factors are important for predicting PMPM cost and are calculated for both the average unit cost per service and the services per thousand. The factor for each age and sex group is the utilization rate or average unit cost for that group divided by the utilization rate for the entire population. These factors may differ by diagnosis grouping. For example, various cancers have very different incidence rates by age and sex, while cardiovascular disease has a fairly constant set of risk factors across individual cardiovascular diagnoses.

Calculation of area factors

If the MCO has widely dispersed locations, it's likely that the unit cost per service will vary by region. Area factors are calculated for unit cost, but *not* for the services per thousand, because:

- the disease management program may promote practice guidelines and protocols that would affect provider practice variation and the service utilization rate, and
- the shifts in age, sex, and diagnosis across regions will account for much of the variance in utilization rates not accounted for by provider practice differences that the disease management program wants to reduce.

Adjustment of cost and utilization statistics

The unit cost per service and the services per thousand are adjusted by the age, sex, and (for unit cost only) area factors. These adjusted statistics are multiplied to get PMPM rates by type of service as described below.

Summarizing the data for capitation rates by type of service

An important task of the baseline analysis is to determine historical disease costs for the population by the various types of service that are covered by an MCO. Analysts derive the following statistics from the MCO's claims and encounter data:

1. *Inpatient* cost and utilization statistics for all ICD-9-CM diagnosis groupings by patient age and sex group:
   a) admission rates per thousand MCO population
   b) average length of stay and variation (range, variance, "skewness")
   c) average cost per case and variation
   d) analysis for each procedure or diagnosis related group (DRG) by patient's Metropolitan Statistical Area (MSA), zip code, and/or county of residence
2. *Outpatient* hospital cost and utilization statistics for covered diagnosis groupings and/or CPT procedure codes:
   a) numbers of services and services per thousand population
   b) average cost per service and variation
   c) average services per patient and variation
   d) analysis for each procedure by patient's MSA, zip code, and/or county of residence
3. *Physician* cost and utilization for physicians sorted by specialty:
   a) average cost by procedure and variation
   b) numbers of services by procedure
   c) analysis by patient's MSA, zip code, and/or county of residence
4. *Nonacute care* (skilled nursing facility [SNF], hospice) cost and utilization statistics for each diagnosis grouping:
   a) admissions rates per thousand population
   b) average length of stay and variation

c) average cost per case and variation
d) analysis by patient's MSA, zip code, and/or county of residence
5. *Pharmaceuticals, medical supplies, and equipment* cost and utilization statistics for each diagnosis grouping:
   a) numbers of prescriptions and prescriptions per thousand population
   b) average cost per prescription and variation
   c) average prescriptions per patient and variation
   d) analysis for each product by patient's MSA, zip code, and/or county of residence
6. For the entire population the analyst would determine:
   a) unique claimants by diagnosis per calendar year (period prevalence)
   b) numbers of patients newly diagnosed with conditions covered by the disease management program (period incidence)
   c) the rate of specific outcomes (health care process, morbidity, and mortality)

Calculation of the cost rate

The service cost and utilization rate for each individual type of service are multiplied and then totaled by major service category (e.g., inpatient, outpatient, physician, drug, etc.) to produce disease-specific cost rates for each category. These can then be added up to produce the overall disease management program cost per member. On a monthly basis, this is the PMPM rate. If there is a capitated arrangement with the MCO, this will be the capitation or subcapitation rate for the CV diseases covered by the contract.

Total program cost

Estimating the total cost of a carve-out or disease management program using the baseline cost of care calculated by the above procedure entails the following steps:

1. Trending baseline claims and encounter experience to account for medical inflation related to:
   a) professional services,
   b) facility use, and
   c) pharmaceuticals and equipment.
2. Calculating a projected cost of services under the new contract by adjusting the trended experience in (1) above for:
   a) known MCO population risks (mainly lifestyle, socioeconomic, and occupational factors), determined using surveys, screening, etc.;
   b) projected medical management savings due to adherence to practice guidelines and utilization review;
   c) supplier contract provisions, such as discounts or fee schedules; and
   d) benefit plan provisions that may be more or less restrictive than those prevailing in the baseline data.
3. Adding general and administrative costs to the projected cost of services in (2) above, including:
   a) net cost of stop-loss or reinsurance (premiums minus payouts);
   b) administrative and infrastructure costs, especially for an information system that monitors cost and utilization under the carve-out or disease management program;
   c) a margin for profit and risk; and
   d) adjustments reflecting financial incentives to providers for meeting managed care goals such as patient satisfaction, control of unnecessary services, and adherence to practice guidelines.

SOURCES OF BASELINE AND NORMATIVE COST DATA

The MCO's own claims and encounter data

The primary data source for a carve-out or disease management agreement is the contracting MCO. In the interest of having a specialist contract that actually saves money, the MCO needs to know what its historical costs have been for the services covered by the agreement. As mentioned above, however, MCO data often have critical limitations.

External claims and administrative data

It's likely that the baseline analysis of disease-specific costs of a particular MCO will need to be supplemented using large external databases of commercially insured or Medicare claims. Analysts can purchase data from commercial or public insurers for a given set of diseases for a geographic region. Often, the data indicates the type of patient coverage under which services were utilized, that is, indemnity or preferred provider organization (PPO) versus point-of-service or HMO.

Alternative normative data

Some health care analyses require norms that reflect broad-based inpatient UB-92 data. Others need data reflecting a consensus on medical practice on the part of expert panels rather than statistical averages of health claims data. Again, it is possible to purchase databases that provide such norms, including the HCIA Length of Stay norms and the leading health care management guidelines used by utilization review firms.

Certain databases provide information that can supplement that obtained from claims data. For example, the Health Insurance Association of America (HIAA) maintains a Prevailing Health Care Charges System (PHCS). This is a database of prevailing unit charges for both CPT procedures and DRGs that enables the analyst to evaluate carrier, hospital and physician fee schedules, submitted charges, allowed charges, paid amounts, and discounts. These comparisons are useful for determining the real value of "reasonable and customary" allowances, PPO discounts, and DRGs, for example. These data also permit the calculation of conversion factors for application of a resource-based relative value scale (RBRVS) to physician reimbursement. The First Databank company maintains a phar-

maceutical database for prescription drug price (average wholesale price or AWP) norms. Available databases and their various functions include:

- *Commercially insured databases.* For analyzing patient-specific cost and utilization data, particularly for ambulatory services at the community level. Certain data suppliers maintain normative data for millions of covered lives.
- *State-maintained inpatient hospital discharge databases.* For analyzing all of the inpatient data for a given region. Rich in utilization detail, sparse in financial detail, sometimes containing charges but not payments. Data may be up to a year old in some states, and is not available in all states.
- *Medicare Standard Analytical Files from the HCFA Public Use Files database.* Medicare Part A and Part B claim database for inpatient, outpatient, physician/supplier, skilled nursing facility, home health agency, and hospice care. This is the best source of data for older populations. Medigap data are available from commercially insured data vendors.
- *HIAA PHCS database.* This is a prevailing charges database at the three-digit zip code level. It can be used to evaluate charges and set unit pricing for capitation.
- *NDDF database.* This is a database of AWP for drugs available from First Databank. It can be used to evaluate unit drug pricing for capitation.
- *HCIA length of stay (LOS) norms.* HCIA Inc. maintains a database of average lengths of hospital stays based on a large national sample of inpatient admissions. The LOS norms are stratified by age, sex, and other factors. HCIA is also a source of raw privately insured claims data, mainly from large, self-insured employers.
- *Health Care Management Guidelines.* This database, used by many utilization review operations, provides "best practices" length of stay and admission rate information, and

benchmarks for inpatient or ambulatory utilization useful in concurrent hospital stay review.

PMPM EXAMPLE FROM ONCOLOGY

Cancer is a specialty area that readily lends itself to carve-out arrangements and disease management because it is not only of long duration (the average survival period for cancer patients in general exceeds five years), but also extremely technical and expensive to treat. Once a patient has been diagnosed with cancer, there can be a significant advantage to letting an oncologist coordinate further care.

Many MCOs now either carve out or share risk with oncologists for some or all cancer treatment. National organizations coordinating regional oncology networks are operating in most major U.S. cities. A recent actuarial project in oncology involved analyzing data on all types of cancer care in a large state in which managed care has high penetration. The managed oncology program aimed to initially cover about 3 million managed care lives under a capitated carve-out arrangement in which all cancer-related care for cancer patients would be coordinated by medical oncologists.

This project was one of the earliest (outside of the mental health field) where a national network of medical specialists developed an integrated delivery system to treat a specific set of diseases—which was to be marketed nationally to managed care organizations. Leading edge analytical techniques were used to develop oncology-specific pricing and risk modeling from commercially insured individual patient claims data.

In this study it was found that the relative cost proportions of major types of service varying by cancer diagnosis category, as shown in Table 2, and the proportion of total cancer costs is attributable to each cancer diagnosis category. The age/sex factors used in estimating disease cost varied significantly by type of cancer. This type of finding suggests the wealth of detail that can be gleaned from patient level claims and encounter data, and which is necessary to support

Table 2 Percent of PMPM costs by cancer grouping (does not include benign tumors)

Service type	Breast	Lung	Colorectal	Lymphoma	Prostate	Ovarian	Other invasive	Non-invasive	Total
Inpatient	24	40	49	38	48	37	54	16	42
Hospital	24	38	48	38	48	37	54	16	41
Other	0	2	1	0	0	0	0	0	1
Outpatient	21	13	11	21	11	15	13	17	15
Hospital	18	11	8	18	10	11	11	11	12
Other	3	3	3	3	1	4	3	6	3
Physician/ professional	46	37	34	32	35	39	27	60	36
Surgery/ anesthesia	13	8	12	6	16	17	11	41	15
Radiation Oncology	10	8	3	3	7	0	3	3	5
Chemotherapy	3	4	5	4	1	4	2	1	2
Other	19	17	14	19	11	17	11	16	14
Drugs	7	8	5	8	5	7	4	5	5
Chemotherapy	2	3	1	3	1	2	1	1	1
Other	5	5	4	5	4	4	3	4	4
Other services	2	2	2	1	0	2	2	2	2
Total	100	100	100	100	100	100	100	100	100
% of Grand total	16	8	7	5	6	3	42	12	100

disease management and carve-out programs under managed care.

Risk and stop loss issues

For specialist groups accepting a PMPM rate it is nearly as important to be able to quantify the risk caused by experience fluctuations as it is to agree upon a fair capitation with the MCO. Although MCOs can offer specialist groups stop loss insurance, large specialist networks dealing with multiple MCOs are generally better off shopping for coverage in the health care special risk marketplace.

Specialist groups may want aggregate stop loss coverage to protect against adverse fluctuation in the total claim amount under the agreement. Aggregate stop loss is probably most advantageous in the first few years of an agreement. Alternatively, the specialist group may want specific stop loss to protect against the impact of large claims. Specific stop loss "smooths" the claim size distribution, making emerging experience more predictable. This may be more appropriate for a group that has several years of experience on which to base pricing.

One of the advantages of using patient level data in a disease-specific analysis such as the oncology project cited above is that the distribution of large claims exceeding particular amounts can be developed for a given population. This enables the analyst to calculate a stop loss premium estimate by age group and in total. Knowing the claim size distribution based on patient level data facilitates the calculation of probabilities that the actual PMPM cost of care will exceed the expected cost by a certain percentage.

It was found in the oncology study that the size of surgical claims was skewed to the left (i.e., most surgical claims were more expensive than the average), while medical oncology claims were skewed to the right (i.e., most medical oncology claims were less expensive than the average), as were radiation oncology claims. This means that actual experienced PMPM costs for a number of contracts for a *package* of radiation oncology, medical oncology, and surgical oncology should be normally distributed around the expected PMPM cost.

This also means that the cost of agreements covering only medical oncology or radiation oncology or both may be far less stable. In addition, projections of PMPM may be less reliable for these services alone than the PMPM for all cancer care. Fluctuations in the three major types of cancer care "balance" one another. This example points to the disadvantage of carving out a very small set of services under a capitated arrangement. The "law of large numbers" means in such cases that fluctuations in a large portfolio of services will be a lower proportion of the expected PMPM rate than in a small portfolio.

If the carve-out agreement is for a case rate rather than a PMPM rate, the breadth of the portfolio of services is less important a consideration because the volume (of services) risk is considerably reduced under a case rate.

REFERENCE

1. Plocher, D.W. "Disease Management." In *The Managed Health Care Handbook,* ed. P.R. Kongstvedt. Gaithersburg, MD: Aspen, 1996, pp. 318–329.

Case Management and Home Health Care: An Integrated Model

Sherry L. Aliotta and Jo-Anne Andre

Case management continues to be valued as an effective strategy in the managed care industry (see box entitled "Defining the Managed Care Players"). A recent study indicated that over 90% of managed care organizations surveyed planned to expand their existing case management efforts or to establish case management programs.[1] Although the goals of the individual programs vary, there are usually some common themes. These themes include increasing member satisfaction, improving quality of care, reducing unnecessary medical cost, and promoting continuity of care.

The role of home health care in the success of case management programs is critical. It is important that home health care organizations recognize their contribution to case management. An understanding of this point can allow home health care organizations to properly position themselves for success in the changing health care arena.

Hospital lengths of stay continue to decline. In the California market, adjusted bed days per 1,000 have declined by nearly 10% in the commercial population and by over 6% in the senior population since 1990.[2] The increasing use of home health care and the ability of home health care to manage increasingly complex patients at home has contributed to this decline.

The ability of home health care to decrease lengths of stay by providing continued care at

the end of an acute care admission is but one area where home health care can make an impact. The increased focus on chronic care management and disease management provides home health care providers with a unique opportunity to impact the demand for acute care. It is important for case managers and home health care organizations to collaborate and create a fully integrated model that truly supports the continuum of health care.

CASE MANAGEMENT AND HOME HEALTH SUPPORTING THE CONTINUUM

There has been much recent discussion of the health care continuum (Fig 1). This concept is especially effective in viewing the management of chronic illness. To illustrate the continuum concept, consider diabetes. At the optimal end of the continuum, the individuals with diabetes would be well educated in the management of

The authors acknowledge FHP/Take Care Staff Model Patient Care Management and Continuing Care Division. Disclaimer: 1) Only Staff Model patients were included in the study although IPA patients were also served. 2) When FHP recently reorganized into a pure contracted care HMO company (FHP, Inc.) and a multispecialty Medical Group (Talbert Medical Management Corporation), the model was changed to reflect the reorganization. 3) Only preliminary results are reported.

Home Health Care Manage Prac 1997; 9(2): 1–12
© 1997 Aspen Publishers, Inc.

Defining the Managed Care Players

The various types of managed health care organizations, once quite distinct in their defined roles, have now evolved to a point where their distinctions have become blurred. The differences have narrowed, making the definition and description of such systems difficult. The following are briefly descriptive definitions of some of the managed health care systems that are encountered in today's market.

—HMOs

An organized health care system that is responsible for both the financing and the delivery of a broad range of comprehensive health care services to an enrolled population. It is the combination of a health care insurer and health care delivery system. The five common models differ in how the HMO relates to its participating physicians.

1. Staff model (closed panel)

   Physicians are salaried by the HMO and may receive bonus or incentive payments based on performance and productivity. Community physicians, except for rarely needed subcontracted specialists, may not participate. Centralized ambulatory care facilities resembling outpatient clinics contain physician offices and ancillary support facilities. Nonphysician services are provided through contracted hospitals or organization-owned hospitals.

2. Group model

   • Captive group

     Multispecialty physician groups exist solely to provide services to HMO beneficiaries (eg, Kaiser Foundation Health Plan is the administrative HMO for the Permanente Medical Groups).

   • Independent group

     Independent multispecialty physician groups contract with HMO to provide services while still providing non-HMO services to its own private patients.

3. Network model

   HMO contracts with many multispecialty physician group practices. Typically groups are compensated by the HMOs on a capitation basis.

4. IPA model

   HMOs contract with an association of physicians to provide services to its members. The IPA is a separate legal entity, but its physicians remain as individual practitioners, retaining separate offices and identities. IPA groups independently established by community physicians can contract with more than one HMO on a nonexclusive basis. Or an HMO can create its own exclusive IPA group and recruit physicians to participate in it. IPAs can be hospital-based or community-based. Most HMOs compensate their IPAs on an all-inclusive physician capitation basis to provide services.

5. Direct contract model

   HMOs contract directly with individual physicians to provide services. Physicians are compensated on either fee-for-services basis or primary care capitation basis. HMOs usually retain most of the financial risk. Physicians have little incentive to participate in UM programs due to lack of group organization.

—PPOs

An organization through which employer health benefit plans and health insurance carriers contract to purchase health care services from a selected group of participating providers. Through UM and use of incentives (varying reimbursement structures), care costs are controlled. A less formal structure may be known as a PPA.

Additional managed care terms

—Capitation

Prepayment for services on a per-member/per-month basis. A primary care physician, association, or facility is paid the same amount of money every month, regardless of whether that member receives services or not and regardless of how expensive those services are.

—Fee-for-service

A straight reimbursement for service is provided. This arrangement can be negotiated with straight discounts or discounts based on volume.

Source: Copyright © 1993, Peter R. Kongstvedt.

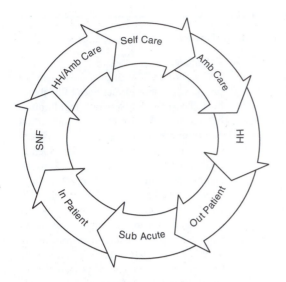

Figure 1. Health care continuum.

their disease and actively managing their care. They would be participating in preventive care and availing themselves of regular medical assessment and treatment and would not require active case management at this time.

These individuals could be experiencing minor educational needs and low-level treatment adherence problems that may have caused exacerbations of their illness. These exacerbations could lead to acute inpatient admission if not controlled. These individuals would be moved to the next progression in the continuum without patient case management. The next level of the continuum could involve the addition of a home health care program to intensify both the education and attention to the treatment adherence problems. The level and complexity of care increases with each step along the continuum. The goal of continuum-based care is to maintain individuals at the most appropriate levels of care. Self-management may not be achievable for all individuals. However, the continuum approach can ensure that individuals are contributing to their care at their optimal level and are receiving the additional support necessary to meet their medical management needs. This new paradigm of health care delivery maximizes the options while improving the quality.

The continuum approach has developed over time and home health care has done much to reshape the paradigm of health care delivery. In addition, there have been significant innovations in alternatives to acute hospital care. Managed health care has spurred many of these innovations. The innovations have been advanced by the evolving sophistication of home care services and the growth in suitable inpatient alternatives to hospitalization. The concept of gradations in acuity and health care delivery options have been reinforced. The choices in alternative delivery settings have evolved rapidly in the past 10 to 15 years. Prior to that the "continuum" was far more limited. Case managers had few options beyond hospitals, nursing homes, and home care. Choices now include specialized tertiary care units (TCUs), subacute units, rehabilitation centers, transitional living centers, board and care homes, assisted living centers, outpatient surgical centers, day treatment facilities, and infusion centers. In addition, the level of home care services has increased in sophistication and enabled them to handle individuals requiring higher levels of acuity.

In tandem with these changes, there has been increased growth in the managed care industry. Enrollment in health maintenance organizations (HMOs) has increased and continues to grow. Managed care has responded with more effective methods of managing the health care needs of its members. Expanding and enhancing case management programs is one method that has been widely employed. One of the roles of case management is to identify care options that are acceptable to the individual, thus increasing the likelihood of compliance with the treatment plan and successful outcomes.[3] Additionally case managers promote quality, cost-effective outcomes by evaluating the individual's health needs and the available options.[3] As case managers searched for better options, the system responded. The result is an expanded continuum focus of care.

The integration of home health care and case management is the ideal model to optimize the goals of continuum of care. In fact, when used effectively, case management and home health care have produced some favorable outcomes. This integration must include some new perceptions on the part of home health nurses and case managers.

RATIONALE FOR INTEGRATION

Traditionally home care nurses have looked at themselves as the "case managers" of their patients. They have been responsible for the coordination of all home-based disciplines and therapies, communication with physicians, and coordination of outside resources. Some have questioned and even resented the addition of the case management practitioner to the health care teams.

However, as the paradigm of health care changes, these same nurses may begin to see the case manager as an ally rather than an enemy. With the growth of managed care, increasing capitation for home health care services, and the expectations of payers to do more for less, many home health care nurses have turned to the case manager to be the coordinating and integrating force with the physician and resources outside the home.

At the same time, the home health care nurse's role of case management within the home setting has greatly expanded as the interventions being employed to reduce hospital and skilled nursing facility bed days and to retain the patient in the least costly and most appropriate level of care have multiplied.

A MODEL OF INTEGRATION

With the variety and sophistication of home care programs available at FHP, a large senior and commercial HMO, the case managers had a wide array of options with which to manage their patients. The case management model had to be extremely proactive in the identification and management of the patients most likely to benefit from their services.

Originating in the staff model, the case management program had the opportunity to work closely with the plan physicians and had access to the data and resources of the health plan. This combination aided in the creation of a model that performed effectively in achieving the desired outcomes.

The ambulatory case management program identified patients for entry on the basis of behaviors rather than diagnosis. In dealing with a large population of chronically ill, frail elderly with multiple diagnoses, it was believed that inclusion for a specific diagnosis only would not accurately identify FHP's target population. An alternative was sought to more traditional diagnostic- or treatment-focused criteria, and criteria of behaviors that indicated a patient was failing in the medical management of his or her chronic illness were looked at. The more "traditional" case management diagnoses, such as head injuries, prematurity, and oncology, were handled by the catastrophic case managers.

Due to the large population of senior members, many of the screening efforts were targeted to that group. Each new senior enrollee was sent a health assessment questionnaire to identify high-risk members. High risk was defined as members who were at risk for a decline in health status that could result in a hospitalization or emergency care. Case management assessments were used to determine those members who were identified as high risk whose outcomes could be positively impacted by their intervention (see the box entitled "The Patient Care Management Process" and Table 1).

In addition to the screening questionnaire, physicians and other members of the health care delivery team were well informed of the services case management could offer, as well as the criteria for entry. The independent practice association (IPA) or staff model plan utilization staff

---

The Patient Care Management Process

Targeting
Case finding
Screening
Problem identification
Planning
Intervention
Evaluation and monitoring

Table 1 Case management assessments

Parameter	Goal	What to look for
Identifiable method for identification and selection of patients for case management	There are written protocols for the types of patients to be followed by case management and how they are selected	Criteria could include: 1. Diagnosis-specific indications such as: a. AIDS b. Spinal cord injury c. COPD, etc 2. Behavioral/functional indicators a. Impairment in activities of daily living (bathing, dressing, etc) that render a patient unable to comply with a medical regimen b. Noncompliance with medical regimen that results in increased use of resources 3. Utilization issues a. Frequent readmissions b. High clinic encounters c. Frequent emergency department use d. Polypharmacy 4. Cost indications a. Over $10,000 ambulatory FFS equivalent b. Over $10,000 inpatient FFS equivalent 5. Screening: Health questionnaires, etc

were key in the identification of the behaviors that indicated a member was managing ineffectively. The utilization staff alerted case managers to members with frequent hospital admissions and provided case managers with the reports needed to identify potential case management candidates. Every individual having any member contact was made aware of the case management program and the types of member behaviors that could indicate a need for case management intervention.

Once the member was identified and entered into the case management program, the case manager collaborated with the members' primary care physician and any other health care team members involved in the members care to accurately define the members' problems. The case manager, member, and health care delivery team developed a plan of care to address the individual's needs. The goals of the interdisciplinary care plan were to create interventions that improved the member's ability to manage his or her own illness and to provide the necessary ongoing support (Fig 2 and box entitled "Multidisciplinary Core Team").

The innovative and flexible home care options allowed case managers to use home care, not just as a posthospital continuation but to stabilize the ambulatory care and prevent hospitalization.

THE INTERVENTIONS

Home health beyond the Medicare model

Although home care has always included the continuum of care that encompassed unskilled through high-technology interventions (Table 2), the focus encouraged by the reality of reimbursement methodologies has traditionally been on the Medicare model. Medicare's criteria of homebound, medically necessary, intermittent, skilled, and physician-ordered services have dominated the growth and development of home care since its passage in 1965. Medicaid and

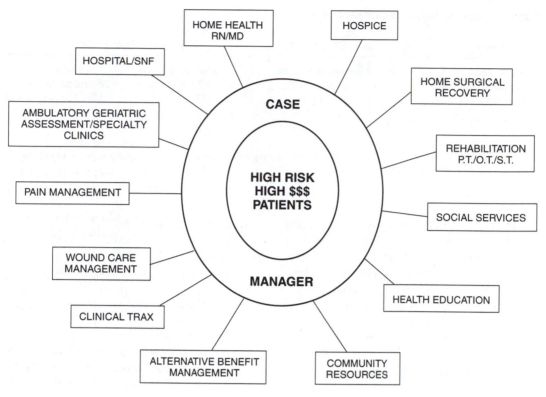

Figure 2. Case manager.

most insurers adopted this model with many insurance companies modeling their benefit plans to mirror Medicare and requiring Medicare-certified home care agencies to provide the care.

Multidisciplinary Core Team

—Core members
    Physician
    Nursing
    Pharmacist
    Social services
    Administrator
    Case manager
—Weekly conferences
—Ad hoc members may include:
    Acute care discharge planner
    Health education
    Member services
    Hospice

In the early stages of managed care the varieties of managed care plans (HMOs, IPAs, managed indemnity, preferred provider organizations [PPOs]) continued to follow suit. However, as managed care began to more closely examine home care cost/benefits, a new set of criteria for home care has emerged (see box, "Multidisciplinary Core Team").

The managed care organization's goal to provide the combination of services meeting the patient's needs at the lowest level of cost caused a revolutionary idea to take hold. Medicare services created in 1965 as a posthospital acute care benefit could not adequately meet the needs of a growing elderly population whose needs were heavily dominated by chronic long-term illnesses rather than short, acute episodes of care.

The new set of criteria for providing home care in a more mature managed care or insurance setting has become provision and payment for those services that are medically appropriate;

Table 2 Continuum of home care services*

Unskilled	Paraprofessional	Skilled	Highly skilled
Homemaker	Home health care aide	Nursing	Ventilators
Companion		PT	Premies
Board and care		OT	Mini-ICUs at home
		ST	
		SW	

*The goal is to use whatever combination of services best meets the patient's needs at the lowest level care and cost whether or not traditionally covered by Medicare.

cost-effective; safe; and accepted by the patient, physician, and family. This opened the door wider for services on both sides of the home care continuum: the unskilled or paraprofessional services and the high-technology services.

A few examples may serve to illustrate this point. FHP in 1992 created a benefit substitution model called "alternative health care." This model included time limited, prior-authorized services in a treatment plan that fell outside the member's covered benefits when they were more cost-effective than the covered benefit.

For example, an elderly patient might be able to receive intravenous (IV) antibiotics for pneumonia at home. This is known to be medically safe and appropriate. However, during the early days of the pneumonia the infection, fatigue, fever, and shortness of breath may necessitate that to be truly safe at home, someone would need to be with the patient, assist the patient to the commode, prepare meals, for example. Should this elderly person live with a caregiver who is at work 12 hours a day and is unable to be at home, other support systems, such as the registered nurse (RN)/home health aide (HHA) combination covered by Medicare, might not suffice. A 12-hour day unskilled companion (non-Medicare covered) could be reimbursed and taught by the nurse to call the agency should the IV infiltrate or other signs and symptoms of complications occur.

At this point the cost-benefit analysis would be done to determine the cost of a 12-hour day companion ($100) and one nursing visit ($70) as compared to the alternative of a hospital stay ($1,200) or a subacute day ($350) or a skilled nursing facility (SNF) day, if SNFs in the area do IVs. Dependent on this analysis and the family/physician considerations, the noncovered care might be substituted for the covered care.

It is clear to see in this example how the home care nurse's role has changed (see the box, "Expanded Home Care Versus Medicare Model"). He or she is responsible for coordinating with the discharge planner, family, and physician; performing the cost/benefit analysis; and providing supervision to a worker less skilled than Medicare would normally reimburse. The nurse also must determine at what point in time this "benefit substitution" should be terminated and a traditional 1- to 2-hour home health visit substituted.

In this paradigm the home care nurse is compelled to know more about health care financing, the family situation, and the supervision of unskilled workers and is able to pass the baton back

---

Expanded Home Care Versus Medicare Model

Medically appropriate
Safe
Cost-effective
Accepted by patient and family
Intermittent
Skilled
Homebound
Medically necessary

to the case manager to coordinate with the physician once home care will no longer be appropriate.

The focus of care becomes not merely the subacute period Medicare reimburses but extends prehospital and posthospital care and focuses more on the resolution of long-term problems, education, and prevention in concert with the case manager.

Hospice

Hospice case management has extended the "home care" role to encompass all settings of care (hospital, SNF, home, ECF, respite facility) and to assume responsibility in the management and coordination of care for the patient/family/ significant other as a unit of care. In this instance the role of the case manager becomes one of case finding for the hospice team so that patients are referred before the acutely dying, terminal phase and assisting with coordination of benefit plans, particularly in the instance of commercial patients where the "Medicare hospice benefit" is not part of the covered benefit.

Hospice nurse case management expands the role to holistically coordinate and plan for all aspects of the family unit of care, inclusive of medical, spiritual, financial, emotional, psychosocial, and environmental. It also extends through the bereavement program for 1 year after the death of the identified patient and may require care coordination with the case manager for those family members demonstrating pathologic grieving, somaticizing of their grief, or the need for social work interventions.

Hospice has received increasing acceptance outside the Medicare model due to its cost-effectiveness obtained primarily through the use of palliative care, abandonment of expensive and useless curative treatment, and substitution of a less costly locus of care (the home) in most instances. In addition, the humane holistic focus of hospice has led to wide acceptance by patients and families who may have clamored for curative measures causing only pain and suffering for their loved ones in the past.

Home visiting physician program

In compiling a menu of services needed to achieve the goal of appropriate care in the most cost-effective setting, it soon became clear that there were issues that could adequately be addressed only by physicians. This primarily was found to be in the situations where essentially homebound patients needed an assessment beyond the level of nursing scope of practice and subsequent intervention to prevent an emergency department (ED) visit and hospitalization.

Although many physicians are uncomfortable without the full armament of technologies available in the hospital, FHP found that good general internists with no more equipment than a portable electrocardiogram (ECG), portable blood chemistry equipment, Fax, pulse oximeter, and mobile radiograph machine could save significant hospital days for the majority of the frail, elderly homebound or chronically ill population.

An example could be the bedbound patient status post-cerebrovascular accident (CVA) developing upper respiratory congestion. A mobile radiograph determines the presence or absence of pneumonia and/or pleural effusion, the physician is able to assess the patient's full medical history and start, prescribe, and administer the first dose of antibiotics at home and return the case for follow-up to the home health nurse.

A second group of patients found to benefit from this program were the chronically truly homebound (ie, those meeting the Medicare definition of leaving home infrequently with very taxing effort), or bedbound. In this instance the physician or nurse practitioner could act as a primary care provider, seeing the patient for periodic assessment without the cost and risk associated with transport to a physician's office by gurney.

One anecdotal demonstration of this program's effectiveness was seen when one of the two full-time home visiting physicians called in sick. All five of the patients he had been scheduled to see that day were hospitalized primarily because they were acutely ill and were seen by physicians who did not know them and their history well enough to intervene at home.

Home surgical recovery

Another innovative program developed by the HMO to use in its arsenal of interventions developed from examining what types of surgical patients typically have 2- to 3-day hospital stays per surgical episode of care. A program was then developed to identify, educate, and manage these patients on a one-on-one basis to enable discharge home straight from the recovery room for 50% of the patients and after a very brief stay for the other 50%.

Both senior and commercial members (about 50–50) were included in this program after prescreening by their physician for comorbidities that might make such an approach unsafe.

The types of surgeries included are listed in Table 3. In this HMO's experience, the general surgery-mastectomy, laparoscopic cholecystectomy, and hysterectomy patients predominated. Given another environment (ie, other home health care agencies that have tried this approach) and group of physicians, however, there would also be enormous potential to genitourinary (GU), orthopaedic, and obstetric/gynecologic (OB/GYN) populations in such a program.

The program consists of:

- a preoperative visit when time allows (ie, the program is notified of the surgery sufficiently in advance);

Table 3 Types of surgical procedures appropriate for home recovery

Regional LOS*			
> 65 Senior	< 65 Commercial	Procedures	Home Recovery ALOS
2.5	2.6	Mastectomy (simple, modified radical, axillary node dissection)	O.P.**
2.8	2.8		
1.8	1.1	Ventral hernia repair, requiring drains or mesh	O.P.
2.1	2.0	Breast implants/tissue expanders	O.P.
2.1	2.0	Breast reconstruction reduction mammoplasty	O.P.
2.5	1.7	Laparoscopic cholecystectomy	O.P.
6.2		Anterior cruciate ligament (ACL) reconstruction	O.P.
2.6	2.0	Repair of rotator cuff	O.P.
1.2	2.3	Hand and wrist surgeries	O.P.
3.6	3.0	Open reduction internal fixation (ORIF) ankle, or wrist	O.P.
2.3	1.8	Acromioplasty-arthroplasty	O.P.
	3.8	Cesarean sections	48 hrs
4.0	3.5	Laproscopically assisted vaginal hysterectomy	23 hrs
4.3	4.0	Total abdominal hysterectomy (TAH)-bilateral sulpinooophorectomy (BSO)	48 hrs
3.2	2.6	Cystocele, Enterocele, and rectocele repair	24–48 hrs
2.1	2.0	Hemithyroidectomy	O.P.
2.6	2.6	Caldwell LUC procedures	O.P.
2.2	1.7	Podiatry cases, including drain removal within 24–48 hours	O.P.

*Average length of stay
**Outpatient

- meeting the patient in the recovery room and reviewing the operative and postoperative courses with the nurse and physician;
- returning home with the patient for usually 2 to 4 hours to teach family members pain control, symptom management, observation for complications, advance diet;
- the same nurse remaining on beeper or call for 24 hours for the patient;
- revisit in the morning and either transfer to home health care or continuation of intermittent visits until drains are removed and patient is returned to the outpatient setting.

It should be emphasized that these are not surgeries that would normally be done outpatient routinely but rather surgeries for which a 2- to 3-day hospital stay would have been, or already had been, authorized.

The complication rate in these patients in over 1,000 cases done is less than 1%, which is significantly lower than the complications seen in hospitalized patients, and patient/physician satisfaction typically is excellent.

Pharmacy case management

The pharmacist played a key role in the case management model. Drug interactions and adverse drug effects due to polypharmacy and the natural physiologic changes associated with the elderly are important case management considerations. Specific questions were asked as a part of the health screening process to identify members with potential pharmaceutical risks. These members were referred to the clinical pharmacist for a review of their medications. The pharmacist looked for potential interactions, drugs with high rates of adverse effects in the geriatric population, drugs that may be eliminated, and opportunities to substitute formulary drugs for nonformulary drugs. The pharmacist's recommendations were reviewed with the member's primary care physician and implemented if the physician was in agreement.

OUTCOMES

The case management program resulted in significant savings. Overall the program interventions saved $4 for every $1 in program costs. Most of the savings realized were the result of the use of home care to prevent or decrease the length of a hospital stay. The savings reported includes the cost of providing home care and other services. In addition, case management was effective in resolving the behaviors that caused entry into case management. In preliminary data analysis, case managers reported resolution rates of over 80% for the problems identified during case management. Case-managed patients spent fewer days in the hospital or SNF during and after case management intervention than prior to case management. Initial satisfaction surveys also provided positive results.

HOW TO FUND/REIMBURSE THE CASE MANAGEMENT/HOME HEALTH CARE MODEL

Even if one believes that an integrated home health care/case management model is optimal for patient care and clinical outcomes, how does one go about funding it?

An essential component of this answer is that the administrative arm of both disciplines must become proficient and knowledgeable regarding the various payment methodologies under managed care.

At this time neither Medicare nor Medicaid (except through state-approved waiver exception programs) is open to funding this type of model. As both are moving toward a managed care orientation through Medicare risk-sharing contracts, state operated or contracted managed care organizations, or simply prospective pay under a new hybrid model this will undoubtedly change. At this time, however, managed care organizations present the best opportunity to work with this model.

It is important to first identify the type of managed care organization providing service, as they span the spectrum, from (Table 4) man-

Table 4 The managed care continuum*

Managed indemnity and service plans	PPOs	POs	HMO IPA model	HMO staff model
Simple precertification of elective admissions Large case management of catastrophic cases Contractual relationship with providers	Selected group of participating Utilization management	Combination HMO & non-network care options Cost control through incentives	Provide a broad choice of physicians Require more effort toward utilization management due to physician independence Assumes risk for cost from HMO Manages care & cost	Great degree of control over utilization of health services Limited choice of employed participating physicians

*Moving from left to right on the continuum: (1) elements of control and accountability are added, (2) complexity and operational overheads are increased, and (3) potential for greater control of cost and quality is achieved.

aged indemnity through an exclusive provider organization.

At this time most managed care falls into the contracted network model (eg, PPO, IPA, physician hospital organization [PHO], Mixed Model). If services are paid on a discounted fee-for-service model, the goal is simply to negotiate appropriate rate structures for covered services, criteria for benefit substitution, and discounted rates for "substituted benefits."

The more complex models involve some form of capitation rate to one or all of the primary players, inclusive of the hospital, the physician group, and the HMO.

Some part of the delivery system may be capped, but typically the premium dollar (commercial or senior risk) is split into several funds varying in their percentages and services they cover. One very common model is to separate the premium into four or five funds. These include:

- Hospice fund: This fund is inclusive of acute care, transitional care, subacute care, SNF care, and facility-based charges for

services provided elsewhere as well as some specific hospital services. In many contracts, home health care, commercial hospital, home medical equipment, respiratory therapist, and home infusion come from this fund.

- Physician fund: This may be a capitation to primary care with a subcapitation to specialists or a capitated pool into which both primary care providers and specialists bill fee-for-service or some other arrangement (i.e., primary care is capped by specialists who are on a discounted fee-for-service). This fund is typically responsible for all professional services. It may include home health, hospice, HME, and home infusion but is less frequently structured to do so unless the physicians lobby for it and the hospital does not have its own agency.

- HMO fund: This fund is typically responsible for marketing, network development, oversight of quality management and utilization management. It is occasionally responsible for home health care, home infu-

sion, and durable medical equipment (DME).
- Ancillary services fund: This fund's responsibility may be shared by all parties and may include, in addition to such services as home health care; home infusion; and durable medical equipment (DME); the services of ambulance, orthotics, prosthetics, and the like.
- A home care services carve-out is inclusive of home health care, home infusion, DME, orthotics, and prosthetics.

Most typically seen are the first two alternatives. It is critical for the home health care agency/case management agency to know where the funding lies in order to prepare a marketing strategy. In all cases, the marketing strategy would focus on the reduction of acute inpatient days and SNF days if the physicians and hospitals are capitated. In these cases at least these two partners, and usually also the HMO, share in the "risk pool" for beddays, and if beddays decrease below contracted averages, money is returned proportional to contracted percentages to each group. For example, if Senior beddays per 1,000 members were below 1,300 by 150 beddays, then the 150 beddays would be multiplied by the hospital per diem rate (ie, $800) and the savings split 40% to physicians, 40% to the hospital, and 20% to the HMO.

The most highly incentivized group to aggressively utilize home health care is, therefore, the capitated hospital which gains from bringing in costs under the capitation and also from the percentage allocated from the shared bedday risk pool.

Physician groups who have been in managed care for a period of time and are more knowledgeable about the financing will also see the advantage of using the case management/home care model presented here. Newer physician groups may see that they are paying 100% of the case management/home health care costs and only receiving a percentage of the bedday savings. Actual numbers need to be put to these formulas to determine and demonstrate the cost benefit to these new physician groups.

While the hospital and the physician group may be capitated and the home health agency positions itself to market to the party with the fund responsibility, the issue of how the home health care agency will be paid must also be considered. The additional consideration of who funds the case management must also be discussed.

If a discounted fee-for-service structure for home health care is negotiated, the critical areas of consideration include actual costs/discipline, charges to Medicare, and percentage of discount to be offered, will a blended rate or a per discipline rate work best, should medical supplies be included in the visit rate and financial consideration as to payment terms and billing requirements.

If capitation is chosen, a past utilization history for the capitated group of members is necessary to appropriately set rates. If this is unavailable, a regional average of use by managed care payers for senior and commercial patients can be used with either risk corridors (ie, over X number of visits/month are paid fee-for-service) or stoploss provisions (ie, once a certain dollar amount is expended it reverts to fee-for-service). While managed care organizations do not tend to look favorably on these provisions, they are essential in an untested market. In addition, fee-for-service should be requested during low enrollment periods to guard against the risk of not being spread over an adequate number of enrollees.

Definition of terms also becomes essential in contracting. Will Medicare definitions be used? Will visits be limited to a certain number of hours or a certain number per day? How is home health defined? How are medical supplies defined and billed? The definitional section and/or amendment can be the key to success or failure in a capitation agreement.

The case management services may also be billed fee-for-service, per member, per month, or on a case-rate basis. Definitions of case management must be determined as to whether they will include screening and case finding or simply management of cases referred and who will be responsible to fund this? It is not unusual to see the HMO fund the service as part of its utilization management (UM) oversight with new plans to teach them UM techniques. As the plan matures, the HMO will typically attempt to transfer the responsibility to the medical group as it more completely delegates quality management (QM) and UM.

An integrated model of home care and case management such as the one presented in this article can present a win-win situation for all involved, both financially and in clinical outcomes and patient satisfaction.

REFERENCES

1. Pacala JT, Hepburn K, Kane R, Kane R. Case management in health maintenance organizations. Final report. In: *Chronic Care Initiates in HMOs*. Washington, DC: Group Health Foundation; 1994.

2. Entoven AC, Singer SA. Managed competition and California's health care economy. *Health Affairs*. 1996;15(1):47.

3. Case Management Society of America. *Standards of Practice for Case Management*. Little Rock, Ark: Case Management Society of America; 1995.

Tutorial: Causal Modeling and Patient Satisfaction

Dale N. Glaser and Barbara Riegel

Human behavior is infinitely complex and researchers have struggled for decades to find the best way of describing, explaining, and predicting actions. Inferential statistics such as analysis of variance may be helpful if, for example, the researcher is interested in determining how a certain treatment (e.g., medication) influences a particular outcome (e.g., blood pressure). Human behavior, however, is typically not so straightforward. In fact, any phenomenon becomes increasingly more interesting if other relevant factors are examined in concert. Such factors may include, but are not limited to: (1) psychological variables (e.g., locus of control, hardiness, perceived stress), (2) physiological factors (e.g., catecholamine levels), (3) behavioral factors (e.g., risky lifestyle), and (4) contextual variables (e.g., time of day or work reporting relationships).

Causal modeling is a statistical technique for examining models in which several variables are considered simultaneously. The purpose of this article is to introduce the concept, the technique, and the interpretation of causal modeling to the new user. In other words, this article is an introductory primer to causal modeling. As a way of demonstrating its usefulness, the technique is applied to health care and issues of quality. A model of patient satisfaction is hypothesized and tested using a combination of hypothetical and actual data.

Quality Management in Health Care 1996; 5(1): 49–58
© 1996 Aspen Publishers, Inc.

Structural equation modeling (causal modeling) is a relatively new technique that has generated a great deal of interest because of its capacity to explore problematic or mathematically impossible puzzles. Structural equation models are simply theoretical models of relationships among variables.[1] In the past, researchers interested in testing multiple relationships might have used one of two related techniques: regression analysis or path analysis. Regression analysis and path analysis are related techniques, as both use correlational data. Regression analysis is a technique that uses categorical or continuous level variables to predict a single outcome variable.[2] Generally, this technique involves the entry of a select number of predictor variables that are thought to be possible predictors of the outcome.

If the investigator has an actual model in mind, path analysis might be used. Path analysis can only be used if the model progresses in a linear, sequential fashion (e.g., one variable causing another). Path analysis is a method for studying the direct and indirect effects of variables thought to cause subsequent variables. Of course, once the factor preceding a variable is identified, then the variable itself becomes an outcome or an effect.[3]

Both regression analysis and path analysis have significant limitations. In regression analysis, a single variable must be chosen as the outcome. As described above, it is easy for any budding theorist to postulate a variety of causes and levels of outcomes. In fact, it is far more difficult to identify a single outcome variable. In path analysis, each relationship must be assumed to progress in a linear fashion, a commonly untenable assumption in everyday life.

Causal modeling allows one to test models with multiple outcome variables and those in which relationships are thought to go in both directions. For example, social support has been shown to decrease emotional stress.[4] But emotional distress has also been shown to decrease social support. Because causal modeling is so useful in mimicking reality, it has been used widely in the sciences (e.g., economics, psychology, sociology, nursing, behavioral medicine). Several recent publications have used this method to investigate group success or failure and its effect on job satisfaction and organizational commitment[5]; consumer satisfaction and perceived quality[6]; participative decision making and job-related strain[7]; job performance, job satisfaction, and turnover[8]; and organizational characteristics, perceived work stress, and depression.[9]

CAUSALITY

It is not the intention of this article to clarify the reasoning behind the term *causal* or the controversy that surrounds the use of the term. As James, Mulaik, and Brett point out in their classic text, *Causal Analysis: Assumptions, Models, and Data,* "Causality is a complex topic, beset by controversy because of metaphysical and epistemological differences among philosophers of science."[10(p.13)] One of the major arguments against presumptions of causality when employing such techniques is that any technique using correlational data cannot aspire to causality. Mulaik counters that argument with this:

These experimentalists claim everyone knows (or should know) that correlation does not imply causation. We may say in rebuttal that, whereas correlation does not imply causation, it is also true that causation implies correlation. It is this which makes the testing of hypotheses about causation possible with correlational data.[11(p.23)]

Whether one views causality as a product of "functional relations,"[10] "probabilistic causality,"[11] or "deterministic relations,"[12] the prevailing notion is that (1) causal analysis is contingent on assumptions about causal direction and (2) these assumptions are empirically or data based. The last point is critical. Guided by prior research and empirical data, the researcher develops and tests a model that specifies causal direction. Hayduk argues that social scientists typically think of one thing as influencing another and there is no reason to abandon causal statements.[1]

TERMINOLOGY

The reader of publications using causal-modeling techniques must become familiar with a new language unique to these applications. That language will be taught using an example drawn from a hypothesized model (Figure 1) of patient satisfaction. The model, based on dummy data, is for illustrative purposes only.

The initial step in applying causal modeling is to develop a *model* that delineates specific relationships among a host of interrelated variables. It is important that the model be empirically based, as causal modeling is ideally a technique for confirming a theory. The validity of the model is reinforced through the inclusion of prior research in which the proposed relationship or relationships were demonstrated. For example, in the development of the consumer satisfaction or perceived quality model, Gotlieb and colleagues investigated a variety of relationships (e.g., between perceived situational control and satisfaction and between expectations and satisfaction) for the purpose of establishing an empirical foundation for their hypothesized model.[6]

Causal modeling can be used in an exploratory manner, however. If a researcher is investigating an area with little empirical verification, he or she can develop a model based on hypothesized relationships among the model variables. In this case, experience and observation would guide model development instead of theoretical evidence. The model shown in Figure 1 is an exploratory model.

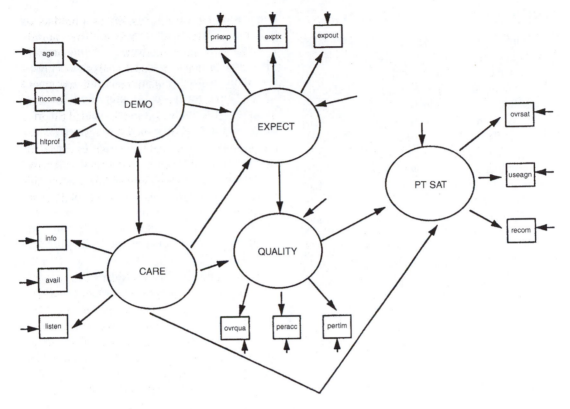

Figure 1. Patient satisfaction model.

Causal modeling involves the analysis of *latent variables.* Latent variables are pure unidimensional concepts or constructs.[12] Such variables typically vary in their degree of abstraction. For example, "emotion," a variable often studied by psychologists, is an abstract construct that requires definition and operationalization before it can be used in a causal model. However, a latent variable such as "economic status" may be more easily used in a causal model.

LATENT VARIABLES

Latent variables can be characterized as *exogenous* and *endogenous.* If a variable has a cause that lies outside of the model (i.e., the variable acts as a cause and not as an effect), it is described as exogenous.[1,12] In the model shown in Figure 1, demographics (DEMO) and care re-

ceived (CARE) are the exogenous variables. We acknowledge that there may be factors that cause or influence the exogenous factors in this patient satisfaction model. However, as this model is solely exploratory and pedagogical in nature, we will call these two variables exogenous.

Endogenous latent variables are those that are hypothesized to be determined or caused by variables within the model (i.e., directly caused or influenced by any of the other variables).[1,12] Patient expectations (EXPECT), perceived quality of services (QUALITY), and patient satisfaction (PTSAT) are the endogenous variables in this model. Arrows in the model specify our hypotheses about which variables are causing other latent variables. An endogenous variable may also influence another endogenous variable in the model. The relationship between patient expectations and perceived quality of services is a causal relationship between two endogenous variables.

MATRICES

The intent of this article is to serve as a primer rather than a mathematical treatise, so the mathematical process for arriving at the structural equations is not discussed. The reader interested in understanding the calculations derived from matrix algebra is referred elsewhere.[1,12,13] Older versions of commonly used statistical packages for structural equation modeling like Lisrel[14] required an understanding of matrix algebra and Greek notation, but such knowledge is no longer essential. There is now a command language developed by the authors of Lisrel called SIMPLIS[15] that is more user friendly. Other programs, such as EQS,[16] were marketed originally without the need for knowledge of Greek notation. One only needs to know the name of the variables to test relationships. However, a cursory review of the literature and the Internet site devoted to structural equation modeling (SEMNET) demonstrates that quite a few researchers still refer to the matrices by their Greek notation.

THE STRUCTURAL MODEL

The structural equation for the latent variables involves the relationships among the concepts. Specifically, these relationships include the (1) relationships between the exogenous and endogenous factors (e.g., DEMO → EXPECT) and (2) relationships between the endogenous factors (e.g., EXPECT → QUALITY). An error variable is associated with each of the endogenous concepts and represents the latent error in the equation. The latent error, analogous to the residual term in regression, takes into account that there is usually some measurement error involved in the development and testing of a model. This error is represented in the model by the lone arrow leading to the endogenous variables (e.g., QUALITY).

THE MEASUREMENT MODEL

Besides the structural (latent variable) model, one calculates a *measurement model*. As Figure 1 illustrates, the latent variables, even though conceptual in nature, are operationalized by what can be termed *observed variables, manifest variables, measures, proxies,* or *indicators.*[12] These indicators are variables that actually measure the construct. For instance, the exogenous factor "care received" is measured by three items: (1) information communicated by nurses (info), (2) availability of the caregiver (avail), and (3) nurse took time to listen (listen). The causal model can be tested with indicators that are single items, as in this case, or with scale scores derived from multiple items (e.g., a 10-item job satisfaction scale). What is crucial is that the items display sufficient reliability and validity. Structural equation modeling statistical packages (e.g., Lisrel) can be used to assess the construct validity of the indicators.[17]

Construct validity is evident when either *convergent validity* or *discriminant validity* are evident. Evidence of convergent validity exists when there is overlap (i.e., correlation) of items on two measures of the same construct (e.g., two separate intelligence tests). Discriminant validity is evident when two tests that measure separate constructs are poorly correlated (e.g., a scale measuring job satisfaction should have a relatively low correlation with another scale measuring anxiety). Thus, the measurement model is used to demonstrate the relationship between the measured indicators and the conceptual latent variable. In the measurement model example, the relationships between the endogenous factors (e.g., patient expectations, perceived quality of services, and patient satisfaction) and their indicators (e.g., priexp, ovrqua, useagn) are shown.

As depicted in the model, each of the indicators has a lone arrow leading toward it. These arrows represent the error associated with the latent variable–indicator relationship. Such errors may be due to measurement flaws (e.g., imperfect reliability), inappropriate specification of the concept–indicator (or concept–concept) relationship, or omission of relevant variables in the overall model. Omissions frequently arise during the course of model development. Given the complexity of human behavior, it is an insurmountable task to arrive at a truly comprehensive model that considers all possible behaviors or variables. But leaving out a variable that is potentially a common cause of two other factors may result in spurious findings. An error such as this is a common violation of the underlying mathematical assumption that errors are not correlated.

PROCEDURE

Once the investigator has sufficiently prepared a model, chosen valid and reliable indicators, and gathered data, he or she is prepared to test the model. The model is tested by estimating the coefficients and testing the goodness of fit of the hypothesized model to the data. Estimation is a product of the hypothesized relationships. For instance, in the example, care received is thought to have both a direct effect and an indirect effect (mediated by perceived quality of services) on patient satisfaction. Patient expectations (EXPECT) are also hypothesized to have an effect on patient satisfaction as mediated by perceived quality of services. The argument could be made that patient expectations may also have a direct effect on patient satisfaction.

Even though theory, common sense, and especially parsimony should drive the development of the model, statistical programs afford the opportunity to test variations of the model in an effort to arrive at the one that fits best. Best fit is arrived at by estimating the fit of the hypothesized model to the actual data. Model fit is tested by a likelihood-ratio chi-square statistic (χ^2).

When developing the model and testing its fit to the data, the advantages of causal modeling over other traditional techniques (e.g., regression analysis) become apparent: (1) solutions for models with multiple indicators can be generated, (2) latent variables can be introduced, (3) estimates of errors of measurement can be entered into the model (e.g., a scale with a reliability coefficient $\alpha = .83$ has an error of .17 that can be entered into the model), and (4) bidirectionality can be assessed (quality causing expectations *and* expectations causing qual-

ity).[18] A distinct advantage of causal modeling is its ability to simultaneously analyze all the factors pertinent to the model (in contrast, path analysis needs to be conducted in a step-by-step, linear fashion).

The data analyzed using structural equation modeling is usually composed of covariance or correlation matrices. (For a discussion of the use of correlations when using covariance structure modeling, see Cudeck[19].) In this example, the correlation coefficient was used as the unit of analysis, even though there are some experts who argue that covariances are more appropriate given that (1) the measured construct is maintained in its original metric and (2) correlations may result in imprecise estimates of the population variances and covariances.[12] However, the use of actual and fictitious data in this article made it problematic to derive comparable covariances. Table 1 provides the correlation matrix that was analyzed and also the syntax used for SIMPLIS (i.e., analysis with Lisrel).

DESCRIPTION OF SYNTAX

The SIMPLIS language allows the researcher the option of using the actual variable name when writing the statistical commands rather than requiring familiarity with Greek notation. This convenience makes structural equation modeling more intelligible to the new user. However, a fundamental understanding of matrix algebra can be especially fruitful when error messages arise, some of which border on the arcane. Alternatively, texts by Hayduk[1] and Bollen[13] may help the new user understand various error messages.

The "observed variables" mentioned in the first line of the command structure (Table 1) are the "indicator variables." Recall that indicator variables are those items or scales actually measured and attributed to the latent variables. A "correlation matrix" is identified as the mathematical unit of analysis. The correlation matrix is then entered into the program triangularly with a designated sample size of 200 to be analyzed. The "latent variables" are the hypothetical

Table 1 Syntax and Correlation Matrix for Patient Satisfaction Data

Observed Variables 'age' 'income' 'hlthprof' 'priorexp' 'exptx' 'expout' 'info' 'avail' 'listen' 'overqual' 'percacc' 'perctime' 'oversat' 'useagain' 'recommen'
correlation matrix

```
1.0
.42  1.0
.33  .52  1.0
.27  .22  .27  1.0
.35  .17  .22  .37  1.0
.29  .07  .14  .42  .48  1.0
.23  .22  .07  .23  .23  .19  1.0
.26  .13  .12  .22  .17  .08  .51  1.0
.25  .16  .22  .18  .19  .22  .44  .50  1.0
.35  .18  .13  .14  .21  .21  .25  .29  .32  1.0
.34  .21  .12  .18  .22  .17  .27  .32  .28  .52  1.0
.33  .23  .22  .13  .17  .16  .26  .33  .29  .62  .65  1.0
.28  .14  .21  .24  .21  .22  .51  .33  .63  .44  .43  .33  1.0
.27  .16  .23  .26  .22  .23  .33  .20  .36  .37  .38  .35  .45  1.0
.26  .18  .24  .29  .18  .22  .33  .33  .52  .35  .32  .36  .58  .65  1.0
```

Note: Sample size = 200.
Latent Variables 'DEMO' 'EXPECT' 'CARE' 'QUALITY' 'PTSAT'
Relationships
'age'=1*'DEMO'
'income'-'hlthprof'='DEMO'
'priorexp'=1*'EXPECT'
'exptx'-'expout'='EXPECT'
'info'=1*'CARE'
'avail'-'listen'='CARE'
'overqual'=1*'QUALITY'
'percacc'-'perctime'='QUALITY'
'oversat'=1*'PTSAT'
'useagain'-'recommen'='PTSAT'
'EXPECT'='DEMO' 'CARE'
'QUALITY'='EXPECT' 'CARE'
'PTSAT'='QUALITY' 'CARE'
Path Diagram
End of problem

constructs. The "relationships" are the linkages between (1) the indicator variables and the latent variables (e.g., income – hlthprof = DEMO) and (2) the relationships between the latent variables (e.g., EXPECT = DEMO CARE). The reader will notice that for each latent variable one of the indicator variables is multiplied by 1 (e.g., age = 1* DEMO). This notation serves to assign a unit of measurement for each latent variable, thus standardizing the measurement process. That is, the unit of measurement in each latent variable equals its population standard deviation. For more information on the SIMPLIS language, see Joreskog and Sorbom.[15] Finally, "path diagram" is entered in the syntax; this recent addition to the Lisrel program provides the user with visual illustrations of the structural model, measurement model, t-values, and modification indices (to be discussed).

Once the syntax is established, the data can be analyzed to assess how well the model fits the data. It is important to emphasize that model development is based on theory, prior research, and observation and carries with it inevitable measurement or specification error. Furthermore, even if an adequate fit of the model is achieved, there may be alternate models or relationships. As Anderson and Gerbing[20] point out, models are never confirmed by data; they are supported or fail to be disconfirmed. Although a given model may fit the data well, other acceptable models may exist.

Generally, a two-step process of analysis is recommended. First the measurement model is tested and then the structural model is tested. Testing of the measurement model involves determining the fit of the indicators with the latent conceptual variables. No relationships between the latent variables are identified at this time. Testing of the structural model involves determining how well the entire model fits the data, including the relationships between the latent variables. It is interesting to note that when test-

ing the measurement model (both for the exogenous and endogenous latent variables), one may actually be performing a confirmatory factor analysis. For example, we have hypothesized that age, income, and health profile best describe the latent variable demographics (DEMO). We can then test this a priori relationship by conducting a confirmatory factor analysis and thereby determine the fit of the indicators to the latent variable. Confirmatory factor analysis is a crucial step in that it establishes the psychometric properties (i.e., reliability and validity) of the constructs.

RESULTS

Figure 2 provides the results of the Lisrel (parameter) estimates for the full model. These re-

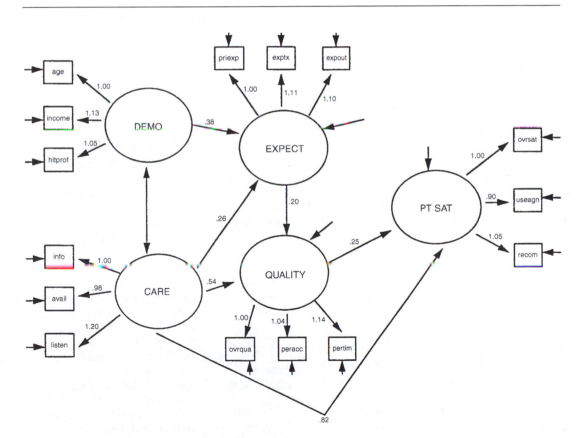

Figure 2. Patient satisfaction model with parameter estimates.

sults are similar to regression coefficients. The significance of each parameter estimate is then tested using a t-test. Parameter estimates include estimates of the relationships between the latent variables and the indicator variables and the relationships between the various latent variables.

Initially, a confirmatory factor analysis was conducted to assess the strength of the measurement model (i.e., relationship between the latent variables and their indicators). Separate estimates were made of the (1) exogenous factors (DEMO and CARE) and their measures and (2) endogenous factors (EXPECT, QUALITY, and PTSAT) and their respective indicators. For the exogenous factors, R^2 was determined for each of the indicators. This statistic indicates the strength of the relationship between the latent variable and the specific scale or item. "Income" had the largest relationship with the demographics construct ($R^2 = .60$) whereas "availability of caregiver" had the largest relationship with the "care received" construct ($R^2 = .55$). All of the indicators had significant t-values (.05 level of significance), indicating that each of the indicator variables was a significant estimate of its respective latent variable. For the endogenous latent variables, expectation of outcome (expout) had the largest relationship with patient expectations (EXPECT) ($R^2 = .51$), perception of timeliness of services (perctime) had the largest relationship with perceived quality of services (QUALITY) ($R^2 = .71$), and likelihood of recommending services (recommen) had the largest relationship with patient satisfaction (PTSAT) ($R^2 = .71$). All of the indicators had significant t-values (.05 level of significance).

GOODNESS OF FIT

Final analysis of the model involves determining how well the model fits the data. Does the model depicting patient satisfaction adequately fit the sample data? Part of the answer lies in the chi-square statistic (χ^2). This nonparametric statistic (normal distribution is not assumed) is employed to assess "goodness of fit."

As opposed to convention, in this application a *nonsignificant* result (i.e., $p > .05$) is desired. One hopes that the hypothesized model does not drastically differ from the actual data. This statistic is fitted for each of the measurement models as well as the full conceptual model (i.e., all latent variables, exogenous and endogenous, and their indicators).

The chi-square was significant ($p = .018$) for the exogenous factors (the measurement model for DEMO and CARE), indicating that the model for these factors differed significantly from the data. However, chi-square statistics are notoriously sensitive to differences when sample sizes are large (approximately 200 and more). Thus, it is not unusual to scan the litera-

Table 2 List of Latent and Observed Variables

Latent Variable	Observed Variable
DEMO (demographics)	age income hlthprof (health profile)
CARE (care received)	info (information communicated by nurse) avail (availability of caregiver) listen (nurse took time to listen)
EXPECT (patient expectations)	priorexp (overall expectation) exptx (expectations based on prior treatment) expout (expectation of outcome)
QUALITY (perceived quality of services)	overqual (overall perception of quality) percacc (perception of accuracy/effectiveness) perctime (perception of timeliness of services)
PTSAT (patient satisfaction)	oversat (overall satisfaction with experience) useagain (likelihood would use services again) recommen (likelihood would recommend services)

ture and find significant differences between the model and the data and yet have a desirable *fit.* This discrepancy occurs when the goodness-of-fit measures are calculated.

The Lisrel printout supplies an abundance of fit measures; the choice of which to use is contingent on sample size, change in number of parameter estimates, and whether the researcher is comparing alternative or nested models. The one most frequently cited is the goodness of fit index (GFI). Even though there is not broad consensus as to what exactly determines a good fit, generally if the index is at or above .90 an acceptable fit of the model to the data has been achieved. For the measurement model of the exogenous factors, the GFI was .97. This result suggests a good fit of the model to the data in spite of the fact that the chi-square statistic was significant. The chi-square was also significant ($p = .026$) for the endogenous factors, but the GFI was .96. It appears that the latent constructs are adequately measured by their indicators.

MODIFICATION TO THE MODEL

The Lisrel printout also provides *modification indices.* If there were problems with the measurement model, for instance, and the item measuring health profile (hlthprof) was found to be more highly correlated with the conceptual variable care received (CARE) than its hypothesized construct demographics (DEMO), then the modification index will indicate this. The modification indices provide an estimate of the decrease in chi-square (keeping in mind that a low chi-square is desired as nonsignificance is sought) that would be achieved if you estimate the new relationship: CARE $\rightarrow$ hlthprofile. However, it is crucial to keep in mind that any modification made to the model must make theoretical and intuitive sense and not be based simply on the statistical output. It does not make sense to arbitrarily modify the model to achieve a decrease in chi-square if the change evolves into a nonsensical morass. Any change in the model, especially if it is data driven, must make sense.

Subsequently, the full structural equation model is tested. For the hypothesized sample model, all of the estimates were significant, with the exception of the path leading from EXPECT to QUALITY (estimate = .20, $t = 1.58$). This finding implies that the hypothesized model needs to be reconsidered, at least the EXPECT–QUALITY relationship needs further thought. As one wants to modify the model based on theory and prior empirical data, such a suggestion may require a literature search or discussions with colleagues.

• • •

The objective of this article was to provide a brief summary of causal modeling and its potential application to patient satisfaction data. The increased popularity of structural equation modeling is indicated by the recent increase in publications based on the technique. But experts caution about the potential abuse associated with this statistical tool.[21] The wholesale employment of modeling applications like causal modeling may be problematic when researchers violate requirements like adequacy of measures, knowledge of structural relations, or theoretically driven models for testing.[21]

Computer software that is easy to use, like SIMPLIS, allows even the unsophisticated user to test models. Just because the technique is new and enticing should not lead researchers to use it when a technique like regression analysis would be sufficient, however. Ultimately, it should be the design and methodology (e.g., data collection, sampling, etc.) that drives the choice of analytic technique. When appropriate, modeling applications make a significant contribution to investigators interested in understanding multifactorial, interweaving, bidirectional relationships. Health care is rife with such relationships, and thus causal modeling would seem likely to be a powerful tool for exploring phenomena such as patient satisfaction with health care.

REFERENCES

1. Hayduk, L.A. *Structural Equation Modeling with LISREL*. Baltimore, Md.: Johns Hopkins University Press, 1987.

2. Cohen, J., and Cohen, P. *Applied Multiple Regression/Correlation Analysis for the Behavioral Sciences*. 2nd ed. Hillsdale, N.J.: Erlbaum, 1983.

3. Pedhazur, E.J. *Multiple Regression in Behavioral Research*. 2nd ed. Fort Worth, Tex.: Holt, Rinehart, and Winston, 1982.

4. Fiore, J., Becker, J., and Coppel, D.B. "Social Network Interactions: A Buffer or a Stress?" *American Journal of Community Psychology* 11 (1983): 423–39.

5. Riggs, M.L., and Knight, P.A. "The Impact of Perceived Group Success-Failure on Motivational Beliefs and Attitudes: A Causal Model." *Journal of Applied Psychology* 79 (1994): 755–66.

6. Gotlieb, J.B., Grewal, D., and Brown, S.W. "Consumer Satisfaction and Perceived Quality: Complementary or Divergent Constructs?" *Journal of Applied Psychology* 79 (1994): 875–85.

7. Jackson, S.E. "Participation in Decision Making as a Strategy for Reducing Job-related Strain." *Journal of Applied Psychology* 68 (1983): 3–19.

8. Birnbaum, D., and Somers, M.J. "Fitting Job Performance into Turnover Model: An Examination of the Form of the Job Performance–Turnover Relationship and a Path Model." *Journal of Management* 19, no. 1 (1993): 1–11.

9. Revicki, D.A., Whitley, T.W., and Gallery, M.E. "Organizational Characteristics, Perceived Work Stress, and Depression in Emergency Medicine Residents." *Behavioral Medicine* 19 (1993): 74–81.

10. James, L.R., Mulaik, S.A., and Brett, J.M. *Causal Analysis: Assumptions, Models, and Data*. Beverly Hills, Calif.: Sage Publications, 1983.

11. Mulaik, S.A. "Toward a Conception of Causality Applicable to Experimentation and Causal Modeling." *Child Development* 58 (1987): 18–32.

12. Bollen, K. A. *Structural Equations with Latent Variables*. New York, N.Y.: Wiley, 1989.

13. Stevens, J. *Applied Multivariate Statistics for the Social Sciences*. 2nd ed. Hillsdale, N.J.: Erlbaum, 1992.

14. Joreskog, K.G., and Sorbom, D. *Lisrel 8 User's Reference Guide*. Chicago, Ill.: Scientific Software International, 1993.

15. Joreskog, K.G., and Sorbom, D. *Lisrel 8: Structural Equation Modeling with the SIMPLIS Command Language*. Chicago, Ill.: Scientific Software International, 1993.

16. Bentler, P.M. *EQS: Structural Equations Program Manual*. Los Angeles, Calif.: BMDP, 1989.

17. Widaman, K.F. "Hierarchically Nested Covariance Structure Models for Multitrait-Multimethod Data." *Applied Psychological Measurement* 9, no. 1 (1985): 1–26.

18. Biddle, B.J., and Marlin, M.M. "Causality, Confirmation, Credulity, and Structural Equation Modeling." *Child Development* 58 (1987): 4–17.

19. Cudeck, R. "Analysis of Correlation Matrices Using Covariance Structure Models." *Psychological Bulletin* 105, no. 1 (1989): 317–27.

20. Anderson, J.C., and Gerbing, D.W. "Structural Equation Modeling in Practice: A Review and Recommended Two-Step Approach." *Psychological Bulletin* 103, no. 3 (1988): 411–423.

21. Brannick, M.T. "Critical Comments on Applying Covariance Structure Modeling." *Journal of Organizational Behavior* 16 (1995): 201–13.

Comprehensive Case Management: Implications for Program Managers

L. Michele Issel

As health care organizations seek ways to provide the least costly service to low income, high-risk patients, the use of comprehensive case management may increase. Case management by registered nurses and allied health professionals, such as social workers, can help control health care expenditures for this type of patient and contribute to improved patient outcomes. Comprehensive case management has been provided for some time by health care organizations in the public sector to outpatients that are both low income and high risk. The organizations' experiences with comprehensive case management can be used to identify ways to better design and manage the program delivery to low-income, high-risk outpatients receiving services in other types of health care organizations.

BACKGROUND

Case management

Despite the growing belief that case management began in 1987, nursing case management has its roots in public health and district nursing, in which the nurse was responsible for the general welfare of patients.[1,2] This early form of case management that required attention to patients' medical and social conditions is today called comprehensive, advanced, and medical-social case management.[3–5] Comprehensive case management differs substantively from the form of case management used in conjunction with clinical or critical paths. While both forms share key elements of monitoring the utilization of services, of coordinating services so that the least costly services are utilized, and of collaboration among health professionals,[6] an additional key element of comprehensive case management is developing trust and support between case managers (CMs) and clients.[5]

Comprehensive case management is a highly complex task, not amenable to the use of critical or clinical paths for two reasons. First, patient problems addressed by a CM are numerous and extremely varied. For example, in the caseload of one CM, there may be a patient who requires assistance in gaining access to a primary care physician, assistance with transportation to prenatal visits, and referral to a substance abuse program, while another patient requires encouragement to stay in high school and needs a referral to a domestic violence shelter. Second, patient problems encountered by CMs require

This article was supported in part by NIH, BRSG, NSS, RR0057991 and the Ed and Molly Smith Centennial Fellowship. Paper was presented at the Sixth National Conference on Nursing Administration Research, St. Paul, Minnesota. Special thanks to the participants for providing interviews and insights into their work, and to David Kahn for comments on previous drafts.

Health Care Superv 1997; 15(3): 39–50

personalized and tailored interventions to affect a change in the medical and social risks experienced by patients. This highly complex and uncertain nature of comprehensive case management has implications for the management of the program. However, little is known about what CMs experience as problems in doing their work.

Studies of comprehensive case management programs provide few clues about how to improve management in order to achieve greater efficiency and effectiveness. This information is important, given that the extent to which the effects of case management might be increased by better management is unknown. Also, most case management studies focus on individual patients and their outcomes, including studies of prenatal case management.[7–9] Thus, the extent to which organizational or managerial factors affect the case management program and patient outcomes is unknown. To begin to address these and similar questions, research is first needed that describes what CMs experience as employees of a comprehensive case management program.

One population that has been case managed by nurses is high-risk pregnant women.[7–9] This population has received comprehensive, outpatient case management that is reimbursed by Medicaid. The potential to receive Medicaid reimbursement has made comprehensive case management of this population financially more attractive and thus more widespread. The elements of comprehensive case management described above are consistent with the Medicaid guidelines for providing reimbursable comprehensive case management services to high-risk pregnant women. Thus, comprehensive case management of high-risk pregnant women can be used as an exemplar of managerial and program issues facing other comprehensive case management programs of high-risk outpatients.

Conceptual framework

Issel developed a model of case management, consisting of patient, CM, program, organization, and community levels of analysis (see Figure 1).[10] The model is grounded in organizational and ecological theories.[11,12] Each level in the model can be analyzed or managed and is affected by factors from other levels. The model shows that community factors such as state regulations, reimbursement constraints from other organizations, and availability of local health and human service organizations can affect health care organizations. In turn, organizational factors such as organizational goals, resources, design, and structure affect case management programs. Both the case management program and characteristics of patients affect the decisions CMs make regarding the use of interventions with patients. Figure 1 shows these relationships among the levels and includes variables derived from findings in this study relevant to a particular level.

STUDY DESCRIPTION

In the study presented here, the CM is the focus of attention, but factors from other levels that affect CMs are identified. The purpose of this study was to identify factors and forces that affect CMs in doing case management. The research question was what factors are perceived by the CM as affecting their ability to do case management.

METHODS

Design

This study was part of a descriptive study of prenatal Medicaid case management programs in Texas, using a purposive sample of CMs. Data obtained from semi-structured interviews conducted with CMs in two local health departments are the focus of this article. The participating organizations were selected to increase the diversity in the sample; the two local health departments represent a mix of rural and urban populations, different lengths of time since implementing case management, and different approaches to implementing case management.

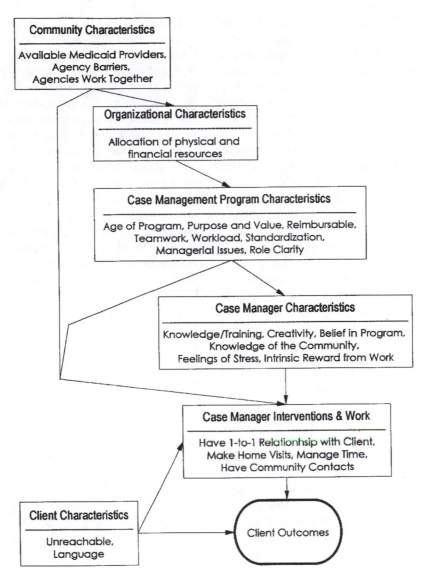

Figure 1. Model of case management with variables derived from current study.

Sample

All staff directly involved in providing comprehensive case management services were invited to participate in semi-structured audio tape–recorded interviews conducted at each site and at the convenience of the participants. Twenty-two participants were interviewed; 13 were from Site 1 and 9 from Site 2, for an overall participation rate of 89 percent.

Each site had a different approach to implementing comprehensive case management. Site 1, with four outpatient clinic sites and over two years of experience with case management, used a team approach to case management, exemplified by weekly meetings with all staff discussing current cases. CMs were either registered nurses (RNs) or social workers. Case management aides assisted CMs in some case management activities. CMs and case management aides jointly followed cases throughout the pregnancy and maintained contact with patients during clinic visits or by telephone. In contrast, Site 2 had only one outpatient clinic and one year of case management experience. CMs were RNs, with the case management aides assigned to each case working with the RN. RNs delegated activities to the case management aides who maintained contact with patients throughout the pregnancy by telephone or home visits. However, case management aides at Site 2 were supervised by the social worker.

Participants included public health nurses, social workers, nurse managers, clinical nurse specialists, and case management aides. The average age of participants was 41 years. Most participants had a baccalaureate degree (41 percent), although 77 percent of participants at Site 1 had a baccalaureate or master's degree compared with 57 percent of participants at Site 2. Participants at Site 1 had been in their current position for an average of 2.1 years and participants at Site 2 had been in their current position for 4.0 years. The average size of the caseload was 33 clients at Site 1 and 29 clients at Site 2. There were no statistical differences between sites with regard to the amount of time participants spent doing case management or the size of their caseload. There was no significant difference between RNs and social workers in educational level or length of time in their position.

Methods

The qualitative method, ethnographic content analysis, enabled the creation of a description of issues involved in doing case management without relying on existing notions of managerial practice or norms.[13,14] Ethnographic content analysis combines semantic content analysis with the ethnographic focus on the meaning of what is said. This method accommodates existing knowledge, specifically allowing for the use

of levels as specified in the model of case management. It also allows for further theory development, specifically through the development of new categories to be incorporated into existing theory.

The interview included open-ended questions that referred to the comprehensive case management of pregnant clients. Included in this study are responses to the questions "What barriers, problems, or issues have you experienced in doing case management" and "Tell me about your case management program." Probes were used to clarify statements and elicit additional information regarding actions taken by participants. Because of the open-ended nature of the interview, statements from throughout the full interview were included in the analysis if the data related to doing the work of case management or management of the program. During visits to each site, interviews were conducted in private offices of participants. Prior to the audio tape–recorded interview, study procedures were explained, participants signed an informed consent form and completed a demographics questionnaire.

Analysis

Interviews were transcribed verbatim and checked for accuracy. Any statement in the interview that described problems or issues was bracketed as a unit of data for analysis. Based on the manifest meaning of statements, initial categories of problems experienced by participants were developed by comparing each new statement to statements already in the category, and a new category was developed when a statement was not similar to a statement within an existing category. Category refinement consisted of constant comparison based on manifest meaning. The final set of categories thus reflects participants' perspective of doing the work of case management. Upon reflection of the model of case management, the final set of categories appeared to group into the levels of analysis, namely patient, CM, program, and community.

Validity was assured by using the manifest meaning of statements and by not forcing data to fit into predetermined categories; rather categories were revised to reflect the interview data. Reliability of the final categories was assured by establishing interrater reliability of coding the statements using 20 percent of statements randomly selected from the total set of data. Three nurse experts who received no special training in coding or the category definitions of statements achieved 70 percent agreement in independently coding the statements.

RESULTS

Although participants answered a specific interview question about problems in doing case management, they also spoke of solutions to the problems and their perceptions about case management. Categories in each of these areas readily grouped into the levels in the model of case management based on a manifest reference to patients, CMs, program, or community. Table 1 categorizes both problem and solution categories.

Problems

Participants talked about difficulties related to clients being unreachable and language barriers. Some clients had no telephones, others moved without forwarding addresses, and others were receiving prenatal care from private providers and therefore were not readily accessible during prenatal visits at the clinic. Language was an issue, given the large portion of Spanish-speaking clients. These were client level problems.

Participants also talked of problems related to themselves and their peers. Problems included a general lack of knowledge about case management and ways to affect or interact with clients,

Table 1. Number and percentage of participants who mentioned each problem and solution category (n = 22)

Level	Problem categories	n (%)
Client	Client unreachable	9 (41)
	Language barrier with client	4 (18)
CM	Not enough knowledge/training	8 (36)
	Don't know the community	4 (18)
	Personal discomforts	3 (14)
Program	Things pull away from case management	19 (86)
	Managerial problems	7 (33)
	Bad office logistics	6 (27)
	Role confusion	5 (23)
	Lack of standardization	3 (14)
	Can't transport clients	2 (9)
Community	Lack of Medicaid providers	5 (23)
	Access is a barrier	4 (18)

Level	Solution categories	
CM	Be creative and efficient	8 (36)
	Make time for case management	5 (23)
	Have one-to-one relationship with client	4 (18)
	Develop agency contacts	4 (18)
	Make home visits	3 (14)
Program	Have different roles	8 (36)
	Cooperate in covering cases	6 (29)
Community	Agencies work together	7 (32)

lack of knowledge about the community and its resources and geography, and a personal discomfort with some aspect of doing case management such that choices about interventions were altered.

With regard to the case management program, several problems were mentioned. One aspect of the most frequently mentioned problem, things pull away from case management, was having a large caseload. One RN aptly described the situation: "There are too many of them and too few of us." Another aspect of this problem was that other clinic and managerial responsibilities had priority, and thus took time away from doing case management. Frequently mentioned aspects were documentation, billing, and paperwork. Some of this problem was duplication of forms, repetitive data collection between visits, and time required to complete Medicaid billing forms, all of which was necessary to be in compliance with Medicaid regulations.

Simply not having enough time for case management was often the consequence of the various factors taking time away from doing case management. Another program problem, managerial problems, included personnel issues and insufficient planning for the case management program. Bad office logistics including inadequate office space, limited number of telephones for CM use, inadequate personnel for language interpreting, and difficulties scheduling clients for clinic visits while allowing a case management contact while the client was in the building. These are examples of how office logistics made it difficult for CMs to do their work. While this was a program-level problem, it can be viewed as a result of inadequate resource allocation by the organization to the program. Role confusion was another program-level problem, especially role distinctions between being a CM and being a clinician, between nursing and social work roles, and between being a CM whose services are Medicaid billable and being a case aide whose services were not billable. Lack of standardization to their work was yet another problem; some participants wanted more consistency within the of-

fice regarding what to do. The last program problem was that they could not transport patients due to issues of liability. This was seen as a problem in light of inadequate mass transit and urgent needs for medical care.

Two major barriers were identified at the community level: lack of Medicaid providers and access barriers. Together these community problems either decreased participants' ability to obtain or delayed their getting necessary services for clients. Lack of physicians accepting Medicaid clients was a problem in these health departments because the health department only provided low-risk prenatal care; occasionally a client became high risk and needed care from a specialist. Access barriers included issues such as lack of community resources, bureaucratic red tape, and lack of collaboration from community agencies or providers in mutually providing services.

Solutions

Solutions mentioned by participants (also in Table 1) also related to CM, program, and community. Overall, more strategies were mentioned by participants from Site 1, which had been doing case management for a year longer than Site 2.

At the CM level, solution categories were personal and seemed to reflect personal philosophies and preferences. Case management personnel made special efforts to arrange their own schedules to assure that they had time designated for case management. Be creative and efficient, a frequently mentioned solution, reflected that participants developed and used personal strategies that aided them in adapting to the barriers and problems they experienced. With time set aside for case management (make time for case management), they could then focus on how to interact with clients. Having personal contact and establishing and maintaining a personal relationship with their clients (have one-to-one relationship) was a solution to either client-level or program-level barriers and problems. Although time and resources made it difficult, CMs preferred to make home visits rather than relying on interactions during the client's clinic visit. This was an important solution because clients would "look good" during a clinic visit, but a home visit would reveal a daily reality for clients that "didn't look so good." Develop agency contact, another solution, involved having a personal contact within an agency to overcome the barriers to access, the red tape, challenging procedures, and impersonal nature of that agency.

Participants also mentioned program factors that made doing case management easier: have different roles for nurses, social workers, and case aides, and share cases and information. The development and use of standardized procedures and role clarity were generally viewed as the responsibility of the program manager. But working together as a team, through meetings, sharing case information, and case responsibility, was viewed as the collective responsibility of the CMs and aides to assure that the program was a success and that client needs were addressed.

One solution applied to the community. Agencies worked together to establish and maintain direct interagency or interprofessional collaboration in managing selected clients. Also, interagency meetings were used to exchange information about resources and current agency policies and services. It is worth noting that to receive approval as a Medicaid case management program, the agency must be engaged in communitywide coordination of services, which presumably requires interagency meetings.

Perceptions

Participants volunteered their perceptions about clients, about being a CM, about the program, and about the community (Table 2). Participants discussed case management from a personal perspective. Some feel overloaded, while others expressed feeling good from case management as a personal benefit or reward that was based on the close relationship they developed with clients and the positive changes they saw in their clients. Others had a sense of expectations that was an awareness of expectations of themselves as CMs, and a discrepancy between what they were able to do in case management and what they or others expected of them.

Perceptions of the case management program were mentioned. They said that case management has a purpose and value; specifically, there is a philosophy or explicit intent to case management, but the benefit to clients from case management was often intertwined with the inherent limitations (has limits). Participants attributed being a team within the office to the case management program. Because the case management program had been in place for two years or less in both sites, most were still wrestling with whether or not and to what extent case management was a new role of them. Some participants mentioned money issues related to paying for case management, with some viewing it as a waste of money and others wanting payment for all activities by both professionals and case management aides to be billable.

Table 2. Number and percentage of participants who mentioned each perception category (n = 22)

Level	Perception categories	n (%)
CM	Feel overloaded, stressed, frustrated	10 (45)
	Sense of expectations	7 (32)
	Feel good from case management	4 (18)
Program	It has value and purpose	14 (64)
	It is (not) new	13 (59)
	It has limits	5 (23)
	It fostered teamwork	5 (23)
	It has money issues	5 (23)
Community	Community characteristics	3 (14)

DISCUSSION

Through interviews, several key points about case management become evident. One solution to getting work done was to engage in various networking activities, both within the program and with community agencies. The extent to which the networking ability of CMs affects their work warrants further attention both in managing programs and in research. Other solutions are consistent with organizational theory. For example, having one-to-one relationships with clients is consistent with the use of high media richness when the task has a high degree of uncertainty and ambiguity.[15] Also, the lack of standardization as an indicator of formalization is consistent with findings from prior research into the relationship between structure and technology, which suggests formalization is needed when the work is high in uncertainty.[8,16]

With regard to the program, dominant themes were the use of teamwork and sharing of the work and workload. The development of a team spirit and sharing the work is a natural consequence of the ambiguity and uncertainty of the work involved in doing comprehensive case management, and can be seen as adaptive and consistent with organizational theory.[11,17] Site differences in mentioning program factors hint at the effect of organization and program on doing case management. For example, the extent of teamwork might have been underreported at Site 1 because the team approach had been in place longer than at Site 2 and therefore was more of an unconsciously used solution. Other site differences were seen; the mention of management and personnel problems and the extent of feeling overloaded at Site 2 might be related to several unfilled staff positions at the time of the interviews, as well as explicit dissatisfaction with the manager. This suggests that attitudes toward the program can be affected by managerial factors. This is consistent with the model of case management that suggests program level variables affect CMs.

Some correspondence between problems and solutions are evident. The problem of role confusion corresponds to the solution "have different roles"; access barriers and need to know the community could lead to develop agency contact and agencies work together. Similarly, some perceptions seem to correspond to problems and solutions: feel overloaded may stem from a variety of CM or program-level problems; feel good is related to have one-to-one relationship with clients; and the feeling of fostered teamwork is a likely result of cooperate in covering cases.

Managerial implications

At the client level, patient needs that are related to social problems underlying their medical problems need to be addressed. Understanding the social etiology of medical problems will be important in the work of CMs and the design of the case management program.[18] Also, clients interface with various providers, such as physicians, laboratory and diagnostic imaging technicians, social workers, and state and federal financial assistance program personnel. Barriers to accessing services within and outside of the health organizations may exist, and client abilities to maneuver across settings and providers ought to be considered.

At the CM level, personnel characteristics such as level of training and attitudes toward case management may affect CMs' work and ought to be considered in selecting and training CMs. Additionally, CMs need information about community resources, training in case management procedures, and guidance in reconciling role expectations and self-expectations, and they may need help with the emotional aspect of the work that arises from taking a personal interest in clients.

At the program level, two recommendations flow from this study. First, the importance of home visits must be recognized and integrated into comprehensive case management programs. CMs said that clients' presentation in the clinic and information obtained by phone are not congruent with the observations made during home visits. Home visits enabled CMs to make a full and accurate assessment of client situations. The program ought to be designed to permit CMs the discretion to do home visits as a means of reducing their uncertainty about their clients. Also, just as health department CMs experienced specific difficulties when their clients received care from private physicians, CMs in other health care organizations may lose contact with their clients if clients change primary providers or are referred to specialty care. This further suggests that CMs ought not be "place bound" nor rely exclusively on phone information, and that there should be adequate resources for making home visits. In other words, the case management program ought to be designed to follow clients regardless of site or setting of care.

Second, teamwork and case sharing within the case management program is necessary, as is role clarity for each employee involved in the team effort. More efficient case management through teamwork requires that the CM's only job responsibility be that of doing case management, so that other responsibilities do not take priority over doing case management.

At the organization level, two implications are noted. First, sufficient resources are needed for personnel and for information systems to exchange information among providers involved with the client. Implied in the perception of case management having a purpose is that the program was consistent with the organization's mission and strategic goals and the professional goals of its personnel. If organizational goals include cost containment, then comprehensive case management programs can be important to health care organizations through utilization management and reduction of client risk factors. Second, while money issues raised in this study were in reference to reimbursement and use of public funds, questions about paying for case management services will surface because case management programs are a cost center and may not be specified as a benefit in health plans.

Therefore, program managers must work with insurance benefits and marketing personnel to make comprehensive case management a desirable health benefit and to include the program costs in the premium. At the community level, the program manager could take the lead in forming coalitions around populations receiving case management and in fostering information exchange, especially about services needed by clients.

Limitations

The results of this study are not generalizable to all case management programs due to small sample size of organizations and participants. Also, there may be recall bias inherent in the data in the interviews. The percent of participants who mentioned a category shown in Tables 1 and 2 should be interpreted cautiously. Because of the small sample size and the nature of this qualitative study, these percentages cannot be generalized to case management programs and are intended only as an indicator of the possible prevalence. Also, additional categories might be identified with a larger sample.

SUMMARY

Findings from this descriptive study of doing the work of case management have contributed to our understanding of factors that can affect the effectiveness and efficiency of delivering case management in different settings. Suggestions were offered regarding ways to design comprehensive case management programs within health care organizations that will benefit both the organization and clients, while making the work of doing case management more efficient and effective.

REFERENCES

1. Zander, K. "The Early Years: The Evolution of Nursing Case Management." *Handbook of Nursing Case Management: Health Care Delivery in a World of Managed Care,* edited by D.L. Flarey and S.S. Blancett. Gaithersburg, Md.: Aspen, 1996.

2. Shamansky, S. "Editorial." *Public Health Nurse* 13, no. 1 (1996): i.

3. Korr, W.S., and Cloninger, L. "Assessing Models of Case Management: An Empirical Approach." *Journal of Social Service Research* 14 (1991): 129–46.

4. Merrill, J. "Defining Case Management." *Business and Health* 2 (1985): 1634–38.

5. Raiff, N., and Shore, B. *Advanced Case Management.* Newbury Park, Calif.: Sage, 1993.

6. Lyon, J.C. "Models of Nursing Care Delivery and Case Management: Clarification of Terms." *Nursing Economics* 11 (1993): 163–69.

7. Buescher, P.A., Roth, M.S., Williams, D., and Goforth, C.M. "Evaluation of the Impact of Maternity Care Coordination on Medicaid Birth Outcomes in North Carolina." *American Journal of Public Health* 81 (1991): 1625–29.

8. Alexander, J.A., and Bauerschmidt, A.D. "Implications for Nursing Administration of the Relationship of Technology and Structure to Quality of Care." *Nursing Administration Quarterly* 11, no. 4 (1987): 1–10.

9. Korenbrot, C.C. et al. "Birth Weight Outcomes in a Teenage Pregnancy Case Management Program." *Journal of Adolescent Health Care* 10 (1989): 97–104.

10. Issel, L.M. "Use of Community Resources by Prenatal Case Managers." *Public Health Nurse* 13 (1996): 3–12.

11. Daft, R.L. *Organization Theory and Design.* 3rd ed. St. Paul, Minn.: West, 1989.

12. Bronfenbrenner, U. *The Ecology of Human Development: Experiments by Nature and Design.* Cambridge, Mass.: Harvard University Press, 1979.

13. Morse, J.M. "Designing Funded Qualitative Research." In *Handbook of Qualitative Research,* edited by N.K. Densin and Y.S. Lincoln. Thousand Oaks, Calif.: Sage Publications, 1992.

14. Tesch, R. *Qualitative Research: Analysis Types and Software Tools.* New York: Falmer Press, 1990.

15. Daft, R.L., and Lengel, R.H. "Organizational Information Requirements, Media Richness and Structural Design." *Organizational Science* 32 (1986): 554–71.

16. Hage, J., and Aiken, M. "Routine Technology, Social Structure, and Organizational Goals." *Administrative Science Quarterly* 14 (1969): 366–76.

17. Thompson, J.D. *Organizations in Action.* New York: McGraw-Hill, 1967.

18. Issel, L.M., and Anderson, R.A. "Take Charge: Six Transformations in Health Care." *Nursing Economics* 19 (1996): 1–8.

Effects of the Program-Management Model: A Case Study on Professional Rehabilitation Nursing

Mary Ann Miller and Laban Darrel Miller

Since 1993 when Cardinal Hill Rehabilitation Hospital in Lexington, Kentucky, a free-standing, 100-bed physical rehabilitation hospital certified by the Commission on Accreditation of Rehabilitation Facilities (CARF), revamped its organizational structure, its nursing staff has functioned without a director of nursing. Under the new program-management design, governance of nursing—just as in governance of other clinical disciplines—occurred under program managers. (At Cardinal Hill there were now seven program managers with professional backgrounds in nursing, physical therapy, and social work.) With this new arrangement, nurses for the first time did not have a director with a singular focus on nursing. Some nurses were now accountable to program managers from other disciplines such as physical therapy and social work.

Cardinal Hill's move to the program-management model involved flattening the clinical management structure by deleting the tier of discipline directors (e.g., the director positions of nursing and physical therapy) and cutting numerous staff positions (see Figures 1 and 2). Cutbacks included the elimination of 28 percent of the RN positions, 18 percent of the licensed practical nurse (LPN) positions, and 19 percent of the certified nursing assistant (CNA) positions. With fewer nurses and no director of nurs-

ing, program managers now faced new challenges in maintaining quality patient outcomes.

ADDRESSING LIMITATIONS IN PROFESSIONALISM

With the belief that many traditionally organized health care institutions will no longer be able to deliver valuable services to their customers,[1] the senior management team at Cardinal Hill implemented the program-management model as a way to encourage greater effectiveness and creativity in organizational planning. The model answered perceived limitations in the traditional discipline-management approach that promoted professionalism but seemed to stifle risk taking and innovation. "I wanted my staff," noted Kerry Gillihan, chief executive officer of Cardinal Hill, "to collectively step out of traditional thinking patterns in order to find better and more affordable ways to serve our customers" (personal interview conducted by L.D. Miller, 27 March 1996).

A primary concern of traditional nursing departments has been the maintenance of established nursing standards. Nursing is considered professional to the extent that nurses adhere to these standards, which are designed to help nurses avoid or manage negligence or malpractice proceedings,[2] achieve autonomy in clinical decision making,[3] maintain a code of ethics,[4] and avoid unnecessary duplication of information.[5]

These standards, as with other disciplines, have served the nursing profession well, but they

Nurs Admin Q 1997; 21(1): 47–54

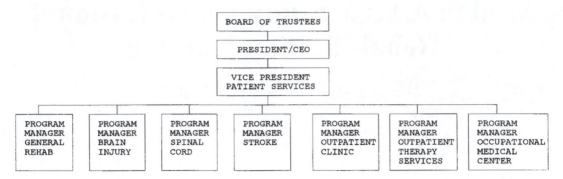

Figure 1. Program-management model. Clinical organizational chart for Cardinal Hill after restructuring in 1993. Support services have not been included in this organizational chart. Over time, most support services will be partially or fully integrated into the new management structure of the programs.

contain an inherent weakness that can limit creative organizational thinking. More specifically, bureaucracies, such as boards of nursing, enforce adherence to professional standards, which cause individuals to think *deductively*. With such thinking, nursing staff tend to force new problems into old pigeonholes. According to Henry Mintzberg, an internationally acclaimed management expert,

> the Professional Bureaucracy is an inflexible structure, well suited to producing its standard outputs but illsuited to adapting to the production of

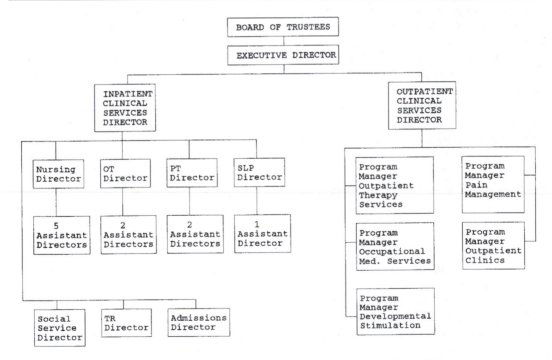

Figure 2. Discipline-management model. Clinical organizational chart for Cardinal Hill before restructuring in 1993. Support services have not been included in this organizational chart.

new ones. Rather than emphasizing the uniqueness of patients' particular situations, a professional nurse is trained to assess multiple symptoms and apply the appropriate, predetermined nursing practices to these situations. Such deductive reasoning converges the particulars to fit generic, standardized frameworks.[6(p.209)]

The alternative to deductive thinking is induction, where specific situations can spin off many new ideas and a situation is not evaluated in terms of predetermined standards. "The fact is that great art and innovative problem solving," says Mintzberg, "require *inductive* reasoning—that is, the inference of new general concepts or programs from particular experiences. That kind of thinking is *divergent*—it breaks away from old routines or standards rather than perfecting existing ones. And that flies in the face of everything the Professional Bureaucracy is designed to do."[6(p.210)]

Working under professional standards, hospital nurses frequently encountered two related, but sometimes conflicting, worlds—a professional world and an organizational world. In addressing this conflict, Cardinal Hill adopted the program-management model in hopes of simultaneously increasing the organizational flexibility and the quality of patient outcomes. "Too often," said Gillihan, "our nurses in the traditional discipline-management model tended to give primary allegiance to their professional world and secondary allegiance to their organization." This, according to Karlene Kerfoot, stifles risk taking and innovative program planning.[7] The new program-management model (which she refers to as "product-line") encourages innovation by forcing more staff to pay attention to finances, teamwork, and other organizational issues.

An example of how the new program-management approach allowed for greater organizational flexibility can be seen in the hospital's new program aide positions. These program aides are qualified to function as nursing assistants (NAs), physical therapy aides, and occupational therapy aides. Cardinal Hill has found that program aides, as compared to the narrower traditional use of NAs, provided a flexibility not possible under the old system. The hospital has found that program aides have been beneficial in terms of reduced overall salary costs, increased levels of responsibility and job satisfaction, and increased use of interdisciplinary teamwork.

SKEPTICISM OF THE PROGRAM-MANAGEMENT MODEL

In the three years since the restructuring, the program-management approach has financially benefited Cardinal Hill.[8] However, an ongoing concern with the implementation of the new program approach has been the hospital's ability to maintain the integrity of professional nursing practices and to ensure benchmark patient outcomes.

A strength of the old discipline-management model was the assurance of professional integrity within each clinical discipline. Cardinal Hill's director of nursing embraced and implemented clinical standards advocated by nursing experts and practiced by many nursing professionals. In the new program-management model, on the other hand, there were no guarantees that program managers, who have an increased span of control, without a singular focus on nursing, would adequately support professional standards in nursing.[9] Some Cardinal Hill nurses doubted the capacity of the new organizational structure to achieve patient outcomes comparable to those of the earlier discipline-management model.

Of the current personnel, approximately 75 nursing employees (RNs, LPNs, CNAs) were on staff for at least six months prior to the restructuring at Cardinal Hill. In a survey conducted three years after the restructuring, in May 1996, these nurses responded on a seven-point scale to indicate whether they thought patient outcomes had improved (7) or worsened (1) under the program-management design. With a 40 percent return rate, total responses concerning patient outcomes averaged 4.5 on the scale. While 44 percent believed patient outcomes had improved under the restructuring, 26 percent indicated that patient outcomes had declined. These statistics suggest that a significant (though only 26 percent) portion of the Cardinal Hill nursing staff still perceived the program-management model as hindering professional nursing practice.

To address the perceptual disparity that existed within nursing, Cardinal Hill used quantifiable data to monitor and shape employees' beliefs about the impact of the program-management approach on patient outcomes. Specifically, the quality of patient outcomes before and after the restructuring was evaluated by comparing functional independent measures (FIM) scores, patient falls, and medication errors.

PATIENT OUTCOMES IN FIM

Cardinal Hill participated in the services of Uniform Data System for Medical Rehabilitation (UDS) to analyze and evaluate progress in patients. A seven-point scale was used in rating various functional areas to track patients from hospital admission through discharge. A patient's progress can be directly attributed to nursing interventions in functional areas such as toileting, bowel and bladder elimination, interaction, problem solving, and memory. Ideally, a patient needing physical rehabilitation would experience a significant positive change in these FIM scores.

FIM scores would not prove a causal relationship, positive or negative, between the program-management design and patient outcomes. But it would suggest a compatibility or incompatibility between the new program-management design and professional rehabilitation nursing care. A compatible relationship would occur when FIM scores in the new management design are equal to, or higher than, the FIM scores prior to the restructuring in 1993.

Five of the six functional areas Cardinal Hill examined using FIM scores supported the compatibility between the program-management model and professional rehabilitation nursing practices at Cardinal Hill. Since the transition to the program-management model, average change scores in FIM increased by 29 percent in toileting, 25 percent in interaction, 13 percent in bladder, and 9 percent in problem solving. When it came to memory function, there was no difference in the FIM change scores. Only in one functional area were the average change scores lower after Cardinal Hill went to the program-management model—bowel elimination scores decreased by 10 percent (see Table 1).

FIM takes into account the effects of average lengths of stay (LOS) on change scores. This relationship is calculated by using a LOS efficiency score (LOS/average change score). This score is significant for the analysis, since Cardinal Hill's average LOS decreased after the restructuring from 21.7 to 20.4 days. Cardinal Hill's LOS efficiency score improved overall by 28 percent after going to the program-management approach.

PATIENT FALLS

Except for several hours of therapy per day, the nursing staff at Cardinal Hill had always had primary responsibility for the well-being of its patients. With the implementation of the pro-

Table 1. FIM-change score differences between the discipline-management era and program-management era

	Toileting	Bladder	Bowel	Interaction	Problem solving	Memory
Difference in change-FIM scores after going to the program-management model	+29%	+13%	−10%	+25%	+9%	0%

gram-management model, a potential threat to patients was introduced when the size of the nursing staff was significantly reduced (by 22%). As one way to ensure the well-being of patients, Cardinal Hill monitored the ability of the reduced nursing staff to prevent patient falls.

Generally, most patient falls at Cardinal Hill have occurred during times of indirect patient care when patients were not receiving therapy, instruction, or assistance in the activities of daily living. The findings indicate that, compared to incidences prior to the restructuring in 1993, there were virtually no changes in the number of inpatient falls since the restructuring event. In outpatient services, the number of falls decreased by an average of 0.5 falls per month. These trends indicate that the program-management model did not adversely affect nursing's ability to prevent patient falls.

MEDICATION ERRORS

At Cardinal Hill, the pharmacy department works collaboratively with nursing in administering drugs. Medication errors can therefore be impacted by services in nursing. Available data seem to indicate a compatibility between program management and accurate drug distribution. Prior to the 1993 restructuring effort, the total number of recorded medication errors averaged 16.55 per month. But since the implementation of the new model, recorded errors decreased to 9.15 per month. This decrease is especially significant since the medication doses per month increased from an average of 31,304 before the restructuring to 42,544 after the event.

Credit cannot automatically be given to the efficiency of the program-management approach for actual decreases in medication errors. According to the Director of Pharmacy, Debra Murphy, Pharm.D., the apparent decrease more likely reflects underreporting and underdocumentation due to time constraints resulting from increased medication doses, organizational changes throughout the hospital, and staff turnover in the pharmacy department (personal interview conducted by L.D. Miller, 12 April 1996). Murphy in-

dicated that Cardinal Hill is currently evaluating the reporting, documenting, and trending processes for medication errors in order to prevent additional errors from occurring.

Regardless of the new structure's impact on medication errors, pharmacists at Cardinal Hill, more than ever, have become integral team players throughout the hospital. "In the new design," said Beth Monarch, Vice-President of Patient Services, "the pharmacy staff became more focused on building teamwork with the program staff and less concerned with identifying who made what error" (personal interview conducted by L.D. Miller, 12 April 1996).

SATISFACTION WITHOUT A DIRECTOR OF NURSING

To compensate for having no director of nursing, Cardinal Hill looked to a part-time nursing clinical specialist to perform several nursing-related functions that were optimally centralized in terms of economies of scale. While this specialist had no governing authority, she supported program managers by staying current in standards of practice, establishing nursing policies and procedures, serving as liaison to the Kentucky Board of Nursing, coordinating hospital-wide nursing float pools, and meeting regularly with nursing coordinators to discuss various nursing issues.

With the new model in place, job satisfaction levels have been maintained or slightly improved among the nursing staff at Cardinal Hill. Turnover rates, for example, have decreased significantly. The numbers of RN and LPN terminations have each decreased by about 43 percent and nursing aide (including program aide) terminations decreased by 17 percent. Nursing employees, however, gave mixed reports concerning their perceptions of job satisfaction—37 percent reported greater job satisfaction, 37 percent reported less job satisfaction, and 26 percent reported the same level of satisfaction.

Cross-functional teams in the program-management model provided the opportunity for staff members to break out of the what Geoffrey

Bellman calls "glass silos" that are built around their disciplinary departments.[10] In general, nurses' overall sense of involvement in interdisciplinary teamwork and patient-related decision making increased. Sixty-three percent of nurses believed interdisciplinary teamwork has increased with the program-management approach; only 15 percent suggested a decrease. Sixty-three percent of surveyed nurses believed their level of involvement in decision making in relation to patient care had remained the same or increased with the new management model.

ADDRESSING SKEPTICISM

For at least the immediate future, Cardinal Hill is committed to the program-management model. "I think it's essential that all our employees accept the new model," said Gillihan. To diminish the skepticism that remains, an intentional effort is under way to change misperceptions. According to Vice-President of Patient Services, Beth Monarch, efforts are being made to present ongoing outcome statistics at management and program team meetings, publish relevant outcome data in the hospital's newsletter, commission a hospital outcomes committee to look at existing and new measurements to evaluate program-management efforts, and evaluate patient satisfaction data before and after going to the program-management approach.

• • •

When the program-management model was first implemented at Cardinal Hill in 1993, the director of nursing position was eliminated and the nursing staff, for the first time, reported to program managers who did not necessarily have nursing backgrounds. While the senior management team has been convinced of the program management model's success in terms of financial effectiveness, the data pertaining to measurements in FIM, patient falls, and medication errors suggest a positive relationship between patient outcomes and the program-management approach.

REFERENCES

1. J.R. Duffy and K.G. Lemieux, "A Cardiac Service Line Approach to Patient-Centered Care," *Nursing Administration Quarterly* 20, no. 1 (1995): 12–23.

2. J. Fiesta, "Failing to Act Like a Professional," *Nursing Management*, 25, no. 7 (1994): 15–17.

3. B.K. Miller, et al., "A Behavioral Inventory for Professionalism in Nursing," *Journal of Professional Nursing* 9, no. 5 (1993):290–95.

4. M.D.M. Fowler, "Professional Associations, Ethics, and Society," *Oncology Nursing Forum* 20, no. 10 Supplement (1994):13–19.

5. L.S. Corpuz and C. Conforti, "Organizing and Documenting Clinical Standards," *Nursing Management* 25, no. 5 (1994):70–72, 74, 76.

6. H. Mintzberg, *Structure in Fives: Designing Effective Organizations* (Englewood Cliffs, NJ: Prentice Hall, 1983), 209, 210.

7. K. Kerfoot, "Today's Patient Care Unit Manager," *Nursing Economics* 11, no. 4 (1993): 246–48.

8. L.D. Miller and B. Monarch, "Restructuring Rehabilitation Services: A Case Study of the Program-Management Model, *Rehab Management* 9, no. 4 (1996): 47–52.

9. M. Peruzzi, et al., "A Community Hospital Redesigns Care," *Nursing Administration Quarterly* 20, no. 1 (1995): 24–46.

10. G.M. Bellman, *Getting Things Done When You Are Not in Charge* (San Francisco: Berrett-Koehler Publishers, 1992).

The Change Process and a Clinical Evaluation Unit at University of Massachusetts Medical Center

Steven L. Strongwater

In 1989, the cost of care in academic medical centers was estimated to exceed that of community hospitals by as much as 30 percent.[1,2] Because of this reality and the well-acknowledged existence of unexplained practice variation, the University of Massachusetts (UMass) launched a series of programs in the late 1980s and early 1990s as part of a formal quality improvement initiative. The goals of these programs were to control expenses and improve the value of services provided. Our quality improvement initiatives, combined with the alignment of external accrediting agencies and financial imperatives, led to the formation of a new department: Quality Management Services (QMS). The mission of QMS was to oversee all UMass quality initiatives as well as Joint Commission on Accreditation of Healthcare Organizations (Joint Commission) preparation; its overarching goal was to improve coordination of such activities. Our efforts at establishing a clinical evaluation unit (CEU) and the new department reflect a desperate and sometimes fragmented way of responding to the new imperative of identifying the right way to push forward organizational change and alter clinical practice.

BACKGROUND

The University of Massachusetts Medical Center is a 381-bed inpatient facility with 30 ambula-

tory clinics located in central Massachusetts. We have several centers of excellence, including cardiac services, public sector psychiatry, cancer, sports medicine, emergency medicine, and trauma. UMass developed one of the first air ambulance services in Massachusetts and is currently running two programs; one in central Massachusetts and the other in the western part of the state, in Turners Falls. UMass was also one of the first programs, in this part of the country, to develop a mobile cardiac catheterization laboratory, which serves eight community hospitals across the state. The city of Worcester has approximately 200,000 residents, and the surrounding towns add another million. We draw patients from throughout New England, including Connecticut, Maine, Vermont, and New Hampshire. Locally, there are two other hospital systems in Worcester. Both have their own selected residency training programs but often utilize UMass house staff and medical students. Many of our faculty admit and care for patients at these hospitals as well.

In 1993, the city of Worcester had eight acute care hospitals. Three have closed. The others have merged to form three systems within the city. Two are community facilities; one is owned and operated by a managed care company and the other is free-standing. The mergers were driven by competitive pressures exacerbated by a reduction in reimbursements from managed care and other payers. There is currently approximately a 60 percent–65 percent penetration of managed care in the Worcester marketplace.

Quality Management in Health Care 1996; 4(4): 30–39
© 1996 Aspen Publishers, Inc.

This article describes the evolution of the UMass Clinical Evaluation Unit through five developmental phases.

PHASE 1: EARLY QUALITY INITIATIVES

Utilization review initiatives (goal: to reduce length of stay and support Joint Commission preparation)

As a consequence of the implementation of a prospective payment system for the Medicare population and the need to involve clinical faculty in cost reduction in 1989, a staff position, the associate chief of staff, was created. As initially conceived, the principal role of the associate chief of staff was to work to reduce the length of stay. To facilitate accomplishment of this goal, the associate chief of staff was named the chair of the Utilization Review Committee and worked closely with the directors of the Utilization Review and Risk Management Departments and the director of the Quality Assurance Program. With attention focused on both length of stay and Joint Commission preparation, it became apparent that support personnel would be needed to guide preoccupied, often indifferent faculty and house staff in this process. Five positions, termed quality management coordinators, were created to support quality management and Joint Commission preparation for 15 medical staff departments.

Gathering physician-specific data (goal: to generate physician involvement)

As the Utilization Review Committee began to meet, it became clear that physician feedback (data) and involvement would be critical. (Focus groups confirmed that physicians would respond best to data.) So began our quest for physician-specific data. Unfortunately, in 1989 and 1990 our hospital systems could not provide the detailed data needed. Only high-level, department-specific, length-of-stay information was available. To motivate physician involvement, a

small grants program modeled after the successful program at the University of Rochester,[3] was developed.

Program for Healthcare Innovations (goal: to promote health services research)

The goal of the Program for Healthcare Innovations (PHI) was to stimulate physician interest in the evolving science of health services research. The vision was to provide seed money, to be given to physicians for creative ideas that might lead to improvements in outcomes and reductions in cost, which would then serve as the basis for external grant support to benefit both the school and the hospital.

A commitment was made by the hospital to fund approximately 13 grants, ranging from $2,000 to $6,000 annually, and to offer administrative support for coordination. PHI planned to allocate grant money and serve as an agency of "technology transfer," disseminating literature-based, proven methodologies to improve outcomes and reduce costs. A PHI steering committee was established, chaired by the chief of staff, and its membership included the chief of surgery and medicine and the director of nursing and quality assurance. Ex-officio membership included the PHI director and the hospital director. A PHI advisory board was also established. Its membership included the dean of the School of Public Health (UMass Amherst campus), the chair of the Central Massachusetts Business Group on Health, the director of the master's of public health program at Clark University, and representatives from a local managed care plan and a local community hospital. Thirteen grants were initially awarded (see box entitled "PHI Grants").

Several important lessons were learned during the first few years of PHI. A decision made early in the program by the PHI Steering Committee was that faculty could not be supported by PHI grant funds, the concern being that if funds were used for faculty salaries, there would be limited accountability and projects might not be completed. This decision proved to be a mis-

PHI Grants

Project Title	Accomplishments
Systematic Plan To Evaluate Appropriateness of Lab Testing	Guidelines established to drastically reduce the use of bleeding times and preoperative lab testing guideline implemented.
Safety and Advocacy of Outpatient Intravenous Heparin Therapy of Lower Extremity Deep Venous Thrombosis	Use of hand-held anticoagulant monitor adopted and treatment guidelines implemented.
Effective and Nutritional Intervention Algorithm on the Use of Parenteral Nutrition in Critically Ill Patients	Approximately 30 patients enrolled; inappropriate TPN costs eliminated, for savings of approximately $700,000.
Nurse–Physician Collaboration: Does It Lead to Improved Patient Outcomes and Status Satisfaction?	Program discontinued.
Assessment of One-to-One Monitoring of Psychiatric Patients on the Medical and Surgical Wards	Incorporation of project into a hospitalwide program, saving approximately $400,000 by implementing new guidelines for patient care.
Evaluation of Respiratory Failure in the Pediatric Intensive Care Unit	Development of appropriate techniques for detection of infections in the Emergency Care Unit.
Training and Credentialing Program for House Staff Procedures	Development of a new program to train house staff for invasive procedures.
Pressure Ulcer QI Auditing: Demonstrating the Clinical and Cost-effective Outcomes of Nursing Interventions for Managing Pressure Ulcer Care	Clinical nurse specialist appointed to manage skin care; reduction of decubitus ulcers documented and AHCPR guideline adopted.
Evaluation of Tympanic Temperatures in Children Less Than Two Years Old in the Emergency Department	Hospital-wide shift to the use of tympanic thermometers for all patients.
Evaluation and Improvement of Warfarin Dosing at UMass Medical Center	Algorithm for anticoagulation implemented.
Surveillance of Postoperative Wound Infection	Development of a program to collect data and understand the rates of postop wound infections.
Drug Dosing in Renal Impairment	Development of sophisticated program to identify and track patients in renal failure who are receiving antibiotics; leading to appropriateness of antibiotic dosing (more than 95 percent) on a hospital-wide basis and a reduction in toxicity.
Indications for Computerized Tomography Prior to Performing Lumbar Puncture	Program discontinued.

take, because faculty were being pressed to work harder on all fronts (service, education, research, and administration) and it became impossible to layer additional responsibilities upon them without some offset of their time. Second, faculty often lacked core competencies needed for health service research. This was problematic in that core statistical and study design support was necessary to ensure that projects would be competitive and could be published in peer-reviewed journals. Another problem was that successful projects were focused more on cost and process improvement rather than on creating new knowledge, the latter being necessary for fundable research projects.

In 1992, therefore, it was decided to reformulate PHI. New leadership was selected to focus on project completion and procurement of external grant support. PHI was separated from hospital operations but still reported to the chief of staff. Despite many successful projects, however, PHI funding was eliminated in 1993, an early casualty of budget reductions.

The DNAs Program (goal: to reduce length of stay and costs)

In 1990, to complement PHI, teams of doctors, nurses, and administrators (DNAs) were convened to work on seven specific clinical projects designed to reduce length of stay and save money. These projects involved kidney transplantation, hip replacement, complicated myocardial infarction, ventilator-dependent patients, cardiac bypass (with and without cardiac catheterization), trauma, and burns. There was a heavy emphasis on the administrative aspects of these programs. Despite valiant efforts, for the most part DNAs were unsuccessful in fundamentally changing the manner in which care was delivered. Length of stay fell slightly, but resource use was not significantly affected.

PHASE 2: QUALITY IMPROVEMENT TEAMS (GOAL: PERFORMANCE IMPROVEMENT LEADING TO COST REDUCTION)

It was approximately at this time that UMass became aware of the results of the National Demonstration Project (see box). Impressed by these results, we became convinced that our best long-term strategy for cost-containment was to apply the principles of continuous quality improvement (CQI). The staff assigned to develop the CQI program were from Decision Support, a hospital-based department composed almost en-

---

The National Demonstration Project: 10 Conclusions

1. Quality improvement tools can work in health care.
2. Cross-functional teams are valuable in improving health care processes.
3. Data useful for quality improvement abound in health care.
4. Quality improvement methods are fun to use.
5. Costs of poor quality are high and savings are within reach.
6. Involving doctors is difficult.
7. Training needs arise early.
8. Nonclinical processes draw early attention.
9. Health care organizations may need a broader definition of quality.
10. In health care, as in industry, the fate of quality improvement is in the hands of the leaders.

Source: Reprinted with permission from D. Berwick, A. Godfrey, and J. Roessner, *Curing Healthcare,* © 1990, Jossey-Bass.

---

tirely of management engineers. In organizing the program, the University of Michigan was visited, and Dr. Brent James from Intermountain Healthcare, Salt Lake City, Utah, was consulted. A Quality Steering Committee (QSC), composed of the hospital CEO, senior hospital associates, the chief of staff, the associate chief of staff, and the directors of the Quality Assurance Program and Risk Management Department, was gathered. Projects defined by the QSC became known as quality improvement teams (QITs).

An institutionwide Quality Council was established to ensure the schools were also involved in quality improvement. The Quality Council membership included the provost, the hospital chief operating officer, and the deans of Biomedical Sciences and the Nursing School as well as the associate chief of staff, elected employees, and quality management coordinators. A CQI strategic plan was developed. The steps included promoting awareness, education, and training; selecting quality improvement teams; defining our customers; defining management expectations; developing performance indicators; involving Human Resources and Information Management; and establishing an effective communication strategy. Milestones for success were defined and tracked by a coordinating group that became known as the "Road Map Group." Our definition of quality was "satisfying or exceeding the valid requirements of our internal and external customers 100 percent of the time."

A rigorous seven-step process was adopted for our QIT projects. Formal training was provided for key managers and administrators. A process for project selection was defined that employed a thematic matrix. Seven initial projects were chosen and a facilitator was assigned to each. Teams included an operating room team, a patient transport team, a patient/discharge/transfer/turnaround time team, a referring physician data team, an improving cash flow from insurance carriers team, a room reservations team, and a paperless hospital systems team. The number of teams to be deployed in the first three years was carefully planned: seven initial projects, a similar number in year two, three times that number in year three, and continued growth thereafter as support permitted. Of the original seven teams, three successfully completed their work. During the process, approximately 35 people were extensively trained in the tools and techniques of CQI. Within approximately three years, we had over 240 QITs. To track the teams, their accomplishments, and barriers to progress, an in-house software program was developed. Teams reported quarterly on their progress.

Interestingly, during the training nonsanctioned or "rogue teams" developed. Our initially well-planned, controlled, rollout of CQI was being overwhelmed by individuals who went through the training program and wanted to begin using their newly acquired skills. However, rather than being viewed negatively by other team members, these "rogues" were generally viewed as furthering QI efforts.

PHASE 3: THE QUALITY MANAGEMENT SERVICES DEPARTMENT

Amidst our 1993 budgetary crisis and dissolution of PHI, the hospital merged the departments of Utilization Review, Decision Support, and Quality Assurance under the direction of the associate chief of staff. The newly formed department was named Quality Management Services (QMS). QMS became accountable for oversight of the institution's quality program as well as Joint Commission preparation. For the first time, all the essential ingredients for a successful clinical evaluation came together: management engineers from Decision Support were able to extract and display data from hospital systems; utilization review nurses, familiar with longstanding system delays, were able to monitor patterns of care; and the quality management coordinators established relationships with faculty and hospital departments. While improving the coordination of activity, the merger also resulted in a reduction of six full-time positions.

QMS reevaluated the quality program at UMass. What was discovered was a growing anti-CQI sentiment. For example, some teams were working on projects for their second year without results and with growing impatience. Most teams did not involve physicians—an obvious problem, as physician involvement was viewed as fundamentally critical to change. Focus groups, held to try to discern why physician involvement in CQI was not occurring, revealed physicians' interesting perspective. They viewed CQI as elitist and exclusionist (because of CQI jargon). They felt the hospital was mostly focusing on cost reductions and not consistently supporting service improvements and that CQI was taking resources away from patient care. They also thought CQI fostered an environment of management by crisis. They could not devote five days to train in CQI (the amount of time of our standard training program for CQI) and were disturbed that CQI provided no reward system for faculty.

To address these concerns, QMS defined five strategic goals:

1. foster more physician involvement and leadership in continuous improvement;
2. develop system changes to support care and meet accreditation requirements;
3. refine the methodology for indicator selection;
4. foster intrahospital health care teams that included physicians; and
5. define, measure, and document outcomes of care.

These new goals were presented to senior management. With their approval, several steps were taken to turn our quality initiatives around. Our strategy to reinvigorate interest in quality and performance improvement included

- reactivating a newsletter developed for PHI;
- deploying storyboards depicting success stories;
- inviting grand rounds speakers;
- scheduling department-specific presentations and semiannual hospital quality forums, with abstract presentations and free lunch; and
- reviving an annual symposium for all area hospitals with national speakers and local abstract presentations.

PHASE 4: SYSTEMS IMPROVEMENT TEAMS

Perhaps the most important step in 1993 was to spend a year researching the needs of various hospital constituencies, including physicians, nurses, admitting and medical records personnel, social services, as well as several other hospital departments, in developing a new quality approach. A group of approximately 20 people, including senior hospital associates, department managers, and physicians, met weekly to try to figure out how various elements of the hospital functioned together, where there was overlap, and what available data could be used for process improvement. We set out to understand if the CQI approach being employed was appropriate for health care or if it needed to be redefined.

Though CQI worked, it had many shortcomings. The success factors for a new model of quality for health care were identified:

- The *program* had to be fast, easy to understand, free of jargon, had to fulfill the needs of the Joint Commission and other accrediting agencies, and had to be creditable to the faculty and multidisciplinary.
- The *process* had to be academically creditable, add value, minimally set the stage for publishable work, and focus on health care, not finance or administration.

The new model sought to build from the positive aspects of the industrial CQI model, while speeding the approach for health care. Interestingly, it was not essential that the new process be supported by senior administration. There was concern that support from senior administration might be viewed negatively. Thus, a permissive environment in which to experiment and move forward was sought. What evolved came to be known as systems improvement teams (SITs).

There are four deliverables for each new SIT: measured clinical and functional outcomes, patient satisfaction, cost, and organizational morale. These measures seek to ensure the best care at the lowest cost, taking the staff involved in providing the care and the patients' needs into account. Improvements or at least stable results must be demonstrated in these dimensions. In contrast to the prior CQI process–driven model, SITs were vision driven. That is, individuals were asked to define what should or could be and plot a course to get there. We attempted to resolve the roadblocks of CQI, such as "data paralysis" (the process of continually seeking new data or to improve the quality of data at hand without making forward progress in solving a problem).

The SIT methodology calls for project completion within three to four months. (Steps in our methodology are outlined in the box entitled "Steps in the Systems Improvement Team Process.") We chose not to abandon CQI teams, as a strategic decision was made that both CQI and SITs were important. Why did we not aban-

---

**Steps in the Systems Improvement
Team Process**

1. Create an environment to achieve
   superiority.
2. Define the "ideal future."
3. Understand the current reality.
4. Plan and implement a change.
5. Measure success.
6. Evaluate performance.
7. Standardize.

---

don CQI teams? First, productive work continued to evolve from some CQI activities and much was invested in the program's development and deployment. Second, SITs and CQI complement each other. SITs result in dramatic change (re-engineering change), but there is still a need for incremental change via CQI techniques after SIT completion.

It is important to note that QMS, through its SITs, is engaged in "process involvement" rather than health outcomes research. SITs may lead to reduced costs, variations in practice, and improved outcomes through improving processes, using existing knowledge, or applying modified delphi techniques to reach consensus about treatment. SITs often generate research questions. Health outcomes research, on the other hand, is much more rigorous and strives to add fundamentally new knowledge to the literature. It is important to understand this distinction, in part because it is often not possible to address outcomes research questions owing to the small sample of patients treated at a single institution (especially for low-volume, high-cost DRGs like transplantation). More often than not, the outcomes research process takes too long (years), given that hospitals need results relatively quickly (within months). Health outcomes research and process improvement (SITs) are complementary approaches but often have different goals. Sharing the expertise of staff involved in health outcomes research, however, can greatly enhance the quality of the work performed in an SIT (e.g., by garnering support

from a pharmacoeconometrician or biostatistician).

PHASE 5: THE CLINICAL EVALUATION PROGRAM

Over the course of the last several years, a comprehensive clinical evaluation unit (CEU) has evolved. The CEU at UMass is composed of key individuals with a unique blend of talents from nursing, finance, management engineering (Decision Support), and the medical staff. The essential elements of our program include competencies in the following (see also the box entitled "Essential Elements of a Clinical Evaluation Unit"):

- *Project selection:* The ability to identify areas of opportunity that are consistent with and supportive of the organization's vision. Project selection is based on many factors, including strategic importance to UMass; the need to improve customer satisfaction (patients and their families, payers, and referring physicians); high-risk, problem-prone, high-volume, or high-cost areas, or the opportunity to affect one of the organizational functions or dimensions of performance (as identified by the Joint Commission).
- *Measurement:* The ability to accurately measure baseline performance in specific dimensions of care (e.g., clinical outcomes,

---

**Essential Elements of a Clinical
Evaluation Unit**

- Project selection methodology
- Process improvement approach
- Definition of measures
- Data collection capability
- Data analysis capability
- Implementation strategies
- Protocol variance measures
- Feedback process
- Integrated information systems
- Data repository

---

patient satisfaction, functional measures of quality of life, costs, and organizational morale).

- *Project approach and plan:* A process to approach the change process and tools to improve the process of care.
- *Implementation strategies:* Strategies for implementing and monitoring newly defined processes of care.
- *Monitoring:* The ability to ensure patient care has been improved or recognize unpredictable results quickly (within hours or days).
- *Organizational oversight:* A structure for reporting to senior management to ensure appropriate dialogue and communications throughout our system.

SITs revisited

We have expended enormous effort in defining the appropriate structure and process to ensure implementation of SITs. For example, prior to any team formation, a meeting with the department chair is scheduled. The chair is asked to identify and inform the team leader of his or her expectations. This simple step has motivated faculty in ways previously not possible. The team's work is presented to the chair; to their department, and quarterly to the Clinic Management Board (hospital board of directors). Support for SITs is provided by facilitators whose role is to drive projects to completion while minimizing meeting time and avoiding disrupting the faculty members' usual activities. One fruitful tactic has been to pair faculty with nurse leaders on each SIT. Typically, the nurse is able to push the process when the physician is otherwise occupied in the operating room or clinic. Nursing is an equal partner in the change process, which further ensures success.

Opportunities to recognize individual and team accomplishments have motivated and further engaged staff. Recent requests for proposals asking for quality and outcomes data have lent further credibility to our efforts because the SIT process automatically demands definitions of

measures and data collection. Developing a trusting environment that permits open communications and some "risk taking" has also been important.

The importance of skilled facilitators cannot be overestimated. These individuals provide the fuel to push SITs along. Not everyone has the requisite skills. Different projects may require different strategies to motivate change. Assigning the wrong facilitator can ensure failure. It is therefore important to share strategies and continue ongoing development efforts for facilitators. Facilitators at UMass meet weekly to discuss barriers and approaches for success. This interaction has been critical and helped move projects along. We are finding that projects, even when completed, never really end; once faculty and staff are engaged, armed with feedback about their outcomes, they use CQI techniques to refine their processes. Facilitators are obliged to disengage during this monitoring and evaluation phase and provide only distant support in order to move on to new projects.

Structural changes at UMass: case management

To assist with the implementation of clinical practice guidelines produced by the SITs, to measure variance in SIT-generated and other protocols, and to assist in the implementation of change, the department of Case Management was created by merging the departments of Social Work and Utilization Review and including several clinical nurse specialists. The merged model of case management is based upon the assignment of a nurse–social worker team to each hospital service (not to a particular location within the hospital).

The merger allowed us to further reduce staffing while improving service. A matrix-reporting relationship for case management between QMS and the director of nursing has had several positive results; the medical staff and nursing staff have been drawn more closely together, which is critical to the new department's success. For example, the Case Management staff remind house staff about clinical protocols, assist in preadmit and discharge planning, and administer patient functional measures and some postdischarge patient satisfaction instruments. The measures are incorporated into clinical data sets to support SITs and ongoing outcomes measurement. Case management is a critical implementation element for SITs. Often Case Management staff are the content experts on the SITs. Their follow-up tracking further ensures compliance.

Physician data reports

Physician data reports were developed to provide explicit feedback to individual physicians regarding their length of stay, utilization of laboratory tests, and overall variable costs. It has not been possible for us to generate these reports from our main hospital system. As a result, we merged information from four data sources: a cost accounting program (Transition Systems, Incorporated), the hospital operating room management information system, and two external data sets—the University HealthSystem Consortium Clinical Information Network (UHC CIN) database and the Massachusetts Health Data Consortium data set. Prior to the distribution of these reports, their content and format were presented to the Utilization Review Committee, the Faculty Practice Plan, and a committee comprising all department chairs. It was advised that these reports be distributed confidentially but that some department- or division-level information be made available to chairs and senior management.

Our first generation of reports distributed in 1993 included a scatter diagram displaying comparative lengths of stay and variable costs for all members of a given department, with the individual identified on the grid. A physician comparative analysis was provided, which included three graphs displaying the aggregate length of stay, average variable costs, and diagnosis-specific lengths of stay and variable costs for up to 15 DRGs. To get around the problem of non–severity-adjusted data, we provided a trend report based on the assumption that costs and length of stay were not likely to change dramatically for a given physician. (Stated differently, over time physicians treating patients who are very, very sick are likely to continue treating patients who are very, very sick.) The physician's performance was compared to the performance of peers as well as to Massachusetts and national data sets.

In recognition of the fact that often physicians rotate on and off clinical services, we provided a "change of attending" analysis. This displayed how often physicians changed from the beginning of an admission to the end of an admission, and it was intended to pre-empt the criticism that the patients used in the analysis were really not theirs. We provided a partial list of test costs, such as the cost of a CBC, BUN, MRI, and CT. A glossary giving definitions of the data and the graphs of the report as well as terminology was provided. Finally, an evaluation form, as well as the phone number of the associate chief of staff, was provided should there be any issues, questions, or comments at the time the reports were received. The chairs were given summarative divisional or departmental data comparing performance.

The impact of the physician data reports by themselves is difficult to assess, as a number of strategies were simultaneously implemented, including the SITs, the case managers, and organization-wide communications regarding the need to be cost conscious. The combined effort, however, has had widespread success. The appearance and content of these reports have improved over time. They now include intraoperative case times by procedure and by surgeon, and special reports are used for psychiatry because of DRG and DSM coding differences.

CEU progress yields improvements

We have compared our financial performance to the best performing UHC hospitals (75th percentile) by DRG using the Clinical Information Network database. Using these data we rank-ordered our performance opportunities from highest to lowest and began to work on the top 10 DRGs through a SIT methodology. Over the past two years, this has resulted in a series of improvements in at least three areas:

1. Clinical outcomes have improved.
2. Utilization has been reduced (the length of stay, the number of diagnostic studies, and pharmaceutical use have all been reduced).
3. Fewer consultants have been used.

In the length-of-stay category, we have seen new protocols for the management of neurosurgical patients, standardized protocols for placement of ventriculostomies outside of the Intensive Care Unit, implementation of same-day admissions for nearly all surgical procedures, and implementation of a variety of multidisciplinary clinical practice guidelines. We have reduced the use of expensive studies, particularly, magnetic resonance imaging, minimized the use of expensive contrast media, standardized the selection and administration protocols for use of antibiotics, and minimized the use of testing for specific diagnoses. We have initiated a regular report (Quality and Performance Report) that organizes several of our outcomes into six major areas (see the box entitled "Quality and Performance Indicators").

The Quality and Performance Report is produced quarterly. This report, however, did not keep pace with management's needs, so a monthly report is produced that displays on a "dashboard" or instrument panel six major indicators of performance: mortality, unplanned readmissions, patient complaints, unplanned day surgery admissions, patient falls, and nosocomial bacteremia. These measures help to quickly pinpoint areas where there are issues or problems that require further intervention.

Over the past two years, we have saved approximately $6 million in clinical resource management. Our average length of stay has continued to decline, while our inpatient admissions have increased. We continue to benchmark our

---

Quality and Performance Indicators

Volume
  Admissions/Visits
  ALOS
  Patient Days
  Vent Days
  OR Cases/Turnaround Time
  Tests/Procedures
  Utilization Review*/
    Avoidable Days/Skilled
    Nursing Facility/Administrative Necessary Day*

Clinical Outcomes
  Mortality
  Unplanned Readmission*
  Unplanned OR Returns
  Unplanned Day Surgery
    Readmissions
  Unplanned Returns ICU
  Surgical Wound Infections*
  Bacteremias*

Drug Usage*
Adverse Drug Reactions*
Blood Usage*
Medical Record Delinquency*
Surgical Case Review*
Autopsy Rate*

Safety/Risk Management
  Patient Falls
  Medication Errors
  IV Infiltrates
  Surgical Counts
  Equipment/Device Occurrences
  Current Malpractice Claims

Satisfaction
  Patient/Family
  Employee
  Referring Physician

Community
Patient Complaints

Performance
  Performance Evaluations*
  Corrective Actions
  Terminations
  Turnover Rates

Financial
  Operating Margin
  Days' Cash-on-Hand
  Current Ratio
  Accounts Receivable Days
    Outstanding
  FTEs Adjusted Occupied
  Net Revenue/FTE
  Variable Cost (Transition
    Systems Incorporated) Per
    Case
  Total Cost/Discharge

*Required by 1995 Joint Commission standards.

performance using a number of external databases, including Medpar, the Massachusetts Health Data Consortium, University Health-System Consortium, and other state databases as appropriate. Patient satisfaction and functional measures (quality-of-life measures) have become a common part of our organizational lexicon.

Because virtually all of the CRM activities and programs, such as the SITs, the seven-step process, our tracking system, and the Case Management Program, were developed internally, reliance on consultants was minimal. Because our work was developed collaboratively, many people are vested in the success of the overall program. Indeed, there was great resentment when a recent consulting group arrived on the scene and tried to undo work in progress.

● ● ●

Our experience at UMass has demonstrated that improvements in outcomes, both clinical and cost, are possible in today's health care environment. Process improvement requires an investment in human resources, measurement instruments, and information technology. Rapid progress can be made when essential elements combine in the appropriate environment. Variation in practice is common and represents a great opportunity to improve care and quality.

Information systems technologies greatly facilitate progress, but enormous progress can be made with rudimentary information. In our case, most advances have been made as a result of individuals discovering new ways of performing common activities. Appropriate information systems support can speed progress and improve efficiency and monitoring, which for us is now largely manual.

Although there may initially be some resistance to imminent change (and there will always be resistance to change), a predictable, structured approach and a demonstrated track record are reassuring and will help garner project cooperation. Involvement of and feedback to senior leaders is essential to ongoing efforts. Data (and their appropriate use), peer pressure, organizational support (by chairs and the CEO), and leadership can successfully motivate change.

What is the right model for other hospitals and organizations? There is no single strategy to facilitate change. At least four generic approaches have been applied successfully at UMass's CEU: CQI, re-engineering, restructuring, and use of focused business initiatives. Each approach is very different. Indeed there are times when one approach may be preferred to another within the same institution. From a clinical perspective, however, there is no substitute for direct physician involvement. The challenge is to develop a program that takes into account the financial and time pressures upon physicians and other health care providers. Ultimately, our experience in establishing a clinical evaluation unit suggests positive movement in the direction of reduction of costs and improvement in customer satisfaction.

REFERENCES

1. Dobson, A., Coleman, K., and Mehanic, R. *Analysis of Teaching Hospital Costs.* Fairfax, Va.: Lewin-VHI, 1994.
2. Kassirer, J.P. "Academic Medical Centers under Siege." *New England Journal of Medicine* 331 (1994): 1370–71.
3. Black, E.R., Weiss, K.D., Erban, S., and Shulkin, D. "Innovations in Patient Care: Changing Clinical Practice and Improving Quality." *Joint Commission Journal on Quality Improvement* 21, no. 8 (1995): 376–93.

PART IV

Case Management in Action: Cases in Profile

Trauma Critical Pathways:
A Care Delivery System That Works

Elizabeth E. Latini

Continuous performance improvement in patient care is of paramount importance to the Robert Packer Hospital, a regional accredited trauma center in rural Pennsylvania. In fall 1991, a care delivery system known as case management was introduced as a mode for achieving this goal.[1] Now, 3 years later, case management has proven a viable means to accomplish this goal and to enhance the quality of care experienced by trauma patients and their families throughout hospitalization.

Case management is defined as the care delivery system that focuses on the attainment of patient goals within a specifically defined time frame, integrating the efforts of all health care team members.[2,3] Case management addresses the entire episode of illness through the use of case management plans or *critical pathways*. These, critical pathways define the anticipated length of stay, delineate desired patient outcomes and goals, and provide directions for care of identified patient care types.[4,5] Because diagnosis-related groups (DRGs) have not been defined for trauma as they have for single-system illnesses, it became evident that development of a trauma critical pathway could not be accomplished based on DRGs. The proposed trauma critical pathway would specifically address the cascade of trauma injury as opposed to a single DRG-related illness.[6]

THE PROBLEM

Trauma patients are members of a unique population who, by their nature, pose difficult patient management situations. Approximately 90% of the trauma patients at the Robert Packer Hospital have sustained blunt trauma, primarily closed-head injury or musculoskeletal insult. A review of the standards defined by the Pennsylvania Trauma Systems Foundation, the State of Pennsylvania, American College of Surgeons, and the Joint Commission on the Accreditation of Healthcare Organizations and the hospital's compliance with them identified common standards that make management of this patient population challenging. For example, multiple injury trauma patients in the intensive care unit (ICU) often had untimely submission of consults, which should occur within 72 hours of admission. Likewise, inconsistent medical record documentation omitted discharge planning, teaching, and family inclusion in planning care.

THE SOLUTION

Based on this knowledge, three trauma critical pathways were developed. Each pathway incorporated biophysical, psychosocial, discharge planning, self-care, environmental, and teaching aspects. All transdisciplinary team members,

Crit Care Nurs Q 1996; 19(1): 83–87
© 1996 Aspen Publishers, Inc.

The author thanks Rosemary K. Sartor, MA. Without her support, this article would not have been possible.

(prehospital, resuscitation, operating and recovery rooms, intensive care and trauma step-down nursing, laboratory, dietary, physical and occupational therapy, rehabilitation, and home care) were integrated in the process. Medical standing orders were written to implement the pathways in a consistent, timely manner. A variation tool was also developed for performance improvement measurement.

FINDINGS

Performance improvement measurement revealed positive trends. Data collection during 1992 and 1993 was accomplished by the trauma clinical nurse specialist, who was the trauma case manager and who reviewed 40% of the trauma medical records. Because of the importance of this data collection, the transdisciplinary trauma team demanded that a more reliable methodology for performance improvement be instituted. Therefore, beginning January 1, 1994, performance indicators regarding length of stay (LOS), appropriate use of the three pathways based on defined protocols, and consultation completion rates were included in the trauma patient abstract form process.

Performance indicators have now become a permanent part of the hospital's trauma registry. Quarterly reports are generated by the trauma registry and trauma clinical nurse specialist on all abstracted patients regarding these indicators instead of a percentage of charts (see Fig 1). LOS within the trauma service patient subpopulations of patients with major head injuries [defined as those head-injured patients with an abbreviated injury severity score (AIS), or AIS of >4][7] as well as patients with major extremity trauma (defined as those extremity injury patients with an AIS of >4) have been positively affected by the implementation of critical pathways (see Fig 1). It is important to note that the average injury severity score (ISS) was less for both trauma patient subpopulations of major head injury and major extremity injury in the years before the trauma service case manage-

ment initiative. Despite this, the average LOS in the ICU, as well as the overall LOS, has remained constant or, in many instances, decreased for these trauma patient subpopulations.

Use of critical pathways

Use of the trauma critical pathways by the transdisciplinary team has been exceptional. Performance improvement review of consultation completion for all three pathways showed an improvement from a low of 22% in 1992 to better than 75.67% in 1994 (see Fig 1 for specifics). Improvement in transdisciplinary team members' ability to place a consult with appropriate disciplines is evident. The transdisciplinary team members are committed to achieving a 100% compliance rate. This high rate is an example of how the data are currently used as feedback, communication tools for the team, and as performance improvement tools. Quarterly reports are presented to the transdisciplinary team members through staff meetings, inservice workshops, and at the trauma multidisciplinary, trauma executive, and morbidity and mortality staff meetings.

After discharge

Following discharge from the trauma center, all patients are mailed a patient/family follow-up survey. The survey has a return rate of 10% to 15%. Positive comments regarding satisfaction with the care a family member received while hospitalized predominate. The trauma critical nurse specialist and primary nurse meet with all trauma service patients, explain the plan of care, and allow family interaction. The trauma critical nurse specialist maintains accountability for family education of head-injured patients and related documentation standards. All trauma patients are discussed at a weekly transdisciplinary meeting. At that time, any patient, practitioner, or system variance that influences the flow of the patient through the system is addressed.

	Total 1992	Total 1993	Total 1994
Average yearly ISS	10.716	10.621*	10.743
Total number of charts reviewed	73	28	294
Number of patient charts meeting criteria	50	19	125
1. 72-hours C.P. used	44	18	109
Percentage	88.00	94.74	87.20
Number of patient charts meeting criteria	2	3	28
2. Head injury C.P. used	N/A	3	19
Percentage	N/A	100.00	67.86
Number of patient charts meeting criteria	23	13	141[†]
3. Musculoskeletal C.P. used	8	12	158[†]
Percentage	34.78	93.31	112.06
4. Consult completed within time frame 1992—24 hours 1993, 1994—48 hours			
Physical therapy	22.75	52.50	88.38
Occupational therapy	22.25	45.24	92.50
Social services	66.25	85.46	90.06
TR	31.25	72.22	75.61
Number of patient charts meeting criteria	5	3	22
5. Family received head injury book	3	3	22
Number of patient charts meeting criteria	8	3	22
6. Received teaching of head injury rehabilitation	8	3	22
7. Major head injured			
Average length of stay	10.6	11.2	13.2
Average length of stay in ICU	3.08	4.47	7.5
8. Major extremity injured			
Average length of stay	12.4	12.34	9.07
Average length of stay in ICU	3.8	5.4	2.67
9. Adequate discharge planning documented (%)	100.00	100.00	100.00

*1st quarter 1993, trauma center closed.
[†]Seventeen additional patients had musculoskeletal pathways used. Of these, 14 were admitted to the trauma service.

Fig 1. Outcome data chart review of trauma patients.

Other outcomes

Trauma case management support has been outstanding. All four trauma surgeons agree that their patients now receive more consistent and timely care. Transdisciplinary team members, including those from physical and occupational therapy, social services, dietary services, rehabilitation, and pastoral care departments, value the prompt consultation and initiation of treatment modalities which promote improved patient outcomes. Registered nurses in trauma care areas cite improved communication and the facilitation of collaboration among disciplines as a pivotal aspect of the critical pathway/case management approach to the patient's hospitalization.

Case management has had a positive impact on cost savings to the consumer. The trauma and finance departments are actively working to interface databases to provide an overall definition of the cost savings to both the consumer and to the trauma center. Although this database can only interface to allow a sampling of, as opposed to overall definition of, this cost savings, a positive relationship can still be observed. In an era of health care reform, this is a strong marketing tool that could positively influence customer use of the Robert Packer Hospital.

• • •

Currently, work is underway for further development of trauma pathways by incorporating daily goals and specific expected outcomes. These additions serve to enhance the present methodology of performance improvement measurement and effectiveness of clinical pathways.

The incorporation of trauma critical pathways into the daily practice of caring for trauma patients at this institution has proven invaluable. The experience of staff members demonstrates that quality patient care can be and is indeed achieved by the use of critical pathways for the management of the trauma patient population.

REFERENCES

1. Latini E, Foote W. Obtaining consistent quality patient care for the trauma patient by using a critical pathway. *Crit Care Nurs Q*. 1992;15:51–55.

2. Zander K. Nursing case management: resolving the DRG paradox. *Nurs Clin North Am*. 1988;23:503–520.

3. Zander K. Nursing case management: strategic management of cost and quality outcomes. *J Nurs Admin*. 1988;18:23–30.

4. Etheridge MLS. *Collaborative Care: Nursing Case Management*. Chicago, Ill: American Hospital; 1989.

5. Etheridge P, Lamb GS. Professional nursing care management improves quality, access, and cost. *Nurs Manag*. 1991;20:30–35.

6. 3M Health Information Systems. *Diagnosis Related Groups: Version 12.0 Definitions Manual*. Murray, Utah: 3M; 1994.

7. Association for the Advancement of Automotive Medicine. *The Abbreviated Injury Scale: 1990 Revision*. Des Plains, Ill. Association for the Advancement of Automotive Medicine; 1990.

Guidelines for Evaluation and Education of Adult Patients with Mild Traumatic Brain Injuries in an Acute Care Hospital Setting

Kathy A. Lawler and Carol A. Terregino

Each year hundreds of thousands of Americans sustain mild traumatic brain injuries (TBIs) from various mechanisms, with an incidence estimated to be as high as 200 cases per year per 100,000 people.[1] The impact on public health is obvious when one considers the large number of patients affected. Currently there is no consensus as to the optimal evaluation and management strategy for mild TBI. Many patients who sustain a mild TBI are initially evaluated in an emergency or trauma department of a hospital. Treatment protocols vary considerably from center to center. A mild TBI is often not diagnosed or addressed until later, when complications draw attention to it.

There are various theories proposed in the literature concerning persistent postconcussion symptoms following mild TBI. For example psychogenic factors including psychiatric disturbances such as posttraumatic stress disorders and affective and somatoform disorders have received considerable emphasis.[2] Other investigators stress the role of legal compensation as a significant contributing factor in the persistence of postconcussion symptoms.[3,4] However, much evidence points to the fact that there are actually underlying neuropathologic changes causing at least some of the postconcussion symptoms, particularly shortly after the trauma. Empirical evidence was provided by Ommaya and

J Head Trauma Rehabil 1996; 11(6): 18–28

Gennarelli,[5] who demonstrated that mild cerebral trauma (concussion) could produce identifiable central nervous system (CNS) lesions in animals. Most early clinical studies failed to find evidence of neuropathologic changes due to the insensitivity of computed tomography (CT) scans in detecting the microscopic changes characteristic of mild TBI.[6] However, more recent clinical studies using magnetic resonance imaging have identified macroscopic CNS lesions (parenchymal) in various cortical sites, especially frontal and temporal lobes, after mild head injury.[7,8] Similarly, a recent study of selected patients with mild TBI and persistent subjective problems, demonstrated temporal and frontal lobe dysfunction on positron emission tomography (PET) scan that correlated with neuropsychological deficits.[9]

It is not uncommon for patients with a mild TBI to have attention/concentration and memory problems for several weeks, months, or even longer following their injury.[8,10,11] However, most of these patients are sent home from the hospital with general advice to "take it easy," with full recovery expected within a few days.[12] Many patients who seem "normal" at discharge report a variety of continuing problems that may be somatic (headaches, dizziness, blurred vision), cognitive (slow or "foggy" thinking, difficulty concentrating, and problems remembering information), or affective (depression, anxiety, decreased frustration tolerance).[13] Patients are often told by their practitioner that they are fine and not to worry, which may have adverse effects. Patients often begin to worry that they are imagining their symptoms, which can lead to further frustration, depression, and anxiety.[14]

Symptoms may also temporarily appear worse due to stress. One way to avoid these secondary emotional complications is to address symptoms early and to provide educational information and reassurance that it is normal to have some of these symptoms lasting a few weeks, months, or longer.[8,15–17]

Early patient education concerning possible postconcussional symptoms may be beneficial in decreasing the incidence of later complications.[15,17] In a well-controlled clinical study, Minderhoud and colleagues[16] showed that postconcussional sequelae were markedly reduced by early treatment, which included information, explanation, and encouragement. Researchers hypothesized that postconcussional sequelae initially have an organic basis, but persistent sequelae after minor head injuries are also caused by psychogenic and especially by iatrogenic factors. These findings suggest that appropriate management and education of mild TBI patients may help to avert symptoms that are of psychological rather than pathophysiologic origin. In spite of compelling evidence from the literature establishing the importance of symptom recognition and referrals, at present many patients treated for mild TBI in hospital settings are typically provided with minimal or no instructions concerning the risk for development of neurobehavioral sequelae or the temporal course of recovery, and referrals are not routinely made.[14,18] In support of previously cited findings, we propose that secondary emotional distress leading to aggravation of postconcussion symptoms, and possibly excessive time away from work or school after mild TBI, could be minimized by early clinical intervention.[17] This intervention should provide educational information, assess the presence of acute neurobehavioral deficits, advise the patient on a gradual and graded resumption of activities, and arrange referrals for follow-up assessment as needed.

DEFINITION OF MILD TBI

The lack of consensus in the definition of mild TBI used in research protocols and the lack of uniform inclusion criteria for mild TBI employed by researchers may account for the inconsistencies in the amount of neurobehavioral recovery reported.[2]

The Mild Traumatic Brain Injury Subcommittee of the Head Injury Interdisciplinary Special Interest Group of the American Congress of Rehabilitation Medicine specified that mild TBI should not include an injury with a posttraumatic amnesia (PTA) exceeding 24 hours.[19] However, very few clinicians routinely assess the length of PTA in any systematic way. Most clinicians and researchers use the reported time of loss of consciousness (LOC) and initial Glasgow Coma Scale (GCS) score to define mild TBI, although several investigators have noted the lack of sensitivity of the GCS within the mild range of impaired consciousness.[2,8] To improve classification and predictions of recovery, Williams et al[20] proposed that it is more accurate from a neurobehavioral standpoint to classify mild TBI patients according to the presence or absence of significant intracranial lesions on computed tomography of the head. They subdivided patients with mild TBI into two groups: (1) an uncomplicated group, which included patients with a GCS score of 13 to 15 and LOC of 20 minutes or less and patients with depressed skull fractures but no evidence of intracranial lesions; and (2) a complicated group, with GCS scores of 13 to 15 and LOC 20 minutes or less and with intracranial lesions as detected by CT scan. This classification system allows the early detection of patients with intracranial lesions who are more at risk for developing neurobehavioral complications and are most likely to require and benefit from more comprehensive examinations and neuropsychological follow-up testing.

Our clinical protocol uses the definition described above of Williams et al[20] for complicated and uncomplicated mild TBI resulting from cranial trauma caused by acceleration/deceleration injury or other blunt mechanisms of injury. This allows us to immediately identify complicated mild TBI patients who have a higher probability of developing persistent symptoms. These patients are automatically referred for follow-up services (see Table 2).

CLINICAL SETTING

This protocol was developed as part of an interdisciplinary mild TBI research project involving the department of emergency medicine, trauma surgery, and neuropsychology within a large urban tertiary care center with a Level I Trauma designation. The focus of this research protocol was to evaluate the relationship among critical clinical parameters, results of CT scanning, and performance on early neuropsychological measures in a large, consecutive series of patients with complicated and uncomplicated mild TBI (Carol A. Terregino, MD, unpublished report). The authors were part of a larger team of investigators who devised a research protocol that includes a brief neuropsychological screening battery described here. The rationale for selecting these tests was based on research that identified the cognitive functions of attention/concentration, speed of information processing, and memory as the primary areas affected by mild TBI.[8,21–24]

PURPOSE OF THE MILD TBI PROTOCOL

The purpose of this protocol is to provide hospital staff in a busy and hectic acute care setting with realistic guidelines that enable them to (1) evaluate the physical and cognitive symptoms of patients with mild TBI; (2) identify patients at high risk for complications due to the specifics of their head injury, to preexisting complications, or to other factors known to correlate with poor recovery (eg, age); (3) provide patients and families with educational information that may help to avoid secondary complications; and (4) make appropriate referrals.

In our experience, the implementation of this protocol has had the added benefit of increasing the awareness and the interest of emergency and trauma staff concerning the cognitive and behavioral aspects of mild TBI. Inservice programs designed to educate staff concerning the neurobehavioral effects of mild TBI have heightened awareness of how important it is to make this relatively minor commitment of time and effort. These inservice programs were designed to train staff to administer and score the evaluation tools in a consistent and reliable manner. Staff then administered the tests while observed by the neuropsychologist to make sure that they followed standardized procedures. In the initial phase of implementing this protocol, we were aided by additional research staff members who were trained to administer the neuropsychological tests. Obviously, perfect compliance is not expected with any practice guideline, and at times emergency staff are too busy for even a short 20-minute cognitive screening evaluation. For those situations, clinical staff were encouraged to prioritize and shorten the protocol to at least include an assessment of any high risk factors (see Table 2) that would necessitate referral for follow-up treatment.

Each day an assigned staff member reviewed the hospital admission list of all patients admitted through the departments of trauma and emergency medicine to ensure that patients with mild TBI who had another primary diagnosis (eg, thoracic, abdominal, orthopedic, or spinal cord injury), were evaluated.

EVALUATION PROTOCOL

The evaluation procedure was designed for patients ages 18 years and older who meet the criteria for complicated or uncomplicated mild TBI discussed above. The evaluation is divided into three parts: medical assessment, cognitive assessment, and assessment of high-risk factors.

Medical assessment

Standard practice at our center includes CT scanning of the head for all patients with acceleration/deceleration injury or blunt mechanism injury that results in LOC or amnesia for the event of injury. In the emergency department, patients with no evidence of intracranial injury on CT scan, a normal neurologic evaluation, and GCS score of 15 are discharged home if a reliable observer is present. Patients without a supportive home environment or under the influence of alcohol or drugs are observed in the department for an extended period. Generally, 4 to 6 hours after presentation or after the effects of intoxicating substances are minimal, however, the specific duration of the observation period is determined by the treating physician. A preprinted instruction sheet with guidelines on activity, diet, analgesics, and periodic wakening for neurologic checks, in addition to warning signs and symptoms, is carefully reviewed by the nurse with patient and family (Fig 1). Patients with a complicated mild TBI or with a normal head CT scan but other significant injuries necessitating further management are admitted.

Cognitive assessment

Impairment of attention, memory, and information-processing efficiency is common during the first few days after mild TBI.[8,21,24] Patients

with mild TBI often have a good outcome,[22,25,26] but persistent impairments have been reported by several investigators.[9,27,28] A mental status examination is not sufficient to capture subtle attention and memory deficits, and it does not allow for adequate documentation of improvement over time. Therefore, neuropsychometric assessments have been recognized as a valuable component of the diagnostic and therapeutic management of mild TBI patients. It is important to realize that although neuropsychological tests are generally more sensitive than routine mental status examinations, they may not be sensitive enough to detect some cognitive deficits. This is especially true for impairments in executive functioning due to prefrontal injury. The high incidence of prefrontal injury in TBI, combined with the fact that it is sometimes difficult to demonstrate impairments in executive functioning with neuropsychological tests, makes it especially important for clinicians to be wary of interpreting success on formal neuropsychological tests as an indication that there are no impairments in executive functioning.

It is also important that clinicians be aware of the fact that there are many factors that may

1. Avoid strenuous activity for at least 24 hours.
2. Eat a light diet for 24 hours following injury.
3. Use aspirin (adults) or Tylenol for headache every 4 hours as needed.
4. The patient should be awakened every 2 hours, day and night, for 24 hours. Deeper than normal sleep (difficulty waking up fully) may indicate a more serious degree of head injury.
5. Call the emergency department (telephone number here) or return immediately for:
   a. Severe or worsening headache
   b. Inability to wake up the patient
   c. Sleepiness or confusion
   d. Unusual restlessness, unsteady walk, or seizures (convulsions, fits)
   e. Trouble seeing properly
   f. Vomiting
   g. Stiff neck
   h. Fever (temperature greater than 100°F by mouth)
   i. Bleeding from nose, mouth, or ears
   j. Trouble controlling urine or bowels
   k. Weakness of arm or leg

Your treatment in the emergency department is only for temporary care. You should see your family doctor or make an appointment for follow-up care as instructed.

Fig 1. Written instruction sheet given to patients who have sustained a concussion or mild TBI. This information is carefully reviewed by the nurse with the patient and family prior to discharge.

cause a patient to perform poorly, especially in an acute hospital setting, and fail a neuropsychological test that has nothing to do with actual cognitive impairments. For example, some patients may be upset because of the accident, worried about injury sustained by other family members or friends, concerned about missing work, distracted by pain, or have poor concentration due to the effects of medication or ongoing activities in the emergency department or the patient's room. Under these conditions, test scores need to be interpreted very cautiously.

Realistically, a cognitive baseline screening evaluation must be short and uncomplicated if it is to be consistently administered in an acute care setting by non-neuropsychologists. It must also be sensitive to the cognitive areas known to be impaired by mild TBI, including attention/concentration, speed of information processing, and learning and memory. We developed a screening evaluation (Table 1) that met these criteria and therefore could be easily administered by a variety of staff (nurses, physicians, students, research assistants, neuropsychologists) after two training sessions with observation/feedback during initial administration of the tests.

Admitted patients are assessed usually within 48 hours of injury and patients being discharged home are assessed prior to discharge from the emergency department. The cognitive screening evaluation takes approximately 20 to 25 minutes and begins with several questions aimed at estimating PTA, which is characterized as a period of disorientation, confusion, and gross anterograde amnesia. This is assessed using the Galveston Orientation and Amnesia Test (GOAT), which measures resolution of PTA and the patient's general level of orientation.[29] According to the standard administration of the GOAT, a score of 75 or greater indicates that a patient is oriented sufficiently to reliably administer other neuropsychological tests. Frequently verbal learning and memory are neuropsychological functions that are at least temporarily impaired following mild TBI.[24,25,30]

Learning and memory are briefly evaluated using the Learning and Memory Subtests of the Neurobehavioral Cognitive Screening Evaluation (NCSE), which requires the patient to learn four words and later tests for recall of the words.[31] A recent study has shown that paragraph-length recall of verbal information is one of the most sensitive neuropsychological tests for mild TBI.[23] Therefore, we included an immediate and 20-minute delayed recall of a paragraph of logically related verbal information from the Rivermead Behavioral Memory Test.[32]

Other areas vulnerable to the effects of mild TBI are attention and concentration.[20,30,33] To evaluate these abilities, we included the auditory Digit Span Forward and Backward subtest from the Wechsler Memory Scale—Revised (WMS-

Table 1. Brief test protocol for screening important cognitive functions of patients with mild TBI in an acute hospital setting

Test	Cognitive function	Time (min)
Auditory Digit Span (subtest of WMS-R)	Concentration and immediate recall of digits forward and backward	4
GOAT	Orientation to person, place, and time; estimate of PTA	4
Paragraph Recall (subtest of Rivermead Behavioral Memory Test)	Verbal memory for logically related information	5
Verbal Learning (subtest of NCSE)	Verbal learning of single words, storage, and retrieval of words	5
PASAT (Series I and II)	Information processing rate, adding single digits presented via audio tape	4

R).[34] To evaluate the frequently affected speed of information processing ability,[30] we used the first two series (Series I and Series II) of the Paced Auditory Serial Addition Task (PASAT), which assess efficiency of information processing under time pressure.[35] This test requires the patient to add a number to an immediately preceding number. The test must be administered using a tape recorder that fits easily into the pocket of a coat so it is always readily available to staff. It is sometimes necessary to eliminate the PASAT from the testing protocol due to the noise level in the emergency department.

Each individual cognitive test has simple scoring directions that are printed on the test form. Criteria are described on the test form that immediately identify failed performance on specific tests. This is done in the form of cutoff scores, based on norms included in the published manual for each test, that denote impaired performance on individual subtests.

The pattern and severity of postconcussion symptoms have been found to have both diagnostic and prognostic significance, and therefore it is important to obtain a thorough and standard measure of these symptoms.[13] Several studies have attempted to specifically evaluate patients with persistent postconcussion symptoms and have found reduced neuropsychological functioning and an inability to resume normal functioning even more than 1 year after injury.[36,37] Patients who report a greater number of symptoms at 1, 6, or 12 months after sustaining a mild TBI may have less adequate neuropsychological functioning than patients reporting few or no symptoms.[38,39] We developed the Postconcussion Symptom Inventory (PSI) with a four-point rating scale (Fig 2) that includes the most commonly reported somatic/physical, emotional, and cognitive complaints.[13] This brief assessment tool is a simple self-report inventory that is very quick and easy to administer, taking approximately 5 minutes of the patient's time, and is scored according to the subjective severity of the symptom from 0 to 3 (see Fig 2). Patients also indicate on the form, using a simple yes/no format, whether their current experience of each

symptom represents a change from their pre-injury state. The inventory covers a wide range of commonly reported postconcussion symptoms, some of which are not directly relevant in the emergency department setting. In the emergency department setting, patients are requested to answer only the relevant items of the inventory dealing with initial physical symptoms such as headaches, dizziness, nausea, and sensitivity to lights and noise.

Assessment of high-risk factors

Research studies have documented a variety of factors that place a patient with a mild TBI at risk for neurobehavioral complications. These include a previous concussion,[40] age 40 or older,[41] preexisting emotional or psychiatric problems,[42] certain demanding occupations,[41] alcohol and/or drug abuse,[12,43] and prolonged PTA.[41,44]

An evaluation of significant high-risk factors consists of a simple structured interview format with a checklist of factors known to be associated with poorer outcomes and increased complications following mild TBI. This simple checklist serves as a "red flag" system to alert staff to patients who should be referred for follow-up services (Table 2).

Educational component

Patients are provided with clearly written educational information concerning the common symptoms of mild TBI, including a description of physical, cognitive, and emotional/behavioral symptoms. To avoid unrealistic expectations and the failure and frustration patients often confront when returning to work and school unaware of possible deficits, we provide them with a realistic but not overly negative view. In essence, recovery may be a prolonged process and may take quite a long time. Appropriate educational information about anticipated problems and recommendations for a gradual return to normal activities may play an important role in outcome by preventing secondary adjustment

Please read each item in the list carefully. Indicate how much you have been bothered by each symptom since your injury. Place an "X" in the corresponding space in the column next to each symptom. In the last column, circle "Y" for yes if your experience of this symptom is different than before your injury and "N" for no if there has been no change.

		NOT AT ALL	MILDLY-IT DID NOT BOTHER ME MUCH	MODERATELY-IT WAS VERY UNPLEASANT BUT I COULD STAND IT	SEVERELY - I COULD BARELY STAND IT	DIFFERENT FROM BEFORE INJURY?	
1.	Dizziness					Y	N
2.	Headaches					Y	N
3.	Nausea					Y	N
4.	Problem with vision blurred/double					Y	N
5.	Sensitivity to light					Y	N
6.	Sensitivity to noise					Y	N
7.	Fatigue (e.g. lower energy level)					Y	N
8.	Loss or decrease in sense of taste					Y	N
9.	Loss or decrease in sense of smell					Y	N
10.	Problems with coordination					Y	N
11.	Sleep disturbance					Y	N
12.	Change in appetite					Y	N
13.	Decreased hearing or ringing in ears					Y	N
14.	Difficulty finding words when speaking					Y	N
15.	Difficulty remembering things					Y	N
16.	Difficulty concentrating					Y	N
17.	Difficulty thinking clearly					Y	N
18.	Irritability					Y	N
19.	Increased moodiness					Y	N
20.	Difficulty controlling impulses					Y	N
21.	Feeling depressed					Y	N
22.	Feeling anxious					Y	N
23.	Quicker loss of temper					Y	N

Scoring: 0 = Not at all
1 = Mildly
2 = Moderately
3 = Severely

Fig 2. Sample of the Postconcussion Symptom Inventory, which is self-administered by the patient and requires approximately 3 to 5 minutes to complete. Each symptom is rated on a four-point scale (0 to 3) according to severity. Patients also indicate whether their experience of each symptom is a change compared with before their injury by circling "Y" for yes or "N" for no.

Table 2. List of questions included in the initial structured interview*

1. Does patient have a previous head injury, loss of consciousness, or neurologic disorder?
2. Is the patient 40 years old or older?
3. Does the patient have a history of alcohol or drug abuse?
4. Does the patient have a psychiatric history?
5. Is the patient a student or involved in a training program?
6. Is the patient scheduled to take any important tests or qualifying examinations in the near future (eg, licensing examination)?
7. Does the patient have a demanding occupation where even mild postconcussion symptoms causing errors may seriously affect job performance or safety (eg, school bus driver)?
8. Does the initial radiologic examination reveal an intracranial lesion?
9. Has the patient had a prolonged period (>6 hr) of posttraumatic amnesia?

*These are aimed at evaluating red flag/high-risk factors in patients who have sustained a mild TBI. If the interviewer circles yes (Y) for any of these questions, then the patient is referred for follow-up evaluation/services to the outpatient mild TBI program so that recovery can be more closely monitored. N = no.

problems and helping to avoid unrealistic expectations and self-blame in the future.[8,15]

Referral for further treatment

In our clinical setting, patients who require follow-up services based on the initial screening evaluation or who later develop problems are instructed (in writing) to call the division of neurology, which has an outpatient mild TBI evaluation and treatment program. Specifically, patients whose performance on the neuropsychological screening battery indicates cognitive impairment and/or patients who have one or more of the high-risk factors listed in Table 2 are referred for follow-up evaluation. In our clinical setting, the neurology consultation service provides a coordinated evaluation of the multidimensional mild TBI symptomatology: somatic, cognitive, and affective. For example, a follow-up neurologic examination for somatic complaints may detect a variety of subtle injuries to the neck or inner ear, which can contribute to headaches and dizziness. Physicians can then evaluate and manage these symptoms before they become chronic. Persistent cognitive and affective symptoms are most accurately assessed through follow-up neuropsychological assessment. It is important to be aware that in many clinical settings, it is more common for physiatrists rather than neurologists to direct

outpatient mild TBI evaluation and rehabilitation/treatment programs.

SUMMARY

The goal of this system is to prevent the development of secondary neurobehavioral complications in patients with mild TBI through early intervention and education. The implementation of this protocol demonstrates the feasibility of evaluating acute neurobehavioral symptoms of mild TBI through a 25-minute evaluation consisting of specific cognitive tests and a self-report questionnaire to assess postconcussion symptoms. Important educational and referral information that describes common symptoms during the first few days and weeks is routinely provided to patients and families. These few preventive measures may prove to be cost-effective in averting secondary complications and avoiding excessive time away from work and/or school.

This protocol may serve as a model for other clinicians who assess and treat patients with mild TBI in an acute hospital setting. The protocol outlined above can be easily modified for use with younger children. We are currently working on such a modification that primarily involves the use of an alternative age-appropriate screening assessment of PTA and cognitive functions in younger children.

REFERENCES

1. Elkind A. Headache and head trauma. *Clin J Pain*. 1989;5:77–87.

2. Binder L. Persisting symptoms after mild head injury: a review of the postconcussive syndrome. *J Clin Exp Neuropsychol*. 1986;8:323–346.

3. Barth J, et al. Neuropsychological sequelae of minor head injury. *Neurosurgery*. 1983;13:529–533.

4. Miller H. Accident neurosis. *Br Med J*. 1969;1:9–19.

5. Ommaya A, Gennarelli T. Cerebral concussion and traumatic unconsciousness: correlation of experimental and clinical observations on blunt head injuries. *Brain*. 1974;95:633–654.

6. Mittl R, et al. Prevalence of MR evidence of diffuse axonal injury in patients with mild head injury and normal head CT findings. *Am J Neuroradiol*. 1994; 15:1,583–1,589.

7. Levin H, et al. Serial MRI and neurobehavioral findings after mild to moderate closed head injury. *J Neurol Neurosurg Psychiatry*. 1992;55:255–262.

8. Levin H, et al. Neurobehavioral outcome following minor head injury: a three-center study. *J Neurosurg*. 1987;66:234–243.

9. Ruff R, et al. Selected cases of poor outcome following a minor brain trauma: comparing neuropsychological and positron emission tomography assessment. *Brain Injury*. 1994;8(4):297–308.

10. Alves W, et al. Understanding posttraumatic symptoms after minor head injury. *J Head Trauma Rehabil*. 1986;2:1–12.

11. Dikmen S, McLean A, Temkin N. Neuropsychological and psychosocial consequences of minor head injury. *J Neurol Neurosurg Psychiatry*. 1986;49: 1,227–1,232.

12. Kay T. Toward a neuropsychological model of functional disability after mild traumatic brain injury. *Neuropsychology*. 1992;6:371–384.

13. Cicerone D, Kalmar K. Persistent postconcussive syndrome: the structure of subjective complaints after mild traumatic brain injury. *J Head Trauma Rehabil*. 1995;10(3):1–17.

14. Kay T. *Minor Head Injury: An Introduction for Professionals*. Washington, DC: National Head Injury Foundation; 1986.

15. Alves W, Macciocchi S, Barth J. Postconcussive symptoms after uncomplicated mild head injury. *J Head Trauma Rehabil*. 1993;3(3):48–59.

16. Minderhoud J, et al. Treatment of minor head injuries. *Clin Neurol Neurosurg*. 1980;82:127–140.

17. Mittenberg W, Burton D. A survey of treatments for post-concussion syndrome. *Brain Injury*. 1994;8: 429–437.

18. Evans R, Evans R. The physician survey on the post-concussion and whiplash syndromes. *Headache*. 1994; 34:268–274.

19. Committee on Mild Traumatic Brain Injury, American Congress of Rehabilitation Medicine. Definition of mild traumatic brain injury. *J Head Trauma Rehabil*. 1993; 8(3):86–87.

20. Williams D, Levin H, Eisenberg H. Mild head injury classification. *Neurosurgery*. 1990;27:422–428.

21. Stewart D, Kaylor J, Koutanis E. Cognitive deficits in presumed minor head-injured patients. *Acad Emerg Med*. 1996;3(1):21–26.

22. Stuss D, et al. Reaction time after head injury: fatigue, divided and focused attention, and consistency of performance. *J Neurol Neurosurg Psychiatry*. 1989; 52:742–748.

23. Guilmette H, Rasile D. Sensitivity, specificity, and diagnostic accuracy of three verbal memory measures in the assessment of mild brain injury. *Neuropsychology*. 1995;9(3):338–344.

24. Hall S, Bornstein R. The relationship between intelligence and memory following minor or mild closed head injury: greater impairment in memory than intelligence. *J Neurosurg*. 1991;75:378–381.

25. Levin H. Neurobehavioral outcome of mild to moderate head injury. In: Hoff J, Anderson T, Cole T, eds. *Moderate Head Injury*. Boston, Mass: Blackwell Scientific; 1989.

26. Dikmen S, Levin H. Methodological issues in the study of mild head injury. *J Head Trauma Rehabil*. 1993;8: 30–37.

27. Bohnen N, Twijnstra A, Jolles J. Persistence of post-concussional symptoms in uncomplicated, mildly head-injured patients: a prospective cohort study. *Neuropsychiatry Neuropsychol Behavior Neurol*. 1993;6(3): 193–200.

28. Stuss D, et al. Subtle neuropsychological deficits in patients with good recovery after closed head injury. *Neurosurgery*. 1985;17:41–47.

29. Levin H, O'Donnell V, Grossman R. The Galveston Orientation and Amnesia Test: a practical scale to assess cognition after head injury. *J Nerv Ment Dis*. 1979;167: 675–684.

30. Newcombe F, Rabbitt P, Briggs M. Minor head injury: pathophysiological or iatrogenic sequelae? *J Neurol Neurosurg Psychiatry*. 1994;57:709–716.

31. Kiernan R, et al. A brief but differentiated approach to cognitive assessment. *Ann Intern Med*. 1987:107: 481–485.

32. Wilson G, Cockburn J, Baddley A. *The Rivermead Be-*

havioral Memory Test. Reading, England: Thames Valley Test Company; 1985.

33. Cicerone K. Attentional deficits and dual-task demands after mild traumatic brain injury. *Brain Injury.* 1995;9:865–875.

34. Wechsler D. *Wechsler Memory Scale—Revised.* New York, NY: Psychological Corporation; 1987.

35. Gronwall D. Paced Auditory Serial-Addition Task: a measure of recovery from concussion. *Percept Motor Skills.* 1977;44:367–373.

36. Yarnell P, Rossie G. Minor whiplash head injury with major debilitation. *Brain Injury.* 1988;2:255–258.

37. Leininger B, Gramling S, Farrel A. Neuropsychological deficits in symptomatic minor head injury patients after concussion and mild concussion. *J Neurol Neurosurg Psychiatry.* 1990;53: 293–296.

38. Dikmen S, Temkin N, Armsden G. Neuropsychological recovery: relationship to psychosocial functioning and postconcussional complaints. In: Levin HS, Eisenberg HM, Benton AL, eds. *Mild Head Injury.* New York, NY: Oxford University Press; 1989.

39. Bohnen M, Jolles J, Twijnstra A. Neuropsychological deficits in patients with persistent symptoms six months after mild head injury. *Neurosurgery.* 1992; 30:692–696.

40. Gronwall D, Wrightson P. Cumulative effects of concussion. *Lancet.* 1975;2:995–997.

41. Alexander M. Mild traumatic brain injury: pathophysiology, natural history, and clinical management. *Neurology.* 1995;45:1,253–1,260.

42. Dencker S, Lofving B. A psychometic study of identical twins dorcordant for closed head injury. *Acta Psychiatr Neurol Scand.* 1958;33(suppl 122):1–50.

43. Dicker B. Profile of those at risk for minor head injury. *J Head Trauma Rehabil.* 1992;7:83–91.

44. Wilson J, et al. Post-traumatic amnesia: still a valuable yardstick. *J Neurol Neurosurg Psychiatry.* 1994;57: 198–201.

The Challenges of Neurobehavioral Case Management

"In the world of case management, difficult cases are common and all in a day's work." That statement seems to be true for most case managers who are involved with the out-of-the-ordinary group medical or workers' compensation cases. However, one neurobehavioral case taught JoAnn, a senior case manager with a national case management firm, how much more complex a case could get. "I was feeling more comfortable with my caseload after five years of experience," says JoAnn, "but it was not until I was assigned John's case that I realized the difference between a difficult case and the complexities of a neurobehavioral case."

THE MECHANICS

The definition of neurobehavioral abnormalities is any abnormal behavior that is contributed by a known or suspected brain injury.

The brain functions in a manner that is influenced by electricity and chemistry in an anatomical structure composed of tissues, nerve cells, and blood vessels. When an insult occurs, changes in the anatomical structure causes disturbances in the electrical and chemical activity. The damages can be irreversible.

In some cases, the consequences of the insult are changes in behavior that interfere with the person's ability to reason, control impulsivity

Inside Case Management 1997; 4(3): 5–7
© 1997 Aspen Publishers, Inc.

and mood swings, exercise judgment, and so forth.

THE CHALLENGE

John is a 24-year-old single male who was involved in a motor vehicle accident and sustained a traumatic brain injury. For the most part, the ICU and initial acute rehabilitation showed typical progress for a ventilator-assisted patient with Glasgow coma 4 and with a five-day coma T.B.I.

It wasn't until the 10th day in the acute rehabilitation unit when JoAnn realized this was like no other case she had encountered. John sustained most of his head injuries to the frontal and temporal areas of his brain. He became combative and impulsive, and would not cooperate with his therapists. His actions and lack of cooperation became difficult for his physical medicine rehabilitation team.

His physiatrist called in a psychiatrist to consult, and John was given some medication to calm him down. But John had a seizure disorder and was allergic to the medication prescribed.

John was also a high risk for wandering and engaging in activities that would endanger himself or others. An attendant was assigned to him 24 hours a day. By this time, John was medicated regularly and was either lethargic or behaviorally challenging for the staff.

JoAnn was under pressure and treading on unfamiliar territory. The insurance company wanted

John to either be treated and show adequate progress or transferred to a less acute (costly) alternative. It seemed to JoAnn that her caseload of 30 patients took a back seat to John's case as she spent hours on the telephone or in person trying to sort out the issues and alternatives.

THE SOLUTION

1. Advice

JoAnn sought the advice of other case managers and clinicians who had dealt with similar cases. The following are suggestions she received:

- Seek a consult with a neuropsychiatrist who specializes in neurobehavioral rehabilitation and neuropharmacotherapy.
- Compile educational materials on brain injury and neurobehavioral rehabilitation appropriate for the patient's family, rehabilitation treatment team, and insurance company representatives.
- Locate a program that specializes in neurobehavioral rehabilitation. (Unfortunately, a program may not be available in your state, so an out-of-state program may need to be considered.)

2. Questionnaire for Rehabilitation Programs

JoAnn also produced a list of questions to ask when researching neurobehavioral rehabilitation programs. This list would be available to the family and others involved when they begin to tour facilities to help them choose the most appropriate program. (See Questions list.)

Few other cases are more challenging for a case manager than neurobehavioral patients. There are many constraints that will frustrate and discourage even the most seasoned case manager: the insurance company may not fund a neurobehavioral rehabilitation program; the acute rehabilitation team may attempt to provide care or refer to a family's referral choice regardless of experience; family members may have their own idea of the kind of care the patient needs, and may choose a program based on non-medical issues.

Because no one in 1997 can cure brain injury or are 100 percent successful in rehabilitation of neurobehavioral complications, there are no guarantees. For a case manager with a neurobehavioral patient, perseverance, flexibility, patience, resources, and knowledge are the key to successfully managing these challenging cases.

Questions to Ask When Researching Neurobehavioral Rehabilitation Programs

1. Is the program licensed by the state in which it operates?
2. Is the program CARF accredited? If so, in what category? Is it in brain injury specifically? What other accreditations has this program received? Is it JCAHO accredited?
3. How many neurobehavioral patients has the program treated in the last year?
4. Who is the medical director? Get the following information: curriculum vitae; where he or she trained; number of years in the brain injury field; number of patients treated in the neurobehavioral field; teaching credentials; affiliations with universities or research programs; and facilities in which he or she practices.
5. Is there a pharmacotherapist available to address medication issues?
6. Who is the clinical director?
7. How accessible is the medical director or clinical director if there are questions?
8. Who are the medical specialists associated with the program?
9. Are there acute care hospitals close by in case?
10. Who is the program director?
11. Is there a case manager assigned?
12. How much contact do the clinical director and program director have with the patient and family?
13. Who is the nurse manager and how many hours per day are licensed nurses available?
14. What are the visitation rules (frequency, limit on hours, weekend or holiday passes, transportation and housing available for the family, and telephone contact)?
15. Who are the people that will be working with the family directly? Get the following information: background, educational level, length of time with program, and length of time in brain injury rehabilitation.
16. Who is in charge of the program at night? How does the staffing pattern change? Does the staff sleep? Is there anyone on call in addition to the staff?
17. What are the staffing plans in case of emergencies (i.e., bad weather)?
18. What is the staff-to-patient ratio?
19. Are there licensed physical, occupational, and speech/cognitive therapists and behavioralists in the program?
20. May I meet some of the direct care staff on my own for a few minutes (not the supervisors or administrators)?
21. How does a program discharge if the discharge location is not in the same area as the program?
22. If the patient is not successful in this program, where is he or she referred?
23. If a patient wants to leave the program, what is the procedure?
24. What type of campus and living facility is there (rural, suburban, city, dormitory, group home, home, hospital, locked unit, open unit, apartments, number of beds per room, private rooms, semi-private rooms, where meals are eaten)?
25. Is guardianship required prior to admission?
26. How is transportation to and from the facility accomplished?
27. What is the distance from nearest major airport?
28. Are escorts available from home to the facility?
29. How is family education handled when the program is in a different state or frequent visits are not feasible?
30. How are family members and insurance case managers involved in patient updates?
31. May I get references for the program from in-state and out-of-state family members?
32. May I get references for the program from other health professionals and insurance case managers?
33. May I get a copy of the program description?

Returning Brain-Injured Clients to Work: A Team Approach

M. J. Schmidt and Mary Pat Murphy

Editor's Note: This is the second article of a 2-part series about returning patients to work after a serious brain injury. Part 1 focused on the steps to follow to return a patient successfully to work. In Part 2, the authors show how a team approach to job coaching can speed the rehabilitation process.

A successful job coach is key to returning clients with brain injuries to work. While one person may be responsible for this process, many brain injury rehabilitation programs recognize the benefit of using a group of professionals in job coaching. This "Team Coaching Model" involves the use of an interdisciplinary rehabilitation team that affords the client the combined skills, talents and interventions of several professionals instead of just one.

Specifically, the team usually consists of two to three job coaches, with at least one physical, occupational, or speech therapist. Together, these people are responsible for vocational evaluation, job development and placement, job training, daily living skill training, transportation training, job adaptation, counseling, and off-the-job community integration.

Under the Team Coaching Model, the process of job coaching is divided into five phases: initial contact of client and job coach; orientation to the job; job training; fading; and job maintenance.

Inside Case Management 1995; 2(4): 1–3

1. Initial contact. Once a suitable placement has been identified, the job coach and client should meet before the first day of work. The client, who may be very anxious, wants to understand the job coaching process and review expectations of the job coach.

At this pre-job meeting, the coach and client may also complete insurance and tax forms, visit the work place, meet with the supervisor, and find out about the work schedule.

2. Orientation. During the first several days, the employer reviews the job tasks. The job coach takes copious notes, and begins the process of task analysis, a systematic ordering of the steps involved in completing the tasks of a particular job.

3. Job training. The job training phase consists of helping the client learn the job. With the help of the job coach, the client uses established strategies, rehearsal, repetition, and feedback to accomplish, and learn the job tasks. During the job training phase, the other rehabilitation team members may help the client to customize the specific strategies and to adapt or to organize his or her new work environment. In addition, the team may opt to incorporate additional reinforcing therapeutic sessions into the client's after-work schedule. These sessions might include transportation training, role play, and developing script cues to help the client interact with co-workers.

4. The fade. Once the client learns the job duties, has established a system of communication with coworkers and employers, and has mastered various activities of daily living which support the job, the job coach needs to prepare the client for eventual independence. This process is known as "the fade."

How and when the fade occurs is determined by the client, the employer, and the job coach. They should review the data that has been collected by the job coach.

The employer or supervisor will meet with the job coach to evaluate the client based on work quality and quantity, and other unique factors that pertain to the client's performance and the job requirements. At this time, the supervisor may take over some of the duties of the job coach and assign tasks, review daily checklists, or answer questions. Now, the supervisor—and not the job coach—will begin to give feedback directly to the client. At this stage, the supervisor must be familiar with the employee's capabilities.

By now, the client should have developed aids such as checklists, signs, pictures, appointment books that serve as cues to help maintain work productivity. With such cues established, the job coach can begin to decrease his or her hours at the job site. Still, the job coach should check in frequently, particularly when the client needs to set up for a new task or has an unusually difficult job load.

5. Job maintenance. Once the client succeeds at working independently, the coaching team devices a maintenance schedule for client, family, and employer contact. The job coach may no longer be needed at the job site. During this time, contact with the client is made weekly for one to two months, then once every month for three to six months. At this time, it could be more cost-effective for the case manager to assume responsibility for these meetings. However, the job coach should agree to return to the case if necessary.

Throughout the five phases, treatment must be consistent. Both job coaches and employers must develop and repeatedly use strategies and therapeutic interventions. They must regularly observe the client's behaviors and collect data. Finally, they must communicate consistently with the client and with members of the rehabilitation team. This means that facilities that provide job coaching should have organized systems of communication and data collection.

Coaches should have access to clinical information, the interventions designed by team members, and the data collected by other coaches. At ReMed Recovery Care Centers, a job coach notebook is created each time a new client returns to work. The notebook contains practical and clinical information required for effective coaching. All of the coaches on the team record data related to the job in this central place.

As case managers, it is important to know how data is collected and how it is updated for client progress. At minimum, case managers should expect a monthly conference with the client and coaches to review all communication, data, and client notes.

SELECTING A QUALIFIED JOB COACH

Because there is no prescribed education or licensure for job coaches, rehabilitation providers can and do use any number of individuals to fill this role.

In some facilities, coaches have a high school diploma and some experience; in others, you may find clinically-trained professionals working as coaches. Similarly, the training and supervision of coaches are highly variable from agency to agency. Coaches are often temporary employees hired to work as a part of a pool or for a specific case; when this occurs, training and supervision are minimal. In other facilities, coaches are permanent members of the rehabilitation team.

As a case manager, it is important to know how coaches are selected, trained, and supervised. At ReMed, coaches are *permanent* employees who are part of the rehabilitation team. They have educational degrees related to the study of people with disabilities. They receive regular on-site supervision. Furthermore, they have received training in brain injury sequelae, strategies, and interventions; job and task analysis; and employer relations. Our job coaches have access to the rest of the rehabilitation team (physical therapist, occupational therapist, speech/language pathologist, psychologist) for support and assistance related to the client's job. They also have access to other job coaches for peer support and idea-sharing, and meet twice a month for case review and training.

THE ROLE OF A CASE MANAGER WHEN A CLIENT RETURNS TO WORK: A CASE STUDY

The role of the rehabilitation case manager in a client's return to work is often key to his or her success. But the division of labor between the job coach and case manager often remains unclear. To better understand these two roles, consider the following case study:

Mr. Smith fell on the ice this past winter, sustaining a subdural hematoma and left-sided weakness. His primary barriers after the injury included: memory impairments for learning new information, impaired gross and fine motor control of the left upper and lower extremity, left hemiparesis, impaired auditory comprehension, and tangential as well as verbose speech. Eventually, he was transferred from an inpatient rehabilitation program to an outpatient program for therapy.

At times, it is the role of the case manager to consider the following questions. Can the individual return to work in his or her previous position? What is the process for that return? Would the client require job modifications or accommodations in his or her place of employment? Or would he require placement in a different or related area? To find the answers to these questions, Mr. Smith's rehabilitation case manager initially contacted the client's employer, his supervisor, and the director of human resources regarding his return to work, potential obstacles, and the role of the job coach.

After an evaluation by the job coach, there was no question that Mr. Smith could not assume his previous position as maintenance supervisor for a large supermarket chain. After all,

his previous job duties included wiring, repairing, and inspecting freezers, air conditioning, and heating units; climbing ladders to the roof; driving from store to store for maintenance and inspections; and surveying fire prevention equipment.

However, Mr. Smith's employer suggested a new position for him, one that was used for employees who returned from work-related injuries. Mr. Smith would work part-time as a clerk, filing invoices and answering telephones. At the initial interview with the job coach, it was projected that job coaching would be required for approximately two months.

When the client began working, the job coach and the case manager talked on the telephone at the end of each week. The case manager made periodic site visits to the client at his home and at work. Eventually, a meeting was held at the supermarket to review the client's progress with the employer. The client, his wife, his immediate supervisor, the job coach, and the case manager attended. While the client was able to complete the filing with 80 percent accuracy, he was slow. He was not able to take phone messages accurately. With the help of his employer and job coach, his job description was modified: rather than answering phone messages, he would shred paper two days per week and file invoices three days per week.

In this particular case, the client continued to participate in outside rehabilitation services for gait and ambulation, driving classes, and medical management for orthopedic pain. The case manager assisted the client in coordinating his work schedule with his rehabilitation program and maintained contact with his physicians and additional team members.

The type and intensity of support required from the case manager varies greatly over time. While maintaining employment is often influenced by many outside variables, it is the case manager's responsibility to assist the client in keeping a job. This means that a case manager may need to communicate with many people during the client's return-to-work process. Indeed, the case manager may be required to advocate to the insurance company for adaptive equipment and ongoing medical support; assess family or parent or significant-other relationships and how they impact on work; facilitate recreation and leisure enhancements; and coordinate counseling for sobriety, stress management, and coping.

For these reasons, the case manager and the job coach need to constantly define and develop a partnership which facilitates the client's independence and ability to work.

Approaching Health and Wellness Issues for Those with High-Level Spinal Cord Injury

Theresa M. Chase

Wellness and health promotion are concepts not often directly associated with the rehabilitation of persons with high-level spinal cord injuries (SCIs). During the acute and rehabilitation phases of treatment, the focus of medical and nursing care is devoted to physiologic stabilization, functional skill development, and training of the patient, family, or attendants in personal care needs. Time and finances are often limited so only the most necessary care is delivered both prior to and after discharge home. Nonetheless, integration of health promotion and rehabilitation has been suggested recently by several authors.[1-7] Voices from the lay literature also indicate a growing demand for access to services that address not only "traditional" disability-related health issues but also general health promotion and fitness strategies.[8] This article will explore the possibilities of including wellness and health-promotion strategies into the rehabilitation course of the high-level SCI patient.

DEFINING HEALTH AND WELLNESS TODAY

The terms health and wellness are often used interchangeably in the literature of health and the popular press. *Wellness* has been defined as a state of being, an attitude more than the absence of illness, an ongoing process.[9] Similarly, the modern day working definition of *health* is no longer limited to "the absence of disease." Rather, dimensions of health now more routinely acknowledge include physical, social, emotional, spiritual, and intellectual health (see Fig 1). *Optimal health,* as described by Hettler,[10] is achieved through the *ongoing* process of self-actualization in each of these five domains. *Health promotion,* therefore, describes all educational, facilitory, and motivational efforts directed toward helping people move toward their unique state of optimal health. The most important behaviors to be encouraged are proper nutrition, stress management, weight control, smoking cessation, physical fitness, elimination of any alcohol or drug misuse, disease and injury prevention, development of social support systems, and maintenance of a regularly scheduled health surveillance plan to monitor health status.[5,11-13]

The person with an SCI can cultivate a wellness-oriented lifestyle by learning to adapt and manage life experiences and incorporate healthful self-care strategies in all aspects of life, emphasizing both disability-related *and* general health-promoting activities. It is also necessary to develop coping strategies that reduce stress, relate to others assertively and flexibly, examine and readjust beliefs and practices to maintain goal-directed wholeness, and seek positive chal-

Top Spinal Cord Inj Rehabil 1997; 2(3): 59–63
© 1997 Aspen Publishers, Inc.

The author thanks Indira S. Lanig, MD, and Sis Theuerkauf, RN, MEd, CRRN, for input and review of this article.

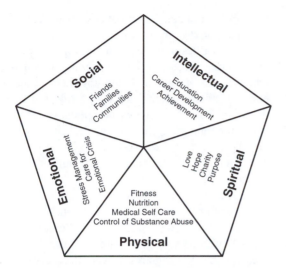

Fig 1. Dimensions of optimal health. Adapted with permission from M. O'Donnell, *American Journal of Health Promotion.* Vol. 1, No. 1, p. 5, © 1986.

lenges.[11–14] To this end, the acute- and post-rehabilitation patient education or patient empowerment process can incorporate specific activities to promote optimal self-care behaviors. Specific attention can be given to modifying health-promoting activities to fit the globally challenging situation of those with high tetraplegia or lower levels of SCI. For example, Lanig[11] notes that *nutritional health* education for those with higher levels of SCI must acknowledge and offer possible solutions for the challenges created by being dependent upon others for food procurement, meal preparation, or feeding. Challenges to eating properly caused by limited or fixed income or caregivers being inclined to rush the feeding process must also be discussed. Tracheostomy tubes, particularly with inflated cuffs, can affect the ease of swallowing or the appreciation of food flavors—thereby influencing appetite or food selection.

Similarly, patient education in *stress management* and *cultivation of social support systems* after onset of high-level tetraplegia can be addressed using the framework of the traditional psychosocial rehabilitation model. This model emphasizes interventions to promote behavioral

and psychologic adaptations to the life situation created by onset of disability. Whiteneck[15] notes that interdisciplinary efforts in this model aim to minimize social handicap in the face of financial disincentives, societal discrimination, environmental barriers, and oftentimes, poor preexisting support networks. For those with high-level tetraplegia, particular attention can be given to teaching mental relaxation strategies and "hands free" social survival skills such as effective communication, assertiveness, and other important life skills. *Intellectual health*—promoting activities—to reduce stress and enhance social skills—can include attention to computer skills training when resources allow, encouragement to use adapted page-turning options, and regular use of library loaned or store-bought audiotaped literature.[16] Academic, vocational, or volunteer work pursuits can be encouraged concurrent with purposeful attention to the fundamentally related issues of reliable transportation, attendant care, and architectural accessibility. *Spiritual development* in the form of meditation, prayer, or expanded consciousness, as well as active participation in one's own healing process can also add to overall health.[17] *Emotional health* is certainly challenged with the onset of an SCI. Development of positive coping mechanisms, and relaxation and stress management techniques, therefore, is valuable; they are tools and skills that can be incorporated into the acute- and postrehabilitation care plan. These life skills, however, are oftentimes neglected aspects of the psychosocial rehabilitation process.[18]

Finally, and perhaps the most perplexing for those with high-level tetraplegia, is the area of optimal physical health. Options for promoting *physical fitness,* in the traditional sense, can be limited or nonexistent for individuals with mid- to high-level cervical lesions. The severity of the disability may tend to overshadow the potential for optimal physical health amidst the physical loss of function. However, while "physical fitness" encompasses the physiologic attributes of cardiopulmonary fitness, muscular strength, muscular endurance, flexibility, and body composition, it also refers to the ability to carry out daily tasks without becoming overly fatigued. For those with higher levels of tetraplegia, therefore, the promotion of optimal physical health can emphasize the following:

- a balanced commitment to maximize functional capabilities in both necessary and discretionary activities of daily living;
- conscientious nutritional health practices to nourish the body; and
- health practices and medical follow-up to minimize the risk of secondary impairments and disabilities.[19]

"Physical activity" exercises for those with high-level tetraplegia can include attention to functional neck range of motion and strength, functional shoulder girdle strength and endurance (if these muscles are present), and attention to optimal wheelchair posture. Some individuals with high-level tetraplegia will incorporate overhead sling functional exercises such as self-feeding, dot-to-dot work, and coloring "within the lines" to promote more controlled movement with their residual proximal upper extremity musculature. Attention to diaphragmatic breath control in ventilator-free individuals with high-level tetraplegia can improve voice volume and control. Voice lessons or singing lessons can be a focused, enjoyable option for some individuals. All of these activities could feasibly become the basis for a "workout" and regularly scheduled throughout the week.

ACHIEVING HEALTH AND WELLNESS GOALS COST-EFFECTIVELY

Because of a prevailing health care industry challenge to contain cost and to do more with fewer personnel, less money, and less time, advocates of health-promotion activities must strive to achieve goals in a cost-effective manner. Demonstration projects and other research-related funded activities should be explored as possible avenues for funding and support. Additionally, collaborative efforts with other community health resources or organizations should be cultivated whenever possible. Equally impor-

tant is a clear understanding of the intended level of impact on the target population.[4]

The most desirable level of impact of a programmatic approach to health promotion is that which yields sustained behavioral changes that enhance health-related quality of life and reduces the risk of secondary complications. Not every rehabilitation clinic or facility, however, has the desire or the resources to comprehensively address all the mentioned health-promotion activities.

Advocates can, however, *systematically* address health-promoting behaviors via one of three basic levels of impact or intervention. Level I consists of awareness programs. Level II consists of lifestyle-change programs. Level III consists of supportive environments for sustained change.[20] Level I awareness-education programs and activities can increase the spinal–cord-injured individual's interest in understanding of health-related topics. Level II lifestyle-change programs utilize action plan oriented didactic sessions coupled with experiential activities over time. Level III supportive environments are used as a means to increase the likelihood of individuals sustaining their commitment to healthy practices. Rehabilitation facilities can provide supportive environments through offering healthy food choices on inpatient menus, in cafeteria selections, and in the selection of routine occupational therapy cooking projects. Healthy role models among staff and alumni can also serve to provide "good health" and "healthy aging" messages.[11] An excellent resource for developing healthy promotion strategies, such as these, within the context of the rehabilitation program is the recently published book, *A Practical Guide to Health Promotion After Spinal Cord Injury.*[4] This resource provides practical patient education activities and materials developed for all levels of SCI.

•   •   •

In closing, rehabilitation services and program management for persons with SCI have developed remarkably over the past two decades. Advances in medical technology and nursing care have ensured a longer life span for those with SCI of all levels. Prevention of secondary disabilities that can arise as individuals age with their SCI is, therefore, of great importance in postrehabilitation health care delivery systems. While the rhetoric of rehabilitation highlights the importance of quality of life issues after onset of disability, the present rehabilitation system of care remains dominated by the traditional medical model in which health is seen as the absence of illness or disease. The incorporation of a health-promotive perspective would lead to a more holistic nature of care, which includes all realms of health. Physiologic functioning would no longer be the single consideration in evaluating the client's health status.[2] Health promotion is consistent with the established rehabilitative practices, which are aimed at helping people with disabilities improve the quality of their lives despite physical problems.[21]

Finally, inclusion of a health-promotion perspective in the rehabilitation care delivery systems must be analyzed both from qualitative and quantitative viewpoints for justification. Qualitatively, questions about quality of life, life satisfaction, and overall healthy lifestyle choices will indicate programmatic impact on the individual. Quantitatively, longitudinal data to demonstrate the cost–benefit ratios over time is the other means of demonstrating favorable program impact. In either case, persons with high-level SCIs deserve health care that attends to the disability-related issues as well as the multidimensional aspects of general health issues noted earlier. A systematic health-promotion program integrated into the traditional rehabilitation model will provide opportunities for self-growth, health promotion, and disease prevention in those with high-level tetraplegia.

REFERENCES

1. Abood DA, Burkhead EJ. Wellness: A valuable resource for persons with disabilities. *Health Educ.* 1988;19(2):21–25.

2. Brandon JE. Health promotion and wellness in rehabilitation services. *J Rehabil.*1985;51(4):54–58.

3. Hodges A. Health promotion and disease prevention for the disabled. *J Allied Health*. 1986;15(4):315–317.

4. Lanig IS. Models, concepts, and terminology. In: Lanig IS, ed. *A Practical Guide to Health Promotion After Spinal Cord Injury*. Gaithersburg, Md: Aspen Publishers; 1996.

5. Marge MM. Health promotion for persons with disabilities: Moving beyond rehabilitation. *Am J Health Promotion.* 1988;2:29–35.

6. Nadolsky JM. Rehabilitation and wellness: In need of integration. *J Rehabil.* 1987;53(2):5–7.

7. Warms CA. Health promotion services in postrehabilitation spinal cord injury health care. *Rehabil Nurs.* 1987;12:304–308.

8. Kailes JI. Midlife criptdom: Getting fewer miles per gallon? *The Disability Rag & Resource*. 1995;16(4):11–15.

9. Travis JW, Ryan RS. *Wellness Workbook.* 2nd ed. Berkeley, Calif: Ten Speed Press; 1988.

10. Hettler, W. Dimensions of Optimal Health. 1977. Patient handout.

11. Lanig, IS, ed. *A Practical Guide to Health Promotion After Spinal Cord Injury.* Gaithersburg, Md: Aspen Publishers; 1996.

12. Pender NJ. *Health Promotion in Nursing Practice.* 2nd ed. Norwalk, Conn: Appleton & Lange; 1987.

13. Spellbring AM. Nursing's role in health promotion—an overview. *Nurs Clin North Am.* 1991;26(4):804–805.

14. Murray RB, Zentner JP. *Nursing Assessment and Health Promotion Strategies Through the Life Span.* 5th ed. Norwalk, Conn: Appleton & Lange; 1993.

15. Whiteneck GG. Outcome analysis in spinal cord injury rehabilitation. In: *Rehabilitation Outcomes: Analysis and Measurement.* Baltimore, Md: Paul H. Brookes, 1987.

16. Hulse KL. Promoting emotional, social, intellectual, and spiritual health. In: Lanig IS, ed. *A Practical Guide to Health Promotion After Spinal Cord Injury.* Gaithersburg, Md: Aspen Publishers; 1996.

17. Barasch MI. *The Healing Path. A Soul Approach to Illness.* New York: Putman; 1993.

18. Butt LM, Lanig IS. Stress management. In: Lanig IS, ed. *A Practical Guide to Health Promotion After Spinal Cord Injury.* Gaithersburg, MD: Aspen Publishers; 1996.

19. Chase TM. Physical fitness strategies. In: Lanig IS, ed. *A Practical Guide to Health Promotion After Spinal Cord Injury.* Gaithersburg, Md: Aspen Publishers; 1996.

20. O'Donnell MP, Harris JS. *Health Promotion in the Work Place.* Albany, NY: Delmar; 1994.

21. People with disabilities. In: Stoto MA, Behrens R, Rosemont C, eds. *Healthy People 2000: Citizens Chart the Course.* Washington, DC: National Academy Press; 1990.

The Effectiveness and Efficiency of an Early Intervention "Spinal Protocol" in Work-Related Low Back Injuries

James M. Alday and Frank J. Fearon

It is a well known fact among medical practitioners that attempting to resolve problematic workers compensation low back injury cases is costly and frustrating. It has been reported that only 10 percent of work-related back injuries account for as much as 80 percent of medical costs.[1,2] Yet in spite of the expense involved, there is very little evidence that the effort is justified by positive outcomes. Several studies have demonstrated an inverse relationship between time out of work due to injury and eventual probability of successful return to work.[3,4] A previous study by the authors evaluated factors that correlated with successful outcomes in the rehabilitation of problematic work-related low back injuries. The most predictive variable of a negative outcome (no return to work and no case resolution) was time out of work.[5,6] This study also identified a dramatic increase in negative outcomes when the worker had been out of work greater than three months, rather than a declining probability of return to work over time. Ninety-two percent of the cases out of work less than three months were resolved successfully, whereas only 40 percent of cases out of work greater than three months were successfully resolved. The only factor found to correlate with outcomes that was unrelated to time out of work was an elevated score on the McGill Pain Questionnaire.[7] The authors concluded that time out

of work may indeed be the single most important factor responsible for the worker developing a "disabled mindset" and subsequent illness behavior. Further, programs designed to intervene in work-related low back cases must address the time issue aggressively if positive results are to be consistently realized. These findings led to the development of a protocol-driven treatment strategy for work-related low back injuries, with initiation of the protocol occurring upon the first physician contact.

The "spinal protocol" integrated the roles of physicians, physical therapists, and case managers in the early management of work-related back injuries. The basic premise is that each discipline must be aware of the impact of time out of work, and actively work toward keeping patients at work or returning them to work as soon as possible. The physician protocol was developed using the guidelines proposed by the Agency for Health Care Policy and Research (AHCPR).[8] The initial physicians involved were the designated company physicians, typically family or general practitioners, or internists. The protocol consisted of maintenance of work status (regular duties or modified, full, or part-time) when possible. Bed rest, if deemed necessary, was limited to less than 72 hours. Prescribed medication included oral nonsteroidal anti-inflammatory agents, specifically cyclobenzaprine while on bed rest. No narcotic or prescription analgesics were to be prescribed if at all possible. A physical therapy referral for "spinal pro-

J Rehabil Outcomes Meas 1997; 1(3): 39–43

tocol" was considered optional at the first office visit, but was mandatory if the injured worker had not recovered within five days of onset. Lumbar spine plain (frontal and sagittal) views were conducted only if a fracture was suspected. The physician protocol is outlined in the box entitled "Spinal Protocol—Physician." If the patient was not progressing within 10 days out of work, in terms of decreased symptoms and improved work status, a referral was made to a spinal specialist (typically an orthopedist or physiatrist participating in the protocol). The spinal specialist evaluation is outlined in the box entitled "Spinal Protocol—Spinal Specialist."

The physical therapy protocol is outlined in the box entitled "Spinal Protocol—Physical Therapy." The basic treatment objective is to minimize symptoms while maintaining activity. Early treatment may be focused on symptom reduction through any effective and appropriate methodology available. However, passive palliative treatment should be limited following the first week to two weeks. An increasing emphasis in the protocol is then placed upon progressive resistive exercise and aerobic exercise. The physical therapist also monitors work ability progression through simple work task assessments (lifting, carrying, pushing and pulling tasks) on a weekly basis. These assessments are used to progress the patient's work status and modify limitations as recovery permits.

Spinal Protocol—Spinal Specialist

Evaluation:
1. McGill Pain Questionnaire
2. Pain drawing
3. Pain history
   - Location and radiation
   - Quality
   - Intensity using Visual Analog Scale
   - Diurnal pattern
   - Aggravating and alleviating factors
4. Review of systems
5. Past medical history
6. Social history
7. Sleep pattern
8. Activities of Daily Living
9. Physical exam
10. Nonphysiologic signs (Hip and Waddell signs)
11. Imaging study review

Evaluation decisions:
1. Further diagnostics?
2. Psychological screen indicated?
3. Spinal protocol treatment indicated?
   If so, any modifications necessary?

Weekly follow-up in Team Conference
Individual patient follow-up with spinal specialist every two weeks or as necessary during treatment program.

Spinal Protocol—Physician

1. Bed rest < 72 hours
2. Medications:
   - Anti-inflammatories
   - No narcotics
   - Cyclobenzaprine while on bed rest
3. Physical therapy referral at ≥ 5 days out of work (OOW)
4. Plain X-rays if fracture suspected
5. Return to modified duty ASAP
6. If not progressing by 10 days OOW, refer to spinal specialist.

The involvement of a case manager can be described as the hinge-point of the protocol. The case manager acts as the communication liaison between the treatment team and the employer and payer. The worker's medical status, treatment schedule, and work status are communicated to the employer weekly. This employer-practitioner relationship is critical to successful outcomes. Employers are assured of a bona fide return-to-work progression and the existence of a defined transitional work program. Additionally, when duties are limited, the case manager provides specific interpretation of these limitations to the employer as it relates to the worker's job. Ideally, the worker continues to perform his or her same job, with those aspects of work that may aggravate the injury modified temporarily.

Spinal Protocol—Physical Therapy

1. Minimize symptoms while maintaining activity
   Week 1:
   - Palliative treatment as indicated (modalities, manual therapy, self-care education)
   - Progress to exercise (progressive resistive exercise and aerobics) as tolerated
   Week 2 (if necessary):
   - Palliative treatment minimized
   - Exercise advanced
   Week 3 and following (if necessary):
   - Palliative treatment discontinued
   - Exercise advanced
   - Lifting capacity exercise
2. Work abilities monitored weekly and advanced as tolerated
   Communicated through case manager

In the event that this is not possible, temporary alternative placement is coordinated with the employer. In essence, the case manager's role is to engage the employer as part of the team seeking to resolve the injury successfully, by not allowing the disabled mindset to develop. The case manager's role is outlined in the box entitled "Spinal Protocol—Case Manager."

The program is facilitated through weekly team meetings at the rehabilitation center involving the spinal specialist, case manager, and physical therapist. The patient's status is thereby monitored continually and communicated to the primary care physician and employer. Addition-

---

Spinal Protocol—Case Manager

1. Weekly communication with employer
2. "Progressive" RTW facilitated
   - Limitations modified weekly or biweekly
   - Worker not left on "limited duty" without specific definition and advancement.

---

ally, in cases where progress is limited due to unabated symptoms, symptom magnification, or noncompliance, a timely referral is made to the spinal specialist for appropriate case resolution. The objective is to insure proper diagnosis, treatment, safe and expedient return to work, or case settlement when appropriate. Prompt action and the avoidance of time delays are the critical elements to successful intervention.

The spinal protocol outlined above was implemented at a regional medical center in Northeast Georgia. Approximately 30 primary care physicians agreed to participate in the protocol. The medical center's outpatient rehabilitation department provided the physical therapy and case management for all worker's compensation back injuries referred by participating physicians. Medical and rehabilitation costs, time out of work, time from injury to rehabilitation referral, total rehabilitation visits, treatment length, and outcomes were tracked on 46 work-related low back injury cases seen in the first six months of protocol implementation, and compared to all low back injury cases seen in the same facility during the same six-month period the year prior to implementation of the program ($N = 49$).

EVALUATING THE DATA

The results of the program implementation are outlined in Tables 1 and 2 and the final box. The patient demographics (Table 1) demonstrated considerable similarity between the two groups in terms of number of discharged cases, age, and gender. Additionally, all cases in both groups were diagnosed as undifferentiated low back pain (nonsurgical), and classified as ICD-9 code 724.2.

A notable difference was seen between the groups in the time since onset prior to initiation of physical therapy treatment. The protocol group averaged 28.8 days with a range of 3 to 86 days versus an average of 173.3 days, ranging from 4 days to over 4 years for the previous year's group. Four patients in the previous year's group had been out of work for over two

Table 1 Demographics

Protocol Group	Previous Year
N = 46	N = 49
Age = 37 (17–63)	Age = 42 (18–74)
Male = 61%	Male = 63%
Female = 39%	Female = 37%

years prior to referral to physical therapy. The removal of these outlying data reduced the mean time since injury to 136 days for the previous year's group, which still indicated a substantial difference between the groups. Treatment length and total rehabilitation visits also demonstrated a substantial difference between groups (36.2 days versus 61.0 days treatment length, and 6.2 visits versus 9.1 visits for the protocol versus previous year's group, respectively). One patient in the previous year's group had 52 visits. With exclusion of this patient's data, the range of the previous year's total visits was 1–27 visits versus 1–15 visits for the protocol group. The difference in total visits was directly reflected in total rehabilitation costs. The protocol group averaged $465.00 in total costs per case versus $682.50 for the previous year.

A very telling indicator of the effect of the protocol was the consistency of tracking out-

Table 2 Results

	Protocol Group	Previous Year
Time from injury to start of RX	x̄ = 28.8 days	x̄ = 173.3 days
Treatment length	x̄ = 36.2 days (1–68)	x̄ = 61.0 days (1–413)
Total visits	x̄ = 6.2 (1–15)	x̄ = 9.1 (1–52)
Rehab costs	x̄ = $465.00	x̄ = $682.50*
RTW	87%	No record

*The previous year's rehabilitation costs were adjusted +3% to equalize for annual charge adjustment.

comes. Lasting return to work was accomplished with 87 percent of the protocol group. In contrast, chart reviews of the previous year's patients revealed inconsistent and often undocumented case outcomes. Therefore, return-to-work rate or final case status was not able to be determined and compared to the protocol group. Follow-up on the protocol noncompliant cases is outlined in the final box ("Protocol Group Results"). Of the six protocol patients who were discharged noncompliant, five of their worker's compensation cases were either settled or had their claims controverted following discharge. Thus the total successful outcome (case closure) of the protocol group was 98 percent.

ISSUES RAISED BY THE REPORT

The implementation of a time-based protocol for treatment of work-related low back injuries and comparison of outcomes to those seen in the same facility the year prior, but without protocol direction, demonstrates several important issues. The first issue is that rehabilitation referral is delayed without protocol guiding direction for primary care physicians. The protocol triggers a mechanism to ensure physician referral in an expedient manner if the patient fails to progress in an appropriate time frame. Secondly, the physical therapy protocol established a functional goal of return to work, rather than a subjective assessment of reduced pain or range of motion gains as primary treatment. The physical therapists were intimately involved in providing work limitation parameters and/or return recommen-

---

Protocol Group Results (Noncompliant)

Of those who did not return to work (RTW):
- 100 percent were discharged noncompliant
- 100 percent were given releases to RTW
- 83 percent settled or had claim controverted

Total Successful RTW/Case Closure = 98 percent

dations to the referring physician and case manager. These recommendations were based upon objective physical performance indicators as opposed to a subjective assessment by the therapist or patient. The result demonstrated a marked reduction in length of time and visits necessary to bring about successful return to work. The reduction in rehabilitation costs is a direct reflection of the protocol's effect on reduction of visits. Notably, an additional cost reduction pertaining to indemnity costs, probably greatly exceeding that of rehabilitation costs, would be reflected in reduced indemnity costs. The combination of reduced medical, rehabilitation, and indemnity costs would make the financial effect of a protocol treatment regimen quite substantial. The most significant effect of the protocol would be the inclusion of case management services within the rehabilitation program. Their inclusion reiterated the need for members of the rehabilitation team to focus upon outcomes and the eventual end result, and recognize the effect of individual decisions upon those outcomes.

The few outlier cases seen in the year previous to implementation of the protocol are notable. Without the watchfulness provided by case management, some cases tend to linger without closure for a variety of reasons. Symptoms may remain unabated, preventing functional progression. There may be constrained or confrontational employer/employee relationships making case resolution difficult. Ultimately the results are reflected in prolonged treatment and unsubstantiated effectiveness. Unwittingly, the clinician facilitates the development of a patient's disabled mindset. Months of unsuccessful treatment can lead to reinforcement of the patient's perception of disability. Additionally, treatment and indemnity costs continue to escalate. The addition of case management with weekly monitoring in the protocol did not result in any outlier cases. Once lack of progress or rehabilitation of the patient is documented, the conclusion of treatment is expedited with communication to all parties involved (physician, employer, payer, etc.).

•   •   •

The implementation of a time-based treatment protocol for acute work-related low back injuries in a regional medical center resulted in earlier appropriate rehabilitation referrals, reduced treatment length, and reduced number of visits (41 and 32 percent, respectively). Rehabilitation costs were significantly decreased (32 percent), and indemnity costs were also likely reduced. The inclusion of a case manager provided structure and an outcomes-based approach for the rehabilitation team, and facilitated an overall 98 percent success rate. The study provides preliminary promising evidence of the efficiency and effectiveness of treating work-related low back injuries by protocol and may limit the development of problematic cases that linger without resolution.

REFERENCES

1. Spengler, D.M., and Szpalski, M. "Newer Assessment Approaches for the Patient with Low Back Pain." *Contemporary Orthopaedics* 21, no. 4 (1990): 371–78.

2. Spengler, D.M., Bigos, S., and Martin, N. "Back Injuries in Industry." *Spine* 11 (1986): 241–45.

3. Waddell, G. "A New Clinical Model for the Treatment of Low Back Pain." *Spine* 12, no. 7 (1987): 632–43.

4. Hrudey, W.P. (Unpublished) Workmen's Compensation Board of British Columbia. Vancouver, B.C., 1987.

5. Alday, J.M., and Fearon, F.J. "Evaluative Factor Correlation to Return to Work Outcome in Patients with Work Related Low Back Pain." Paper presentation, American Academy of Orthopedic Surgeons Annual Conference, Specialty Day, New Orleans, LA, February 1994.

6. Alday, J.M., and Fearon, F.J. "Preventing the 'Disabled Mind-set'." *The Isernhagen Work Report* (Summer 1994): 1–4.

7. Alday, J.M., Fearon, F.J., and Farr, S. "Psychological Factor Correlations to Return to Work in Industrial Low Back Injury." Paper presentation, American Academy of Orthopedic Surgeons Annual Conference, Specialty Day, Orlando, FL, February 1994.

8. U.S. Department of Health and Human Services. *AHCPR Clinical Practice Guidelines #14: Acute Low Back Problems in Adults*. Publication #95-0642. Washington, DC: Government Printing Office, 1994.

HIV Continuum of Care: Challenges in Management

*Robin I. Goldenberg, Stefanie H. Bell, Jacqueline Wright,
Sharon E. Brodeur, Mary Ann Turjanica, Loretta Beckman,
and Nancy Warker*

In the face of the increasing complexity and cost of care for patients with human immunodeficiency virus (HIV) infection, it becomes increasingly beneficial for a health care system to have in place a collaborative care system to maintain high quality and acceptable cost for its services. Inova Health System (IHS) is a large, not-for-profit, multifaceted system in Northern Virginia, comprised of three hospitals, urgent care centers, long-term care facilities, home health care agencies, and behavioral science facilities. In addition, IHS and Inova Home Health (IHH) have enjoyed a long-standing close working relationship with Hospice of Northern Virginia (HNV). The system recently developed ways to integrate the continuum of care from hospital to home.[1] However, further integration and collaboration between home health care and hospice emerged due to the evolution of the HIV infection and changing patient care needs. This article will examine the various transitions of care and the growing role of home health care and hospice, as well as an assessment tool for appropriate patient placement in these two agencies.

The continuum of care model is based on three levels of management: disease-state management, individual case management, and linkage management (Fig 1). Each level has its own array of challenges. The primary challenges for individual patient case management are the in-

teractions and adverse effects of medication treatments, effective and individualized prophylaxis, and a consistent program for the detection of opportunistic infections (OIs). Linkage management involves deciding when to transfer between operating units, such as between home health care and hospice, and collaborating to present a "one-stop shopping" choice for the managed care consumer market. The disease-state management component acts as an "umbrella" for the other levels of management and focuses on the overall planning of treatment, facilitating transitions, increasing patient satisfaction, decreasing average length of stay, and containing costs.

DISEASE-STATE MANAGEMENT

Disease management programs are viewed as viable options for ensuring that clinically appropriate care is delivered in the least costly setting throughout the spectrum of a chronic illness. It is a concept driven by cost-reduction imperatives, yet one that addresses the necessity of providing high-quality care. Embedded in the disease-management model are concepts and tools, such as clinical protocols and pathways, patient education, case management, outcome measures, and access to a comprehensive continuum of care.[2,3]

The need for HIV disease management has increased because antiretroviral drugs and progress in the management of OIs have modified the course of disease progression and conse-

Home Health Care Manage Prac 1996; 8(6): 1–10

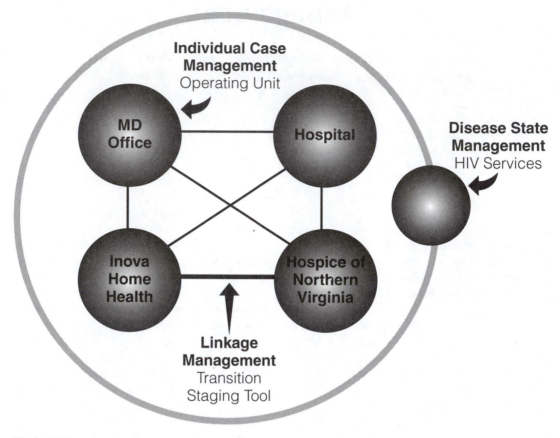

Fig 1. HIV continuum of care.

quent care plans. Rather than rapidly progressing to death, the HIV-infected patient copes with a slowly progressive chronic disease that can last for a number of years and requires numerous and complex treatments in a variety of health care settings. IHS established the Office of HIV Services in 1988 to provide disease management and primary care to HIV-infected residents of Northern Virginia with CD4+ counts below 500. It has provided comprehensive medical care, psychosocial services, and case management for over 500 HIV-infected patients.

Patients are referred to the Office of HIV Services from the region's health departments, substance abuse programs, physician offices, and hospital discharge planners. The program relies on a strong interdisciplinary team (IDT), which includes the physician, nurse practitioner, nurse case manager, social worker, substance abuse counselor, and nutritionist. The disease management of HIV patients provides proactive coordination and management of care across all health care settings and through the complete life cycle of the disease, from infection to death.

Once a patient is admitted to Inova's HIV Services, a nurse case manager initiates a care plan in concert with the social worker, patient, and significant others. The care plan addresses all aspects of the person's life, including medical and mental health needs; nutritional status; financial needs and entitlements; substance abuse issues and spiritual needs; as well as the basics, such as housing and food. Since the care plan is the nurse manager and patient's guide for the coordination of care, the patient meets with the nurse manager monthly—and other members of the interdisciplinary team as needed—to monitor the care plan and make adjustments as necessary.

The nurse manager assesses the patient's health on each visit, providing routine care and arranging laboratory tests and other diagnostic studies as specified under clinical protocols authorized by the patient's physician. If drug or alcohol addiction issues have been identified, the substance abuse counselor will work with the patient to become involved in a treatment program. Approximately 60% of HIV Services patients have a history of past or present substance abuse; thus referrals to county addiction treatment services or programs such as Inova's Comprehensive Addiction Treatment Services (CATS) are facilitated by the substance abuse counselor.

Individual and family counseling and support groups are provided by the social work staff. Since depression is frequent in this population, a psychiatric service is available for patients who require assessment and possibly psychotropic medication.

The HIV Services nurse case manager is responsible for integrating services and providing comprehensive and seamless care. This is accomplished by arranging for care in the most appropriate, cost-effective setting and by facilitating the transition from one setting to another. Hospital admissions often can be averted when the nurse case manager identifies a decrease in the patient's ability to care for himself or herself and subsequently makes a referral to home health care services. When hospital admission is inevitable, the nurse manager supports the patient and the acute care team by providing historical information upon admission, assisting in communication with the patient and family, and initiating discharge planning at the time of admission.

As the HIV-infected patient deteriorates to advanced disease, the HIV Services nurse manager explores with him or her and their families options for end-stage care. The patient is given information about inpatient and outpatient hospice services, about home care and extended care capabilities, and about palliative care versus aggressive treatment. Wherever the choice of health care setting, the nurse manager continues to oversee the coordination of care until death. After a patient's death, the care manager works with the family to provide assistance as necessary regarding burial resource referrals and bereavement needs.

As a person progresses through the course of HIV infection, he or she is cared for in a variety of health care settings. Proactive disease management should result in decreased use of costly settings, such as the emergency room or hospital.[4] The Office of HIV Services has reduced the average inpatient length of stay of its patient population from 8.59 days in 1994 to 7.93 days in 1995. Additional data are being collected on the number of hospital admissions in the last year of life, patient perceptions of quality of life, and appropriate prophylaxis of opportunistic infections. Patient satisfaction surveys conducted for the past 3 years reveal an exceptionally high level of patient satisfaction with the program.

INDIVIDUAL CASE MANAGEMENT

A true continuum of care recognizes the existence of "phases" of HIV infection beyond simply life with asymptomatic HIV infection to acute illness and finally to chronic illness. The different phases are treated by the different operating units of the continuum—physician's office, hospital, home health care, and hospice—to address issues such as education, counseling services, drug treatments, support of medication compliance, home nutritional support, and end-of-life assistance. The roles of the care providers in each setting are vital to maintaining continuous and seamless care.

Each Inova Health System operating unit deploys a multidisciplinary team to ensure that the specific needs of HIV+ patients are addressed. Some services provided by the team are unique to a particular operating unit. Other services, however, are provided across all settings and can be tailored to the specific needs of the patient.

Start of care

Typically the management of HIV+ patients in Inova's continuum of care begins with referrals from any of several outpatient sources, such as referrals from public health, Inova's Office of HIV Services, or physicians. In the outpatient setting, care focuses on institution of and compliance with antiretroviral therapy, institution of prophylaxis at appropriate CD4+ counts, earliest possible detection of OIs, and counseling.

Antiretroviral therapies

One of the most challenging aspects of health maintenance and promotion is the use of antiretroviral therapies. These therapies inhibit the enzyme reverse transcriptase. The institution of azidothymidine (AZT) at CD4+ counts of under 500 has been the mainstay of therapy. AZT treatment requires surveillance for potential hematologic, hepatic, and pancreatic toxicities. The subsequent availability of other reverse transcriptase inhibitors has offered additional alternatives under specific circumstances, such as AZT intolerance, but with greater risks of pancreatitis, severe peripheral neuropathy, and hepatic failure. This relatively limited armamentarium of therapies, however, centers the efforts of outpatient management on juggling antiviral combinations, addressing adverse effects and drug-drug interactions, and surveying for OIs.

The protease inhibitors indinavir, ritonavir, and saquinovir have recently been approved by the US Food and Drug Administration (FDA) as a new class of drugs. While they offer the potential for significant patient benefit, they also have added a layer of complexity to the management of antiviral therapies.[5] The deployment of antiretroviral therapy will probably escalate to a level analogous to cancer chemotherapeutic regimens, relying on varying multiple-drug combinations with their own new sets of potential adverse effects and interactions. Patients under the care of experienced physicians and their case management systems may well experience more significant survival benefits from these regimens than those already documented.[6]

Prophylaxis for opportunistic infections

In contrast to needs for individual tailoring of antiretroviral therapy based on varying tolerances to medications, duration of treatment, and use of prior agents, considerably more uniformity exists in the area of OI prevention regimens. Such regimens typically address prevention of exposure, prevention of the first episode of OIs, and prevention of disease from OI recurrence.[7] A number of factors has gone into those recommendations and practices, including the immunocompromise level at which an OI is likely to occur; the severity, cost, and mortality of unprevented infection; and the cost, efficacy, adverse effects, drug-drug interaction, and quality of life impact intrinsic to preventive regimens.[8] Individual tailoring is required when a patient's prior experience with an infection (eg, herpes simplex) or comorbidities (eg, pregnancy) suggests a high likelihood of recurrence or complications.

For some QIs there is uniform agreement: trimethoprim-sulfamethoxazole (TMP-SMX) is the preferred preventive agent for pneumocystis carinii pneumonia (PCP), begun at the time of detection of CD4+ counts less than 200. That consensus notwithstanding, the usefulness of TMP-SMX is impaired by significant allergenicity, and second line prophylaxis is frequently required.

In contrast, prophylaxis for other OIs is more controversial and requires individualization. The initiation of fluconazole, for example, to patients with CD4+ counts of less than 200 has the advantages of efficacy and the simplicity of a daily regimen; unfortunately, it is prohibitively expensive for some patients, and the emergence of fungal resistance is an increasing problem. Because of the complexity of multiple-drug regimens, compliance and quality of life concerns, expense, and toxicities, decisions about prophylaxis of herpes simplex, cytomegalovirus, disseminated Mycobacterium avium infections (MAC), and toxoplasmosis are necessarily determined on an individualized basis as well.

Thus, even in the face of relative consensus, a given patient may be taking a unique variety of medications that will change over the course of time. This requires individual and independent case management. The need for close surveillance for medication tolerance, compliance, adverse effects, and outcomes of these regimens again suggests the role for fluid communication among care providers at varying levels of the continuum.

Detection of OIs

Regular outpatient follow-up in the physician's office, clinic, home health care setting, or hospice is targeted at a number of issues in HIV case management, primarily the prevention of OIs. Other important issues include

- ongoing education and counseling as the patient's quality of life changes and evolves (eg, assessment of medication tolerance and health status, travel risks, household pets, occupational issues);
- assessment of nutritional status and candidacy for nutritional intervention;
- physical examination to detect new findings and to review existing pathology and devices (eg, central line insertion sites);
- monitoring of CD4+ counts as a measure of the efficacy and toxicity of antiretroviral therapy and as a marker for the institution of specific prophylaxis measures;
- patient candidacy for emerging therapies and investigational research protocols; and
- multidisciplinary reinforcement of medication regimens and patient reeducation for early recognition of signs of OIs.

Since the most common cause of unexpected early deaths in patients with HIV infection is from OIs that potentially are preventable and reversible, successful individual case management depends on the continual education of patients and on the transition of patients to the appropriate level of care. Rigors, protracted fever, cough and/or shortness of breath, abdominal pain, vomiting or refractory diarrhea, severe headache, seizures, slurred speech, and dizziness are all symptoms requiring early medical attention.

All can reflect medication adverse effects, drug-drug interactions, or more severe clinical findings of OIs, and their timeliness of diagnosis can make the difference between home health care and hospitalization, between acute care and invasive care, and between survival and death. Whether primary care is delivered by physicians, nurses, or nurse practitioners, nowhere is communication along the continuum more crucial to maintaining patient quality of life than in facilitating timely recognition of intercurrent OIs.

Acute care

As a patient's immune system continues to decline, even the most diligent compliance, educational efforts, and collaborative management ultimately cannot prevent the need for hospitalization. The advent of opportunistic infections, wasting syndrome, or more insidious conditions (eg, refractory diarrhea, progressive neuropathy, malignancy, or dementia) may well require inpatient care. At this point, Inova's care system requires the collaboration of the physician's office, home health care, or hospice with the hospital's multidisciplinary team. The patient's focus of care shifts from "living with HIV disease," during which he or she may exhibit few or no symptoms of illness, to managing life and career around the effects of these associated disorders.

In the acute care facilities, a multidisciplinary committee of caregivers—which includes physicians, hospital, home health care and utilization review nurses, nutritionists, social workers, chaplains, and care managers from Inova's HIV Services—meet weekly to address the myriad issues that accompany the care of AIDS patients. This approach has benefited not only the patients, but also the caregivers in helping to focus the direction of care and to address problems that arise. The rounds also provide an avenue to share information and research results with team members. This uniting of disciplines allows for anticipatory planning and continuity of care when the patient leaves the hospital and moves on to home health care, hospice, or a skilled nursing facility.[1]

The physician's role necessarily centers on diagnostic efforts, coordination of multiple consultants' recommendations, balancing of potential medication adverse reactions and drug-drug interactions, and offering direction at some point on end-of-life decisions. However, yet another challenge arises as an individual patient may or may not deem the physician as playing a meaningful role in providing emotional and social support.

The provision of nursing care is obviously central to achieving the goals of hospitalization. Though the provision of acute care may sometimes be relatively straightforward (eg, administration of antimicrobial therapy for a specific OI), the collateral benefits of a patient's trust in his or her nurse caregiver may transcend the actual value of the "nursing care" per se. Frequently, patients or their families are more comfortable soliciting advice or broaching difficult ambulatory issues with their nurses. Opportunities for the multidisciplinary team to intervene or advise commonly arise from questions regarding living conditions, career, finances, and insurance that are posed to the nursing staff. Depending on a patient's familiarity with, prior experience with, and trust in his or her nursing caretakers, those issues may be either addressed at the bedside or passed on to other members of the team to address.

Ongoing counseling and education

The realization that counseling is necessarily an ongoing feature of HIV disease management is crucial to health promotion and quality of life for infected individuals. However, the content of the counseling necessarily requires adaptation to varying patient insight, degree of illness, and changes in available treatment options. For example, information presented at the initial visit may well require repetition shortly thereafter, centering on reassurance, discussion of the efficacy of therapies and the realm of research efforts, and on health promotion and partner protection. Candidacy for vaccination against hepatitis B, pneumococcus, and influenza A may also be determined at this time as early steps in health promotion.

As the course of disease progresses, however, multidisciplinary counseling efforts need to continue, successively addressing job and quality of life retention; prophylactic measures for OIs; compliance with medication regimens; education regarding signs and symptoms of OIs; and, later, presentation of options for disability, assisted living, and terminal care.

Home health and hospice care

After drug regimens, prophylaxis, and OI detection are initiated, the HIV patient will eventually have need for the services of traditional home health care, hospice, or both. If it is the patient's first OI, then traditional home health care's aggressive therapy—with the desired outcome being "wellness" or at least "back to baseline"—would be the appropriate choice. If, however, the patient contracts an OI for which the burden of self-care is too great and the outcome would likely be fatal, then hospice would be the appropriate choice. The home health care team consists of a registered nurse in an area of specialty practice, rehabilitation staff, and personal care service providers. The focus is rehabilitative, restorative, or maintenance treatment in the home. The hospice team consists of the physician, nurse, social worker, chaplain, certified nurse assistant, volunteers, dietitian, and specialized therapists. The focus for the hospice team is on enhancing the quality and integrity of life through symptom control and comfort measures.

Depending on the stage of the disease, IHH and HNV provide differing home health care services. Home health care and hospice are not mutually exclusive. If a patient primarily is cared for by home health care, he or she still may access consulting services on pain control and symptom management from hospice. In return, a hospice patient may be seen by a home health care nurse to receive services such as blood transfusions. Generally the patient will be most involved with home health care in the beginning stages of the disease and with hospice in the end stages of the disease. Hospice incorporates more social services to include the patient's significant others to address end-of-life issues. Almost all patients will start with traditional home health care and transition at some point to hospice.

The goals of home health care therapy include OI treatment or palliative treatment or both to minimize symptoms associated with the OI. Management of a long-term venous access device often is critical to the patient's long-term anti-infective therapies and ongoing potential need for hydration and intravenous (IV) pain management. Home health care may include one or more of the following:

- IV therapies, providing teaching for the care of long-term venous access devices;
- nutritional assessment and supplementation (as by total parenteral nutrition, TPN);
- OI prevention (eg, pentamidine aerosol therapy for PCP, in some TMP-SMX–intolerant patients);
- OI treatment (IV ganciclovir for cytomegalovirus [CMV] infection);
- wound care and skin care;
- laboratory specimen retrieval;
- transfusion of blood products and administration or monitoring of biologic response modifiers (ie, CD4+ counts);
- instruction to enable the patient to maintain complex oral medication regimens and pain management techniques; and
- home health care aide visits for personal hygiene.

The key factor to successful home health care management is effective discharge planning to identify the appropriate resources necessary to maintain the patient's safe care at home. This plan involves accurate assessment of the patient by the home health care nurse to identify needs such as social service intervention for enrollment into federal payer programs, personal care services, social workers, or intervention from physician or other allied health professionals. The plan also includes assessment for possible provision of income for food, clothing, or shelter. The home health care nurse also may iden-

tify the appropriate time when intervention from hospice or extended care facilities may need to be considered.

The key factor to successful hospice care management is recognizing the limitations that the disease imposes on quality and quantity of life and to involve the patient and his or her significant other to achieve satisfactory closure. This includes comfort and symptom management, social services, and spiritual guidance. These services can be intermittent or around the clock, and can take place at home, at a nursing home, or at an extended care facility.

LINKAGE MANAGEMENT

As the focus of HIV care has increasingly moved to the home health care setting, the exact point of transition from traditional home health care to hospice care has presented a challenge. HIV disease has an unpredictable course, with periods of stability punctuated by acute phases. The care varies from aggressive treatment involving complex IV therapy regimens to supportive treatment involving symptom management and psychosocial and spiritual care. The primary needs of any given patient may oscillate between home health care and hospice during the progression of the disease. This unpredictable course historically has led to a lack of coordination in care plans. Health care agencies with different philosophies and different areas of expertise provided duplication of care, resulting in decreased patient satisfaction due to multiple caregivers.

In addition to meeting patient expectations, agency collaboration has become increasingly necessary to meet the needs of today's managed care environment. Reducing costs of services and improving patient outcomes while ensuring patient and family satisfaction has become paramount. The common barriers adding to the complexity of care in the continuum involve payer requirements for "one-stop shopping"; preferred provider status; combination federal, state and local program membership; and indigent care. Additional barriers include agency-specific skill expertise and patient resistance to acceptance of terminal care as well as misconceptions of some physician, insurance case manager, or discharge planner referral sources. In view of these barriers, each agency is faced with growing constraints affecting its overall financial viability.

Staging tool

Recognizing an opportunity to strengthen a care continuum for the HIV+ patient requiring shared services, representatives from IHH and HNV established a task force composed of RNs, a social worker, chaplain, physician, pharmacist, and nursing managers. The objective was to develop a clinical pathway indicating a predictable course of care for the patient with HIV infection. Due to the variability of disease progression, however, clinical pathway development proved to be difficult. Although IHS continues to work toward the development of clinical paths, IHH and HNV created an interim staging tool as a means to meet the overall goal of providing seamless service between the two facilities.

The purpose of this tool was to provide case managers, field staff, and other allied health professionals with a method to select systematically the appropriate agency or agencies providing a smooth transition between home health care and hospice settings. The task force identified key categories in which patients can be evaluated for disease progression using standardized assessment tools. Each category was then assigned a "stage" indicating treatment care requirements, physiologic changes, and overall adjustment to illness and poor prognosis. The patient received an overall "score" indicating the agency most suitable for an individual patient's case management. As illustrated in Table 1, if the total score is 16 or below, the patient is primarily managed by IHH, using HNV as a consultative service as required (eg, chaplain and social worker visits or skilled nursing for pain assessment and management intervention). If the total score is 17 or above, the patient is managed primarily by HNV with intervention assistance by IHH as required for provision of complex parenteral therapy.

Upon completion of the tool, the task force approached the Office of HIV Services for testing. A review and trial were conducted to ascertain if appropriate services were being provided to their patients. Twenty patient medical records were reviewed using the tool. The stage of each patient was identified and an assessment made of the appropriateness of placement.

The tool demonstrated a 90% accuracy rate in identifying home health care/hospice-appropriate patients. Based on the performance of the tool in a preliminary trial, both agencies elected to proceed with a coordination of care agreement. This agreement defines the specific role of each coordinating agency. Each agency is identified as either the primary (contracted) agency or secondary (contracting) agency based upon the specific tool stage identified. The critical components of the care agreement include information regarding financial billing responsibilities, specific service provision, contact personnel, and case conference schedules. The agreement is used as a working document to indicate specific services, thereby decreasing the duplication. Upon referral, this document is created and sent to each agency.

A CHANGING LANDSCAPE

IHS seeks to strengthen the HIV continuum of care by smoothing the transition of care among settings. The key to a dynamic, changing, effective continuum lies in communication among the three levels of management. Although each level must face its own array of challenges, the greater challenge lies in the communication of the developments at each level so that the other levels can adjust accordingly.

For example, individual case management is ever changing due to research findings and new treatments that need to be incorporated into the development plan. Recently Kitahata et al[6] demonstrated an association between physician experience in managing acquired immunodeficiency syndrome (AIDS) patients and median survival, noting an apparent survival advantage of over 1 year in patients cared for by physicians with great-

Table 1 IHH/HNV transition staging tool

Category	Score 1	Score 2	Score 3	Suggested consultations
1. IVS	• Prophylactic	Score 2 • Active treatment infection • No complications	Score 3 • Active treatment infection • Significant actual/potential complications	Suggested consultations HNV RN and MSW available for psychoso-cial issues and goal clarification for patient and family
2. CD4 count	200 > 51	50 → 10	< 10	
3. Karnofsky[9]	80–100	50–80	< 50	Score 2 or 3 Nursing assistant help: From Inova if Inova case managed From HNV if HNV case managed
	Functioning: Normal activity with effort; some signs/symptoms of disease (or better)	Requires considerable assistance and frequent medical care/or cares for self but unable to carry on normal activity or active work	Disabled; requires special care and assistance (or worse)	
4. Dementia	Fast 1: No dementia present	Fast 2–4: Forgets location of objects/subjective work difficulties. Decreased ability to perform complex tasks (eg, handling finances)	Fast 5 or >: Ranging from requiring assistance in choosing clothing to totally disabled	Score 2: Hospice MSW support to deal with reactive issues Score 3: HNV MSW/volunteer support for family
5. Support systems	Present, adequate. Allowing patient to stay in situation of choice	Present, experiencing increasing stressors	Absent, no support systems in place and/or available	Score 1: Hospice MSW available to plan for future needs Score 2: HNV MSW to identify needed resources and encourage use of personal/family resources Score 3: HNV MSW to identify and refer to needed resources and provide emotional support
6. CNA	Not required	< 20 hours/week	> 20 hours/week	Score 2 or 3: CNA from Inova if Inova case managed or from HNV if HNV case managed
7. Perception of illness	*Normative responses to diagnosis/prognosis through effective coping mechanisms: stable*	*Difficulty coping with diagnosis/prognosis: anger anxiety and/or depression present*	*Coping mechanisms failing: suicide/euthanasia ideation present*	Score 2: HNV MSW to increase support symptoms/counseling Score 3: HNV MSW for counseling; coordinate physician intervention for antidepressants/psychotherapy

continues

Table 1 Continued

Category	Score 1	Score 2	Score 3	Suggested consultations
8. Spiritual support	Chosen spiritual support in place	Chosen spiritual support not in place	Life history/resolution not effected	Score 1: HNV chaplain coordinates support Score 2: HNV chaplain coordinates or provides support or both
9. Pain	Uncomplicated: *Good prognosis* for control	Stage 2 Edmonton[10]: *intermediate prognosis* for control—unknown pain mechanism; 60–300 mg oral morphine equivalence; abnormal cognition	Stage 3 Edmonton[10]: *poor prognosis* for control—Neuropathic or mixed mechanism; incidental; > 300 mg morphine equivalence; psychological distress present; rapid tolerance; history past/present substance abuse	Score 2: HNV IDT available for assistance in management Score 3: HNV case manages
10. Weight	*Stable:* no or minimal weight loss	*Moderate loss:* decrease 10% lean body mass in 3 months	*Profound loss:* Decrease 10% lean body mass in < 1 month	Score 2 or 3: HNV dietitian consultation

Courtesy of Inova Home Health and Hospice, Springfield, Virginia.

est experience in treating AIDS.[6] This finding will most likely require consideration not only in the individual management processes, but also in the disease management process.

Recent studies have confirmed the advantage of viral load studies over CD4+ counts as predictors of AIDS outcomes and as markers for efficacy of therapy.[11] Any developments positively affecting HIV patient care must be incorporated in the individual plan of treatment. These valuable tools must also be communicated to facilities involved in disease and linkage management and assimilated into those programs. Successful linkage management between home care and hospice depends on continued communication and collaboration as well as further development of staging tools or pathways for other illnesses.

The challenges ahead for disease management lie in incorporating state-of-the-art medications and changes in transition processes into the overall care plan. All of the factors affecting individual case management and linkage management must be addressed. These factors are

- promise for significant prolongation of and improvement of quality of life;
- questions regarding the traditional CD4+ determinations as measures of immune competence and of antiretroviral efficacy;
- potential changes in the frequency and symptoms of OIs; and
- changes in the lifetime cost of providing care and in the locations of that care.

As patients and providers alike gain increasing experience with the impact of these changes, communication will become even more important. Removing barriers to multidisciplinary collaboration and maintaining a fluid continuum of providers will remain crucial to the quality of patients' lives.

REFERENCES

1. Turjanica MA, Ardabell TR, Schiffer NA, Poirier M, Brodeur S. A multidisciplinary, multifaceted HIV program: Linking the resources. *Nurs Admin Q*. 1994;18(2):41–45.

2. Newell M. *Using Nursing Case Management To Improve Health Outcomes*. Gaithersburg, Md: Aspen; 1996.

3. Dubois RW, Kosecoff J, Michelson LD. Disease management: The maturation and application of health services research. *Comp Ben Manage*. Summer: 1995:20–29.

4. Mauskopf J, Turner BJ, Markson LE, Houchens RL, Ganning TR, McKee L. Patterns of ambulatory care for AIDS patients and association with emergency room use. *Health Serv Res*. 1994;29(4):489–510.

5. Cotton DJ, ed. Optimism rises on combination therapy and protease inhibitor data. *AIDS Clin Care*. 1996;8:1–23.

6. Kitahata MM, Koepsell TD, Deyo RA, Maxwell CL, et al. Physicians' experience with the acquired immunodeficiency syndrome as a factor in patients' survival. *N Engl J Med*. 1996; 334:701–706.

7. Kaplan JE, Masur H, Holmes KK, Wilfert CM, et al. USPHS/IDSA guidelines for the prevention of opportunistic infections in persons infected with human immunodeficiency virus: An overview. *Clin Infect Dis*. 1995;21(suppl 1):S12–S31.

8. Kaplan JE, Masur H, Holmes KK, McNeil MM, et al. USPHS/IDSA guidelines for the prevention of opportunistic infections in persons infected with human immunodeficiency virus: Introduction. *Clin Infect Dis*. 1995;21(suppl 1):S1–S11.

9. Mor V, Laliberte L, Morris JN, Wiemann M. The Karnofsky performance scale: An examination of its reliability and validity in a research setting. *Cancer*. 1984;53:2002–2007.

10. Bruera E, Macmillan K, Hanson J, MacDonald RN. The Edmonton staging system for cancer pain: Preliminary report/ Cross Cancer Institute. University of Alberta, Edmonton, Canada. *Pain*. 1989;37(2):203–209.

11. O'Brien WA, Hartigan PM, Martin D, Esinhart J, et al. Changes in plasma HIV-1 RNA and CD4+ lymphocyte counts and the risk of progression to AIDS. *N Engl J Med*. 1996; 334:426–431.

An Interdisciplinary Problem-Based Practicum in Case Management and Rural Border Health

Marion K. Slack and Marylyn M. McEwen

Problem-based learning (PBL) is a method of instruction that uses a client problem as a stimulus for identifying learning issues in the basic and clinical sciences and for learning problem-solving skills.[1,2] The most important benefits of PBL are thought to be the structuring of knowledge for use in clinical contexts, the development of effective clinical reasoning processes, the development of effective self-directed learning skills, and increased motivation for learning.[3] Hence, PBL explicitly addresses issues related to learning as well as content and responds to concerns that students often cannot recall or use scientific information in the context of client care.[4] It is also believed to promote continued learning after formal schooling is completed and to promote continued life-long learning in real-world practice.

Although PBL is thought to promote learning in real practice situations, as described in the literature, it typically does not involve real clients, even when it is incorporated into clerkship experiences. The learning continues to involve case descriptions or simulated clients that are carefully structured to meet learning objectives and are presented to students who then use a clinical reasoning process to address the client's problems.[5] This article describes a community-based practicum in which students of pharmacy, nursing, social work, and public health use PBL to

provide interdisciplinary case management services to clients of a community health center.

STUDENT OBJECTIVES

Students from nursing, pharmacy, social work, and public health are eligible to participate in the practicum. All students are graduate students except the pharmacy students, who are completing the clerkships required for a doctor of pharmacy degree. The students live in a rural community for 10 weeks during the summer; usually the students live together in a rented house or condo. Each student has a disciplinary preceptor or advisor, and students receive credit for the practicum through their disciplinary programs. The practicum was developed as part of an interdisciplinary rural health training grant.

The following student objectives for the practicum apply to both case management and interdisciplinary teamwork:

- apply multiple disciplinary theoretical and conceptual frameworks to practice in a rural community;
- develop and maintain an interdisciplinary team;

Fam Community Health 1997; 20(1): 40–53
© 1997 Aspen Publishers, Inc.

The practicum experience described in this article was developed as part of Rural Interdisciplinary Training Grant ID1-86-6004791 from the Bureau of Health Professions of the Public Health Service.

- function as an interdisciplinary team member and articulate each discipline's contribution to an interdisciplinary team;
- maximize disciplinary and personal contributions to solving client problems;
- recognize the cultural context of health-related behaviors to develop and provide culturally relevant care;
- identify when case management is an appropriate method of meeting the health needs of clients;
- evaluate the outcomes of interdisciplinary case management relative to accessibility, availability, and acceptability of care; and
- establish case management services in their agency or institution if appropriate.

PRACTICE SETTING

The practicum is located in Santa Cruz County in southern Arizona, a county the size of Rhode Island with a population of only 30,000. Nogales, Arizona, and Santa Cruz County are located on the international border between the United States and Mexico. The neighboring Mexican city of Nogales, Sonora, has a population of at least 150,000 and possibly as high as 400,000. The population has mushroomed as people have immigrated to the border region to work in the *maquiladora* plants (the *maquiladora* plants are twin plants with manufacturing in Mexico and distribution from the U.S. side of the border). The consequences to the Nogales, Arizona, community have included increased environmental pollution, heavy traffic across the border, high unemployment, and increased demand for health care services and social services in a rural county with limited resources.

The community health center is the practicum site, and students provide case management services to pregnant women eligible for the Healthy Start program (Healthy Start is a federal–state program aimed at improving pregnancy outcomes) who are currently followed by the *promotoras* (also known as lay health educators or community health workers). The clients of the Healthy Start program who students follow are often at risk because of their socioeconomic status and cultural and language background but do not have complex or high-risk medical conditions. Pregnant adolescents and clients with high-risk medical conditions are followed by a nurse case manager. About half the clients are Spanish speaking only, and few have completed high school. Most are recipients of Arizona's version of Medicaid.

PROBLEM-BASED PRACTICUM MODEL

The learning methods, content, and sequence of activities, identified as the critical components of an instructional model,[6] are shown in Table 1. The practicum begins with an orientation because time is limited, because the students are providing services to actual clients, because the environment is unique (a rural community with a large Spanish-speaking population located on an international border), and because students have a wide variety of backgrounds and knowledge of rural and border health care, case management, and interdisciplinary teamwork. Further, students typically have limited or no knowledge of the cultural issues of health care, nor have they provided care in a border setting where a substantial number of the clients are citizens of another country.

Case management is defined in this practicum as a delivery model for providing patient-focused care. It is based on a care process that includes a comprehensive patient assessment, a problem list, care plan development based on the problem list, implementation of the plan, and evaluation of the interventions. Core case management activities include client advocacy, coordination of care, and individualized education.[7] Clients are involved in the entire process from the assessment through the evaluation of outcomes. They collaborate with the case manager to identify culturally relevant realistic interventions so the services provided solve the problems that the client considers important.

Students receive interdisciplinary team training concurrently with their clinical training. In

Table 1. 10-Week problem-based practicum learning model

Week	Content	Activities
1	Orientation to the practicum	
	Identification of objectives	Group discussions of the readings
	Readings related to rural, border health, interdisciplinary teams, case management, *promotoras**	Team-building activities
	Interdisciplinary database	Work through the documentation needed for an example case
	Identification of case load	Review cases with site coordinator† and *promotoras*; make shadow home visit with a *promotora*
2	Initiation of home visits	Make home visit with a *promotora*
	Interdisciplinary case management seminar	Attend seminar, present cases, participate in problem solving
	Self-directed study	Locate references, interview experts
3–8	Follow-up home visits, weekly case management seminars, self-directed study	Same as week 2
9	Close with clients, case management seminar	Review cases with site coordinator and *promotoras*
10	Write report on case management, including evaluation of team	Meet with team members to discuss report; self-directed synthesis and writing.

Promotoras are lay health educators who provide case management services to pregnant women at risk for poor outcomes because of their socioeconomic status and language and culture.
†The site coordinator is the director of nursing services at the community health clinic.

this practicum, we differentiate interdisciplinary from multidisciplinary teams. Multidisciplinary teams have a team leader who establishes the team goal; then team members contribute their particular expertise toward attaining the goal. Each person works in parallel with little awareness of others' work. Interdisciplinary teams work toward a goal established through an egalitarian process that incorporates findings and recommendations from all team members. Team members may contribute both based on their individual abilities and experience and on their disciplinary expertise.[8]

Students are asked to purchase a reference book on working as a group (*Learning through Discussion*[9]) that specifically outlines how the group process works, criteria for developing an effective group, and the roles and expectations of group members. At the weekly seminars, time is allowed for the faculty member with expertise in teamwork (the social work faculty member) to check in with the team and facilitate additional team exercises as appropriate.

The *promotoras* are considered members of the interdisciplinary team. *Promotoras* share their clients' knowledge and beliefs about health and illness, religion, family structure, and geographic and economic access barriers. All are issues in providing culturally relevant case management. The *promotoras* facilitate student entree into the community subculture by teaching students Spanish and by interpreting attitudes, values, and behaviors. They also participate in the case management seminars, make home visits with the student, and are available for consultation.

The case management seminar is a core component of the practicum. It provides a forum for the students to present their clients and to engage in the problem-solving process with other team members, faculty, and other health care providers. The seminar also provides a safe environment for students to deal directly with cultural problems that, if left unattended, may contribute to frustration and affect quality of care. Cultural conflicts are analyzed, and ways of reducing cultural impositions or strong enthnocentric practices are identified.

The faculty roles are those of coordinator, disciplinary advisor, consultant, and coach. They manage the logistics of the practicum, including coordinating student schedules across disciplines and with the schedules of the practice site, setting the schedule for the practicum, and so on. The faculty team, consisting of a faculty member from pharmacy, nursing, social work, and public health, attend the weekly case management seminars. Faculty provide both coaching and consultation. For example, when a question arose concerning the symptoms of eclampsia, the nursing faculty member provided information about the symptoms and their interpretation. However, the student was also referred to the primary care physician for further information and consultation. In addition, disciplinary faculty provide individual feedback and grade the students from their discipline.

CLINICAL REASONING PROCESS

The components of the clinical reasoning process are usually identified as patient data, problem synthesis, hypothesis generation, and an inquiry strategy.[10] The practitioner forms a problem synthesis based on initial information, generates several hypotheses that might account for the data, then uses an inquiry process to obtain additional data to narrow the range of hypotheses. The process is repeated until a diagnostic decision is made and a treatment plan formulated. When students learn the process in the classroom, they are presented with a patient problem and asked to generate possible hypotheses that will account for the data. The hypotheses serve as a source of learning issues. Through self-directed study and research, students learn the basic or clinical sciences required to understand how the hypothesis does or does not account for the data. Students then re-evaluate the data and discard or generate new hypotheses.

The practicum is designed to support students' learning of the clinical reasoning process. The seminar is structured so that a student presents the problem synthesis for each client, formulates a problem list, describes the proposed interventions, and seeks feedback and consultation from other members of the interdisciplinary team. The students make four visits to each client, which supports the iterative nature of clinical reasoning; that is, it allows the student an opportunity to apply what they have learned during self-study to the client's problem. The weekly case management seminars also allow for review and synthesis of what has been learned and for evaluation.[11]

The interdisciplinary database also facilitates development of the clinical reasoning process by providing a supportive framework; hence, it represents a core component of the PBL practicum. The database is an adaptation of the Omaha System,[12] which is a structured, comprehensive approach to community health practice, documentation, and data management. It provides standardized language to describe problems, interventions, and responses to treatment. Intended for use in conjunction with the medical record, it provides a tool for integrating clinical data with personal and financial data from the client's perspective. The Omaha System was specifically designed to meet the requirements of the problem-oriented record.[12,13]

The relationship between the interdisciplinary database, the clinical reasoning process, and student learning issues is shown in Table 2. The intake summary and the subjective and objective data of the SOAP note (a documentation system

Table 2. Relationship between the interdisciplinary database and the clinical reasoning process*

Database component	Component of the clinical reasoning process[†]	Learning issues
Intake summary (subjective and objective data of SOAP note)	Clinical impression (subjective and objective data needed for problem synthesis)	Type of information, sources and reliability of information, therapeutic communication skills
Problem syntheses[‡] 　Environmental 　Psychosocial 　Physiologic 　Health behaviors	Problem syntheses and hypotheses (explanations that guide inquiry, derived from working with a particular population in a specific practice setting)	Relationship between health and environmental, psychosocial, and behavioral factors; physiology; disease processes; developmental processes
Diagnosis (problem statement on which intervention is based)[§]	Diagnostic decisions (the most likely working hypotheses to explain the client's problem)	Why diagnosis was made, alternative diagnoses
Interventions 　Health teaching, guidance, and counseling 　Treatments and procedures 　Case management 　Surveillance	Therapeutic decision making (decisions based on beliefs concerning the appropriateness and effectiveness of a particular intervention for a specific client)	Types of interventions, when intervention is appropriate, relative effectiveness and cost, client's ability to manage intervention, cultural and social issues related to implementation, mechanisms of action
Evaluation (subjective and objective data on effectiveness of intervention)[ǁ]	Data analysis and hypotheses (explanations for why an intervention was or was not effective)	Inherent effectiveness of intervention, factors affecting effectiveness, alternative interventions

Note: SOAP = subjective and objective data, assessment, and plan.

*The clinical reasoning process encompasses the cognitive skills required for client evaluation and management delineated as hypothesis generation, inquiry strategy, data analysis, problem synthesis, and diagnostic and treatment decision making.[11]

[†]The components of the clinical reasoning process are derived from the discussion of clinical problem solving in Barrows and Pickell.[10]

[‡]The problem syntheses and treatment categories are from the Omaha System of documentation for community health nursing.[12]

[§]The diagnosis is represented as assessment in the SOAP note and is a formal statement of the problems, which in the Omaha System[12] includes a baseline evaluation of knowledge, behavior, and status.

[ǁ]Barrows and Tamblyn[11] and Barrows and Pickell[10] did not explicitly include evaluation in the clinical reasoning process. Outcomes are evaluated related to knowledge, behavior, and status that correspond to the baseline evaluation.

based on subjective and objective data, assessment, and plan) provide a format for the student to describe the client and form a clinical impression and problem syntheses. The problem syntheses are not restricted to the physiologic domain and may describe data in the domains of the environment, health-related behaviors, or the psychosocial domain.

The database is holistic and outcome oriented. It supports the reasoning process by linking the data, the resulting diagnosis and baseline status, the intervention, and the outcome. It also supports a holistic view of the client by requiring a comprehensive review of the client's situation on multiple dimensions. It enables students to identify both existing problems and potential problems and to select appropriate interventions. In addition, by using standard language, it facilitates communication between professionals and disciplines and, hence, interdisciplinary teamwork.

EXAMPLE CASE

The clinical impression and problem synthesis for a client are shown in Table 3. After reviewing the medical record and talking with the *promotora*, the student presented the clinical impression and identified late entry into prenatal care as the problem synthesis during the case management seminar. The group then generated possible hypotheses to explain why this client did not seek prenatal care earlier in her pregnancy. Hypotheses were generated that reflected economic, cultural, transportation, knowledge, and immigration and citizenship issues. Students discussed each of the hypotheses and what they knew about the issue. Because the *promotoras* and practitioners from the clinic also participated in the case management seminar, students obtained information immediately on the cultural issues related to accessing service. Students

also discovered that the clinic provided transportation, although the client may not have known that it was available.

Learning issues related to immigration and citizenship and qualifications for Medicaid appeared more complex, and students arranged for outside experts to speak to the group. At the following case seminar, the social worker from the clinic spoke to the students about Medicaid, eligibility for Medicaid, how to apply, and so forth. The speaker also described the sliding fee scale available at the clinic and eligibility for primary care services through a state-funded grant program. A second speaker provided information on immigration issues. Following the speakers, the students and *promotoras* presented their clients. For the sample case, the student presented additional data from the home visit indicating that the client was a Mexican citizen but a legal resident of the United States. Her husband worked as a welder when jobs were available. Therefore, she was eligible for Medicaid but did not want to apply because use of Medicaid could jeopardize her subsequent application for citizenship. Additional information from the client

Table 3. Example problem* with hypotheses and learning issues

Hypotheses	*Learning issues*
Immigration and citizenship status	Definitions of legal resident, citizenship, process of application
Hesitancy to use clinic services because providers do not speak Spanish, lack cultural sensitivity, have poor client interaction skills, and so forth	Language, cultural expectations, client interaction skills, clinic policy and procedures
Lack of access to transportation, either public or private	Community transportation resources
Cultural beliefs and practices about pregnancy that do not encourage early prenatal care	Culture and pregnancy
Lack of financial resources to pay for care ·	Availability of health insurance, sliding fee scales, qualification for Medicaid
Lack of knowledge about how to obtain health care services	Eligibility of client for services at the clinic, procedures for making appointments

*Clinical impression: 42-year-old woman, gravida 7, para 6, 20-week pregnancy, Spanish-speaking only, has just visited the clinic for the first time. Problem synthesis: Late entry into prenatal care.

indicated that she had never received prenatal care before she felt the infant move, that all her infants had been healthy, that she had no trouble getting to clinic appointments, and that she was satisfied with the care she received at the clinic. As a result of this information, hypotheses concerning the use of clinic services and cultural issues related to services were ruled out. However, cultural beliefs and practices about pregnancy and lack of knowledge about the importance of prenatal care appeared to influence the client's decision of when to seek care. Transportation was ruled out as a barrier to obtaining care based on the client's statement that she had no trouble making her clinic appointments. Therefore, late entry into prenatal care appeared to be related to immigration status, cultural beliefs and practices regarding pregnancy, lack of knowledge, and lack of financial resources.

Based on the problem-solving process that involved both the client and the interdisciplinary team, interventions were identified that were appropriate and effective. By learning about immigration and Medicaid and obtaining additional information from the client, an appropriate referral for a sliding fee scale was made, rather than instructing the client to apply for Medicaid. The intervention was sensitive to the client's goal of obtaining U.S. citizenship and created conditions that facilitated the use of prenatal care services. Referral to Medicaid would have increased the likelihood that the client would not seek care until she had an acute problem or delivery was imminent.

OUTCOMES

Learning outcomes are evaluated on several dimensions, including the development of interdisciplinary team skills, attitudes toward working with lay health educators, and evaluation of the experience through focus group discussions. Clinical skills specific to case management are evaluated by discipline. For example, the pharmacy students are rated on a 15-scale instrument that contains scales related to general effort (eg, reliability in attendance to assessment, prioritiz-

ing care goals). Each scale has five levels, from poorest anticipated level of performance to best anticipated level of performance. The best anticipated level of performance is considered superior (S, or 90% to 100%), and pharmacy students have consistently performed at this level at the end of the practicum. Other students have performed at comparable levels.

Global changes in the students' reasoning process are evident by the end of the practicum. Students become much more proficient in differentiating relevant and irrelevant information and in presenting a coherent, concise clinical impression. The types of hypotheses that the students generate also differ significantly from the beginning to the end. In the beginning, students tend to generate hypotheses that are specific to their discipline; for example, pharmacy students generate medication-related hypotheses, and nursing students generate developmental or physiologic hypotheses. At the end of the practicum, their hypotheses are much broader and not restricted to their discipline.

In the focus groups, students indicated that their ability to work with professionals from other disciplines had changed, and they recognized that patient problems are interrelated and benefit from various disciplines. They thought they could better refer patients for help and coordinate care. One student stated, "It reinforced my belief that working with other professionals as a team is more effective than turf wars in helping clients. I love this model!" Students liked being part of a case management team; they believed they learned about aspects of health other than just the physical aspects. Students thought that working with a lay health educator contributed significantly to their skills, particularly in working with a cultural (Hispanic) minority.

When asked to rate the effectiveness of their interdisciplinary team, the increases in average ratings on a seven-point scale generally showed the six students in the first group had learned to work together as an effective team. Items showing a gain included agreement on goals (3.5 to 5.6), recognition and use of member resources (4.2 to 6.0), establishment of procedures (3.5 to

4.6), and use of agreed-on approaches for solving problems (3.8 to 6.2). Items with less change—trust (5.2 to 5.4), participation in leadership (5.3 to 5.6), and communication (4.7 to 5.1)—were relatively high at the beginning of the training and showed less gain (from 0.5 scale unit to 1.5 scale units). Hence, the students' ability to work as an interdisciplinary team appeared to improve substantially during the clerkship.

A final student outcome that should not be ignored, although no systematic data were collected, is the personal growth experienced by the students. Conversations with the students who participated in the clerkship indicated that they experienced a great deal of personal growth. For one student, it was a matter of recognizing her strengths—that she was a natural teacher and that she liked working with people. As a result, she thought she would explore practice options for underserved people, including rural residents. The clerkship allowed another student to reconnect with his cultural heritage and to value his culture.

PROBLEM-BASED PRACTICUM VERSUS CLASS LEARNING

While the major features of problem-based learning (information from the client, problem synthesis, multiple hypothesis generation, inquiry, data analysis, and decision making) are clearly used in the interdisciplinary problem-based practicum, there are substantial differences between the practicum and problem-based classroom learning. First, the primary purpose of the problem-based practicum is to provide client care and ultimately to improve the client's health status and reduce the client's risk for poor outcomes. In contrast, the primary purpose of problem-based classroom learning is to structure the learning environment so that students learn the basic sciences in the context of a problem situation and learn the clinical reasoning process.

As noted by Barrows and Tamblyn,[11] PBL with real clients necessarily limits the content of learning. Real clients may not be available when the student is learning about a particular disease

state. Further, available clients may present with complexities or unrelated problems that confuse the student. In this practicum, variation in clients is limited and availability ensured by having students select clients from a restricted population of pregnant women eligible for case management with the *promotoras*. Therefore, most of the clients have similar problems such as low income, cultural beliefs that affect their behavior, limited or no English skills, and uncertain immigration status, although the number of problems per client may vary. In addition, some of the restrictions imposed on the content of the problems by using real clients are overcome by having students present and discuss their clients in the case seminar so that students learn about the clients of other students as well as their own.

The content of this particular practicum also differed substantially from problem-based classroom learning. Rather than a focus on physical disease, physical assessment, and medical treatment, the practicum focus was on primary and secondary prevention and risk associated with the environment, psychosocial factors, and health-related behaviors. Thus, a much greater emphasis is placed on establishing and maintaining a positive client–provider relationship that involves the client in problem identification and enhances the potential for client progress. Clients are not likely to discuss their use of herbal remedies and prescription drugs they purchased in Mexico if they do not trust the students. Students are also exposed to problems that may have multiple causes so that management of the problem is complex. The solution to the problem of the client not seeking early prenatal care may require multiple interventions such as education about the advantages of early care and what to expect at the clinic, addressing the client's concerns about immigration status, locating a means of transportation to the clinic, and so on.

Also, because the learning occurs in a real-world situation, the problems appear about equally divided among diagnostic problems, care management problems, and evaluation problems, whereas problems in classroom learning tend to focus on diagnosis. The relative emphasis on management or evaluation compared to diagnosis seems to depend on the problem. For example, identifying a diagnosis of income inadequate to purchase necessities is less problematic than identifying strategies or resources for managing the situation. Some discussion and consultation with multiple people in the community may be required to mitigate the problem. In contrast, students tend to have little or no knowledge of immigration status, and considerable discussion and learning may be required before the student can determine if immigration status is contributing to or causing the client problem.

As well as limiting the content of the learning, provision of care to real clients probably requires faculty to serve as consultants, a role generally avoided in classroom learning, to ensure high-quality client care. The student may lack knowledge of or may have failed to identify symptoms that indicate an urgent problem, for example, the symptoms of eclampsia discussed previously, or the student may not recognize which of several problems should receive priority. For example, a client with no food in the house needs immediate assistance with locating the food bank.

Content learning is also influenced by the need of students to learn skills related to client care such as documentation skills. In this practicum, each student completes a database that includes a comprehensive assessment of the client on multiple dimensions and a SOAP note for each home visit. While the database is structured to support the student's development of clinical reasoning, completing the database requires substantial time and limits the time available for self-directed learning related to diagnosis, management, or evaluation.

Another disadvantage, according to Barrows and Tamblyn,[11] to having students learn with real clients is the demands the student places on the client. In some clinical settings, clients may be subjected to repeated questioning and multiple examinations by students. We have attempted to minimize multiple student contact problems by having one student per client; however, a student could request that a student from a different discipline see the client with him or her if needed and if acceptable to the client. For instance, a social work student may accompany a nursing student on a home visit. Otherwise, consultation with other disciplines or other students occurs during the interdisciplinary case management seminar.

A related disadvantage is the demands that student learning needs place on the practice site, including requirements for an appropriate meeting place for student case seminars or team building activities that does not impinge on the ability of the practice site to provide care to clients. The difficulty may be particularly acute in rural areas that have limited facilities. We are fortunate to have access to the facilities of an Area Health Education Center (AHEC), which has meeting space that we can use. In addition, students may have an impact on the practice site's personnel. For example, students try to visit each client four times within the 10-week practicum. Ordinarily, the *promotoras* would not visit the same client more than once or twice in the same time period, so students place extra demands on the *promotoras*. The *promotoras* also take time to attend the case management seminars; however, the negative impact is limited because it provides an opportunity for the *promotoras* to obtain consultation on difficult cases and provides a means for them to continually develop their problem-solving skills.

DISCUSSION

While substantial differences exist between the problem-based practicum and problem-based classroom learning, our experience with the practicum indicates that interdisciplinary case management and PBL work well together and create an optimal learning environment for the student. Case management is a service delivery model in which multiple perspectives are required for optimal client outcomes; thus the process of problem-based learning works with and enhances service delivery. Further, the documentation required to deliver case management supports the clinical reasoning process so all aspects of service delivery and PBL work together in a coherent whole. Therefore, the learning experience should be more powerful and more efficient than PBL added into a less supportive environment.

PBL is also nonelite,[4] so that lay health educators and local practitioners participate and benefit from the learning process. PBL facilitates learning by everyone. One lay health educator summed up the experience of working with students as follows: "It was really rewarding. It was an all-around learning experience. Students learned from the *promotoras*, the *promotoras* learned from the students. Students learned from the client, the client learned from the students, and the *promotora* also learned from the client. We all learn from each other."

In addition, PBL is an integrated approach to learning and problem solving that reflects problem solving in the real world. Students learn to solve real-world problems with real clients because the process includes cultural, environmental, psychosocial, and behavioral issues. They also develop learning strategies that can be used to continually improve their practice skills after formal education is completed; they learn to assume responsibility for their own learning.

The limitations to the generalizability of the practicum described here as a learning model should be recognized. The environment and content of the practicum are unique. The community is located on an international border in a rural area; the training is through interdisciplinary teams, and the students are mentored by *promotoras*. Therefore, the learning outcomes could be due to the uniqueness of the learning environment rather than to PBL. An additional limitation is the necessity for extensive faculty commitment to learning about interdisciplinary teams and PBL and then learning how to make them work together. Most faculty have not had experience with either technology, and the structure of most academic environments does not facilitate interdisciplinary faculty work.

●   ●   ●

Our experience with the interdisciplinary practicum in rural border health indicates that PBL is a viable framework for facilitating learning in a practicum and that it is compatible with the care of clients. Further, students' knowledge and skills are integrated, so that application to future practice is promoted.

REFERENCES

1. Albanese MA, Mitchel S. Problem-based learning: a review of literature on its outcomes and implementation issues. *Acad Med*. 1993;68:52–81.

2. Dolmans DHJM, Gijselaers WH, Schmidt HG, Van der Meer SB. Problem effectiveness in a course using problem-based learning. *Acad Med*. 1993;68:207–213.

3. Barrows HS. A taxonomy of problem-based learning methods. *Med Educ*. 1986;20:481–486.

4. Walton HJ, Mathews MB. Essentials of problem-based learning. *Med Educ*. 1989;23:542–558.

5. Schwartz RW, Middleton J, Nash PP, Witte FM, Young B. The history of developing a student-centered, problem-based surgery clerkship. *Teaching Learning Med*. 1991;3:38–44.

6. Gagne RM, Briggs LJ. *Principles of Instructional Design*. New York, NY: Holt, Rinehart, & Winston; 1979.

7. Slack MK, McEwen MM, Carter JT, Brueckner R. Case management delivery model for pharmacy. *Am J Health Syst Pharm*. 1996;53:2860–2867.

8. Slack MK, McEwen MM. Pharmacy student participation in interdisciplinary community-based training. *Am J Pharm Educ*. 1993;57:251–257.

9. Rabow J, Charness MA, Kipperman J, Radcliffe-Vasile S. *Learning through Discussion*. Thousand Oaks, Calif: Sage; 1994.

10. Barrows HS, Pickell GC. *Developing Clinical Problem-Solving Skills*. New York, NY: Norton Medical; 1991.

11. Barrows HS, Tamblyn RM. *Problem-Based Learning: An Approach to Medical Education*. New York, NY: Springer; 1980.

12. Martin KS, Scheet NJ. *The Omaha System: Applications for Community Health Nursing*. Philadelphia, Penn: Saunders; 1992.

13. Weed LL. New premises and new tools for medical care and medical education. *Methods Inf Med*. 1989;28:207–214.

Clinical Pathway Across Tertiary and Community Care After an Interventional Cardiology Procedure

Karen Doran, Barbara Sampson, Ruth Staus, Cathy Ahern, and Donna Schiro

THE STORY

Mrs Y is a 68-year-old woman who transferred to a tertiary care center from a rural hospital 2 hours away. She was experiencing increased exertional angina and taking an average of five nitroglycerin tablets a day. Her family practice physician referred her for further evaluation and medical treatment.

Despite having had an angiogram and percutaneous transluminal coronary angioplasty (PTCA) 3 years ago, Mrs Y was upset and afraid about undergoing angiography and possible angioplasty again. Her emotional response was heightened because her family could not be with her before the procedure. Mrs Y had a successful PTCA of the right coronary artery. In the recovery phase, Mrs Y was anxious and unable to concentrate on the educational materials presented. She fell asleep during the teaching videos. She could not identify needed lifestyle changes and admitted that she had not followed the recommendations after the first procedure more than 3 years ago. Mrs Y was discharged to home on her second hospital day with medical follow-up by her community family physician.

THE TECHNOLOGY EXPLOSION FOR INTERVENTIONAL CARDIOLOGY

Mrs Y's health care experience is not unique. Interventional cardiology procedures, which are highly technical in nature and require expensive equipment and highly trained staff, are generally done in large tertiary care centers located in metropolitan areas. As a result, many patients travel considerable distances for treatment. This distance creates problems in providing emotional support by family members during hospitalization, securing accurate and timely communication between health care personnel, and providing educational follow-up after the patient's discharge.

The six types of interventional cardiology procedures for coronary artery disease (CAD) include (1) PTCA, (2) directional coronary atherectomy (DCA), (3) rotational coronary atherectomy, (4) transluminal extraction catheter (TEC) atherectomy, (5) laser atherectomy, and (6) stents. Interventional cardiology was born in September 1977, when Andreas Gruentzig, MD, performed the first PTCA in

J Cardiovasc Nurs 1997; 11(2): 1–14
© 1997 Aspen Publishers, Inc.

This article was made possible by the efforts of the representatives from the Health Bond and Abbott Northwestern Interregional Cardiovascular Collaboration project team whose participation was funded in part by the Robert Wood Johnson Foundation-Pew Charitable Trust national initiative, Strengthening Hospital Nursing: A Program to Improve Patient Care.

Zurich, Switzerland.[1] Since that initial procedure, the number of angioplasty procedures completed has skyrocketed. In 1979 about 2,000 angioplasty procedures were performed in the United States.[2] By 1988 PTCA accounted for more than half of revascularization procedures, exceeding the number of coronary artery bypass graft (CABG) procedures performed.[3] In 1988, 235,000 angioplasty procedures were completed in the United States, and by 1990 more than 300,000 were performed.[4]

In 1980 only about 5% of patients with CAD were candidates for PTCA because of rigid investigational indicators and technology.[2] Ten years later, PTCA is performed on patients who have high risk factors, including advancing age, prior bypass surgery, poor left ventricular function, multivessel disease, and acute myocardial infarction.[5] Major difficulties or limitations of PTCA include difficulty in dilating eccentric lesions, abrupt closure of the coronary artery, and high restenosis rate of 30%–40%.[6] The introduction of atherectomy addressed some of these issues. In 1987 the first successful atherectomy removed atherosclerotic tissue from a coronary artery.[7] Atherectomies are accomplished in several ways, including cutting, pulverizing, or vaporizing the plaque with a thermal laser. Another device is the coronary stent, which was introduced in the 1980s and approved by FDA in 1992 for emergency use. In 1994 FDA approved the Palmaz-Schatz for selected patients.[8] The number of older patients undergoing invasive cardiac procedures continues to increase. In 1980, according to data from the Registry of the Society for Cardiac Angiography and Interventions, the percentage of patients older than age 60 undergoing catheterization was 33%, but by 1990, that figure had risen to 58%.[9]

INTERVENTIONS AND STRATEGIES

A group of nurses from one urban and three rural hospitals representing various health regions met in Mankato, Minnesota, in 1992 to discuss issues and concerns surrounding the transfer of patients with cardiac problems. To gain the patient and family perspective, interviews with 27 patients and their families were completed and medical charts were reviewed. The main themes from the interviews and chart reviews centered around education, documentation, rehabilitation, communication, and continuity. These themes were used to develop a Cardiovascular Interregional Program to address the problems and needs of cardiac patients who travel to a tertiary care center for medical, surgical, or procedural treatment. The patients in the program are diagnosed with ischemic cardiac disease, with or without myocardial infarction, and require interventional procedures, such as PTCA, stent, or atherectomy; bypass surgery; or medical treatment with an adjustment of medications.

The three processes used in the Cardiovascular Interregional Program to promote education, documentation, rehabilitation, communication, and continuity are (1) Phased Clinical Pathway titled "Heart Health Care Patterns," (2) Heart Health Care Notebook, and (3) Tertiary and Community Care Manager Roles.

The program was funded through a Robert Wood Johnson Foundation-Pew Charitable Trust national initiative, Strengthening Hospital Nursing: A Program to Improve Patient Care. In addition, each of the four hospitals supported the program administratively by adjusting the workload of the care managers; approving time for travel and meetings; and providing secretarial, research, and data entry resources.

CLINICAL PATHWAY

The hospitalization course for patients undergoing interventional cardiology procedures averages 1–5 days. Most of this time is spent preparing the patient before the procedure or observing for complications after the procedure. The increase in the number of high-risk patients undergoing invasive cardiac procedures has led to the need for more aggressive nursing management. One way to provide this care is by using clinical pathways. The critical path method (CPM) was developed in the mid-1950s as a way to manage large, complex projects. CPM was first used to manage the annual maintenance work in an oil refinery.[10] CPM was also used in the construction and engineering fields to coordinate the work of hundreds of separate contractors working on the same project. During the early 1970s concepts related to medical critical paths were discussed and researched by some health care providers, but the environment for implementation was not receptive.[10,11] In the mid-1980s, Zander[12] reported the first use of the CPM concept in the delivery of patient care at the New England Medical Center in Boston.

A clinical pathway is a tool that outlines all of the components of care for a "typical" patient with a particular diagnosis.[13] It is a way of visualizing the patient care process.[11] Pathways, regardless of the diagnosis they represent, should have the following elements: (1) be multidisciplinary including health professionals from nursing, cardiac rehabilitation, dietary, respiratory therapy, social service, and home health care, as well as physicians; (2) provide a framework for communication among health care team members; (3) provide a means for documentation of patient care and progress; (4) serve as a staff education and orientation tool; and (5) clarify the "big picture" by making all health care team members and the patient aware of the overall plan of care.[11,14]

SPECIAL CONSIDERATIONS IN DEVELOPING AN INTERVENTIONAL CARDIOLOGY CLINICAL PATHWAY

Although the use of the clinical pathway has been shown to decrease patients' length of stay and increase the effective and efficient use of health care resources,[15] these tools are primarily concerned with an acute illness episode occurring in a hospital. Although the days in acute care affect the patient, most of the recovery period and adjustment to lifestyle changes happen outside the tertiary care hospital setting.

The clinical pathway, called "Heart Health Care Patterns" (HHCP), spans the entire continuum of care from the acute hospital episode through outpatient cardiac rehabilitation and community-based medical care. In addition, the pathway communicates data to other health care providers and directs the flow of patient progress through expected outcomes. This phased clinical pathway links tertiary and community care over 1 year, providing time for the patient and family to adapt to change and develop a trusting relationship with the community care manager.

The 12-month period is divided into four phases: (1) the acute phase, (2) the recovery phase, (3) the rehabilitation phase, and (4) the enhancement/maintenance phase. The acute phase begins when the patient enters the health care system and concludes when the patient is discharged from the tertiary care center. The length of this phase is from 1 to 5 days for the patient undergoing interventional therapy. Most patients have an acute myocardial infarction or unstable angina. The recovery phase begins the day after discharge from the tertiary center and ends when the patient starts outpatient cardiac rehabilitation. During this time, the patient is at home and begins to reflect on events that occurred in the previous week(s) and their impact on daily living. This phase typically lasts 1 week to 10 days after discharge from the tertiary care center. The rehabilitation phase starts with participation in outpatient cardiac rehabilitation and ends with completion of phase 2 of cardiac rehabilitation. During this phase, the patient has medical evaluation and participates in a prescribed exercise program. The patient also receives cardiac risk factor modification education counseling and behavioral interventions. The enhancement maintenance phase begins with the completion of phase 2 of the cardiac rehabilitation phase and ends with the anniversary of the acute event. This phase usually lasts from day 46 to day 365. This is the time for reinforcement of lifestyle changes and for incorporating these changes into daily living.[16]

The 12-month clinical pathway integrates Gordon's Functional Health Patterns[17] and the Omaha System.[18] Gordon's Functional Health Patterns serve as the organizing framework through which patients are evaluated holistically. Gordon designates 11 health patterns: (1) the health perception–health management pattern, (2) the nutrition–metabolic pattern, (3) the elimination pattern, (4) the activity–exercise pattern, (5) the sleep–rest pattern, (6) the cognitive–perceptual pattern, (7) the self-perception–self-concept pattern, (8) the role–relationship pattern, (9) the sexuality–reproductive pattern, (10) the coping–stress tolerance pattern, and (11) the value–belief pattern (see Table 1).

Within Gordon's framework, categories from the Omaha System Problem Classification Scheme (OSPCS)[18] provide a tool for assessment, intervention, and outcome. The Omaha System consists of 44 defined and numbered problems that can be linked to nursing diagnoses. The OSPCS includes problems involving sleep and rest patterns, bowel function, emotional stability, circulation, integument, pain, nutrition, abused adult, income, residence, prescribed medication regimen, spiritual distress, respiration, substance use, human sexuality, physical activity, and personal hygiene. Each problem was modified to include specific areas to be assessed that are relevant to the care of cardiac patients. For example, for the OSPCS category of pain, patients are assessed specifically for chest pain. Each of the categories in the OSPCS has a problem classification number, which is a mutually exclusive number assigned to each category for identification within the Omaha System nomenclature. The number 26, for example, corresponds with the category of integument.

Table 1. Functional Health Patterns

Functional health pattern	Examples
Health perception–health management	Perceived pattern of health
	Health risk management
	General health care pattern
Nutrition–metabolic	Patterns of food and fluid intake
	Food preferences
	Condition of skin, hair, mouth
Elimination	Bowel and bladder function
	Routines for bowel elimination
Activity–exercise	Activities of daily living
	Pattern of exercise and activity
Sleep–rest	Patterns of sleep, rest, and relaxation
	Aids used to sleep
Cognitive–perceptual	Vision, hearing, taste, touch, or smell
	Presence of pain and methods to manage pain
	Memory, language, and decision making
Self-perception–self-concept	Attitude about self
	General emotional pattern
	Body image
Role–relationship	Major roles and responsibilities
	Social relationships
	Satisfaction or disturbances in relationships
Sexuality–reproductive	Female reproductive stage
	Satisfaction or dissatisfaction with sexuality
Coping–stress tolerance	Capacity to handle stress
	Modes of handling stress
Value–belief	Values, goals, or beliefs
	Quality-of-life decisions

Source: Reprinted with permission from M. Gordon, *Nursing Diagnosis: Process and Application*, © 1987, McGraw-Hill.

The Omaha System includes a problem rating scale for outcomes. Patient knowledge (K), behavior (B), or status (S) is assessed within the OSPCS categories. A 5-point Lickert-type scale is used for measuring outcomes (see Table 2). The number indicates the patient's condition in the area being assessed, with the highest number denoting an optimal state of wellness and the lowest number denoting the most negative state of wellness.

The Patient Outcome Score consists of the problem classification number; the letter K, B, or S; and a rank number of 1, 2, 3, 4, or 5. As described in Table 3, which is an example of the phased clinical pathway for health perception–health management, a patient in the acute phase who is afebrile and whose groin site after sheath removal is flat and dry would receive the score of 26 S5 under number 1 on the acute phase of the HHCP. The number 26 corresponds to the OSPCS category of integument, S corresponds with the assessment of patient status, and the number 5 indicates no signs or symptoms (see Table 4).

The clinical pathway provides baseline scores that serve to guide practice. The initial assessment score generated by the tertiary care manager provides a baseline for the community care manager. When the score falls below the predicted number, the community care manager focuses on that area as a priority when initiating contact with the patient. In the case of Mr M, a 41-year-old male who experienced six hospitalizations between the community and tertiary hospital in 19 days, the Omaha scores helped to establish priorities regarding his status and con-

Table 2. Omaha System: Problem Rating Scale for Outcomes

Concept	1	2	3	4	5
Knowledge The ability of the client to remember and interpret information	No knowledge	Minimal knowledge	Basic knowledge	Adequate knowledge	Superior knowledge
Behavior The observable responses, actions, or activities of the client fitting the occasion or purpose	Not appropriate	Rarely appropriate	Inconsistently appropriate	Usually appropriate	Consistently appropriate
Status The condition of the client in relation to objective and subjective defining	Extreme signs and symptoms	Severe signs and symptoms	Moderate signs and symptoms	Minimal signs and symptoms	No signs and symptoms

Source: Reprinted with permission from K. S. Martin, and N. J. Scheet, *The Omaha System: A Pocket Guide for Community Health Nursing*, p. 38, © 1992, W.B. Saunders Company.

Table 3. Heart Health Care Patterns

Health pattern	Dates ___ Acute phase hospital phase	Dates ___ Recovery: post phase	Date ___ Recovery: rehabilitation phase	Date ___ Recovery: enhancement
Health perception/health management (safety)	1. Patient remains free of infection from interventions (26 S5). Score ___ Intervention scheme:	1. Patient remains free of infection from interventions (26 S5). Score ___ Intervention scheme:	1. Patient remains free of infection from interventions (26 S5). Score ___ Intervention scheme:	1. Patient remains free of infections from interventions (26 S5). Score ___ Intervention scheme:
	2. Provider assesses for home and physical environment (3 S5). Score ___ Intervention scheme:	2. Provider assesses for home and physical environment (3 S5). Score ___ Intervention scheme:	2. Patient will report environmental barriers (3 K3). Score ___ Intervention scheme:	2. Patient will identify hazards and have a partial plan (3 K4). Score ___ Intervention scheme:
	3. Provider assesses for health financial needs (1 S5). Score ___ Intervention scheme:	3. Provider assesses for health financial needs (1 S5). Score ___ Intervention scheme:	3. Provider assesses for health financial needs (1 S5). Score ___ Intervention scheme:	3. Provider assesses for health financial needs (1 S5). Score ___ Intervention scheme:
	4. Provider assesses for evidence of abused patient (16 S5). Score ___ Intervention scheme:	4. Provider assesses for evidence of abused client (16 S5). Score ___ Intervention scheme:	4. Provider assesses for evidence of abused client (16 S5). Score ___ Intervention scheme:	4. Provider assesses for evidence of abused client (16 S5). Score ___ Intervention scheme:
	5. Patient has no S&S of personal hygiene needs (38 S5). Score ___ Intervention scheme:	5. Provider assesses for personal hygiene needs (38 S5). Score ___ Intervention scheme:	5. Provider assesses for personal hygiene needs (38 S5). Score ___ Intervention scheme:	5. Provider assesses for personal hygiene needs (38 S5). Score ___ Intervention scheme:

continues

Table 3. Continued

	6. Provider ensures medications are safely administered (42 S5). Score _____ Intervention scheme:	6. Client takes medication as ordered and recognizes some side effects (42 B3). Score _____ Intervention scheme:	6. Client takes medication as ordered and recognizes most side effects (42 B4). Score _____ Intervention scheme:	6. Client takes medication as ordered and recognizes side effects (42 B5). Score _____ Intervention scheme:
Health perception/health management (lifestyle modification for hypertension, smoking, diabetes)	1. Provider will evaluate patient's lifestyle, identify risk factors, and communicate to patients. Risk Factors: _____	1. Patient will attain 39 K3 and 39 B3. Score _____ Intervention scheme:	1. Patient will attain 39 K4 and 39 B4. Score _____ Intervention scheme:	1. Patient will attain 39 K5 and 39 B4 for smoking and hypertension. Score _____ Intervention scheme:
	Patient will obtain 39 K2 level by discharge. Score _____ Intervention scheme:		Cardiac rehabilitation providers will update teaching materials for lifestyle modification and provide resources to assist patient.	Community care manager will reinforce lifestyle modifications and refer to appropriate resources.

Courtesy of Cardiovascular Collaboration Project, Healthbond, and Abbott Northwestern Hospital, Mankato and Minneapolis, Minnesota.

Table 4. Integration of Gordon's Health Patterns and the Omaha System

Health pattern	OSPCS	Specific assessment	Concept	Patient score
Health perception/ health management	Integument Residence Income Abused adult Personal hygiene Prescribed medication regimen Substance use	Infection Home safety Finances Medication safety	Knowledge: The ability of the client to remember and interpret information	1 = no knowledge 2 = minimal knowledge 3 = basic knowledge 4 = adequate knowledge 5 = superior knowledge
Cognitive/ perception	Pain	Cardiac pain	Behavior: The observable responses, actions, or activities of the client fitting the occasion or purpose	1 = not appropriate 2 = rarely appropriate 3 = inconsistently appropriate 4 = usually appropriate 5 = consistently appropriate
Value/belief	Spiritual distress	Support		
Activity/ exercise	Circulation Respiration Physical activity	Cardiac rhythm BP Cardiac devices CHF Activity restrictions	Status: The condition of the client in relation to objective and subjective findings	1 = extreme signs and symptoms 2 = severe signs and symptoms 3 = moderate signs and symptoms 4 = minimal signs and symptoms 5 = no signs and symptoms
Nutrition/ metabolic	Nutrition	Diet		
Coping/stress tolerance	Emotional stability	Coping skills		
Role/ relationship	Role change	Family and work		
Sleep/rest	Sleep/rest	Sleep pattern		
Sexuality/ reproductive	Sexuality	Sexual activity resumption		
Elimination	Bowel function	Last BM Methods to relieve constipation		

cerns that he and his family expressed when transferred between the two hospitals. As a result of seamless communication between the tertiary and community care managers, involvement with the patient and family occurred within minutes of transfer. Mr M had high scores for appropriate management of symptoms and entry into the emergency medical system but showed lower scores in coping ability. Both the community and tertiary care managers reinforced the patient and spouse's need to express frustration and insecurities about future events and ability to survive.

Mr M stabilized and the focus areas were then communicated to home health care and cardiac rehabilitation. The scoring system provided a systematic and specific assessment that helped to measure and evaluate progress.

The content validity was established by using the Omaha System,[18] Functional Health Patterns,[17] and a panel of experts. A Spearman rank correlation coefficient was calculated using the group mean and median scores to determine whether a similarity existed between the actual patient outcome scores determined by interviewing and assessing the patient and the expected patient outcome scores predetermined by the expert panel. A high positive correlation existed between the expected patient outcome scores and the group's median scores ($r_s = .99$) as well as the group's mean scores ($r_s = .99$).

Interrater reliability was established by having the nurse care manager and associates who assisted in data collection compare scores from a written case study and a taped interview. An interrater reliability coefficient of .93 ($n = 3$) was determined.

Patient knowledge

Patients undergoing interventional therapy are hospitalized for an acute episode of a chronic disease, CAD, that requires lifetime treatment. During short hospitalization, the patient has less time for inpatient education and is preoccupied by worries of survival, pain, and discomfort. These circumstances are not conducive to learning.[19] PTCA patients tend to have little concern about their cardiac disease because of short procedure time, short hospital stay, potential of immediate relief of symptoms without undergoing open heart surgery, and minimal time away from work or other activities.[20] In a 1992 investigational study using interviews of 14 PTCA patients, Gaw[20] found that patients undergoing PTCA often consider themselves cured and are

therefore not motivated to modify lifestyle risk factors when they return home. According to one patient: "All I know is that I'm going to have the 'balloon job' that I've heard so much about. I'm glad all I have to do is lay there and when it's over, I'll be cured of all this [heart] trouble."[20(p70)] Tosone, Marcley, Thielen, and Vyhlidal[21] reported that, after a successful atherectomy, the typical patient will focus on his or her improved cardiac status and may feel he or she no longer has a heart problem or heart disease.

Murphy, Fishman, and Shaw,[22] in a study that used a structured educational program to identify coping methods and knowledge retention of PTCA patients, found that knowledge of cardiac risk factors and modifications was forgotten within 6 months of the procedure. Patients undergoing PTCA, atherectomy, and stents must learn that the procedure is not a cure for heart disease but a way to relieve symptoms.

The short length of stay, coupled with the higher risk to patients undergoing invasive cardiology procedures, was a point of concern in developing a pathway. The HHCP bridges the gap between the hospital and the community by providing patient education over four phases. The first phase provides information the patient needs to administer self-care safely after discharge from the hospital. Examples of information provided in the first phase include assessment of groin site; when and how to obtain medical care; activity following procedure; and medication information including name, dosages, and purpose. As the patient progresses to phases 2, 3, and 4, more information is provided with an increase in sophistication. Initially, the patient is expected to list risk factors in phase 1. By phase 4, the expected outcome is for the patient to solve problems related to risk factors and learn how they relate to coronary artery disease (see Table 3).

Cardiac health care notebook

A cardiac health care notebook was developed for the Interregional Cardiovascular Project. The notebook, a three-ring, 2½-inch folder, is for the patient to record information related to his or her health problems, dates and times of visits to the physician or clinic, dates of hospitalizations, and a current list of medications. The notebook has educational information related to diet, exercise, stress, heart disease, and risk factors. Extra plastic pockets store additional handouts and medication cards. The patient and family are encouraged to refer to the notebook for health-related questions. The patient should bring this notebook to future outpatient visits at the physician's office and to cardiac rehabilitation. The notebooks are updated as appropriate by the health care providers.

Nurse care managers

Clinical pathways are only tools and require a care delivery system to implement them. The care manager provides the interventions of education, rehabilitation, communication, and monitoring. Nurse care manager roles include tertiary care manager and community care manager. The role of the care managers is to provide optimal communication with the patient and other health care providers, to decrease duplication of tests and procedures among agencies, to increase efficiency, to develop the priorities of nursing diagnoses, and to provide consistent nurse interaction with the patient and family.

The tertiary care manager's role is performed by a cardiovascular clinical nurse specialist who enters the patients into the project. The tertiary care manager is informed by the community care manager via phone of the patient's name, age, physician, hometown, reasons for referral, and priority issues for the patient and family. The tertiary care manager also is informed of interregional patients by a computer-generated report from the admitting department. Within 24 hours of arriving at the tertiary care center, the patient and family are contacted by the tertiary care case manager. The patient is given information as needed and given written materials in the health care notebook. The tertiary care manager notifies the community care manager of the patient's arrival, status on admission, changes in condition, and current plan of care. The information is provided to the community care manager via a direct phone call or an answering service message, depending on the time of day and whether the receiving care manager can be reached by phone. The tertiary care manager also completes an assessment of the patient, which is documented in the clinical pathway along with a nursing discharge summary. A discharge summary is provided over the phone, and a copy is mailed at time of discharge from the tertiary hospital. The discharge summary includes a list of significant hospital events, a review of the functional health patterns, and a list of priority nursing diagnoses and follow-up requirements for the patient.

The community nursing care manager role is performed by nurses who worked in a variety of areas including nursing administration, cardiac rehabilitation, home health care, and cardiovascular nursing. The community care manager contacts the patient at home within 24 hours of discharge to discuss any concerns, to provide support, and to set up a time to assess the patient. The visit takes place in the patient's home, at the hospital, in conjunction with the clinic visit, or over the phone. At this time, teaching materials received at the tertiary care center are reviewed with the patient. The nurse assesses the patient's knowledge, status, and behavior levels according to the clinical pathway. This time is also used to encourage the patient and family to comment on care and to ask questions. Patients are given reinforcement of the teaching that was initiated at the tertiary hospital. Follow-up appointments with the physician are reviewed.

The first visit held in the home allows for a more complete assessment of the home for safety factors, including uncluttered stairs with rails, safe rugs, and adequate heating and cooling. The home also creates a relaxing and less threatening atmosphere for the patient and family.

Often the visit provides the base for a trusting relationship. This relationship deepens over the year, enabling the patient to discuss issues and concerns honestly and openly that affected his or her feelings and ability to change lifestyle behaviors. This trusting relationship allows the nurse to support the patient. During the first month, weekly phone calls are made; then the calls are made as needed for the rest of the year. The interventions of the community nurse care manager during the year assist the patient to increase knowledge level and improve behavior and status as outlined by the phased clinical pathway.

Role of community care manager in cardiovascular interregional project case study

Mr T is a 76-year-old retired farmer admitted to a small, rural hospital after experiencing intermittent chest pain for more than 12 hours. He was stabilized with an acute myocardial infarction and transferred to the tertiary care hospital for further evaluation and medical treatment.

Mr T was entered into the Cardiovascular Interregional Project and was seen by the tertiary care manager. Mr T had a temporary pacemaker inserted for symptomatic bradycardia while in the tertiary hospital and underwent coronary angioplasty of the right coronary artery and the left anterior descending coronary artery. The tertiary care manager assessed Mr T and provided follow-up according to the HHCP pathway. A discharge summary was provided to the community care manager that showed priority areas for substance use (behavior and knowledge), physical activity (knowledge), prescribed medication regimen (knowledge), emotional stability (behavior and knowledge), and nutrition (behavior and knowledge).

The community care manager (CCM) telephoned Mr T within 24 hours and discussed immediate problems related to presence of pain, shortness of breath, and emotional status. During a home visit the following day, the CCM reviewed with Mr T and his wife the information in the cardiac health care notebook, answered questions, and offered support. Mr T was concerned about his "arrest" at the tertiary hospital and required clarification and psychologic support. Other areas of concern for Mr T and his wife included diet, exercise, medications (especially nitroglycerin), and smoking cessation. He was unclear about his next visit to the physician. The CCM reviewed these areas and provided special emphasis on medication side effects, signs and symptoms of congestive heart failure, and ways to affect cholesterol (both low-density lipoprotein and high-density lipoprotein). Mr T was provided with telephone numbers of the CCM, an appoint-

ment was made with his family physician, and transportation arranged for cardiac rehabilitation.

Mr T was contacted weekly and, during one follow-up call, Mrs T related that her husband had talked about some slight chest discomfort he experienced during exercise. He did not want to take nitroglycerin, so he rested until the feeling passed. The CCM talked with Mr T about therapeutic benefits of nitroglycerin.

A month after discharge from the tertiary hospital, Mr T experienced shortness of breath. He checked his pulse and discovered a rate of 40 beats per minute. He was hospitalized for 2 days for minor adjustments in his medications and the addition of a diuretic. Because Mr T promptly recognized his problem and called his physician, his hospitalization was brief.

Subsequent weekly, then biweekly, phone calls indicated that Mr T was actively participating in cardiac rehabilitation, maintaining his weight, and not smoking. His cholesterol remained high, although he said he was following his diet.

Two months after discharge from the tertiary hospital, Mr T contracted the flu and an ear infection. His cardiac status was stable and did not require additional medical support. The next month, Mr T had increased weight by 2 pounds and developed swelling in his feet. The CCM reviewed by telephone the signs and symptoms of congestive heart failure, ways to reduce swelling, and when to notify his family physician.

The CCM contacted Mr T once a month to assess his status and to offer support and reinforcement of information. Mr T said he checked his pulse and weight daily but sometimes had problems finding his pulse. He was instructed to check his carotid pulse. During one of the monthly calls, Mrs T reported that her husband was becoming lax in his exercise program. The CCM spoke with Mr T and encouraged him to reserve a scheduled time for walking every day.

Six months after discharge from the tertiary hospital, Mr T experienced some episodes of angina and was started on a nitroglycerin patch. He did not experience further problems with chest pain. He was not smoking but was finding it hard to maintain a low fat diet and exercise regularity.

The CCM continued to call Mr T every month. Reinforcement was given for exercise, good nutrition, and side effects of medications, and the signs and symptoms of congestive heart failure were explained.

Mr T completed his year in the Cardiac Interregional Program according to the HHCP clinical pathway. In 1 year, Mr T's assessed scores on knowledge, status, and behavior levels were equal to or above the predicted scores with the exception of decreasing his cholesterol level. He informed the CCM that he knows the types of foods to eat, but he does choose, at times, to "cheat." He has continued a regular exercise program, has not smoked in 1 year, takes his medications as prescribed, and monitors his pulse and weight daily. Mr T and his wife have the knowledge, skills, and community resources to lead healthier lives.

The length of stay for patients undergoing a PTCA, atherectomy, or stent ranges from 1 to 5 days. During this time, the patient is preoccupied with the procedure, is sedated, is experiencing pain, and is exposed to information directly related to the procedure. There is a lack of readiness to learn and an inability to absorb information concerning medications, risk factors, pain control, diet, and exercise. The phased clinical pathway spans 1 year from the acute episode of illness. It incorporates formal follow-up and reinforcement by the community care manager. Through this system, patients such as Mrs Y, Mr M, and Mr T have the support to live a healthier lifestyle.

● ● ●

REFERENCES

1. Gruentzig A. Letter to the editor. *Lancet.* 1978;1:263.
2. Hartzler GO. PTCA in evolution: why is it so popular? *Cleve Clin J Med.* 1990;57:121–124.
3. Bain DS, Ignatius EJ. Use of percutaneous transluminal coronary angioplasty: results of a current survey. *Am J Cardiol.* 1988; 61:3G–8G.
4. Topol EJ, Ellis SG, Cosgrove DM, et al. Analysis of coronary angioplasty practice in the United States with insurance claims data base. *Circulation.* 1993;87:1,489–1,497.
5. Hartzler GO, Rutherford BD, McConahay DR, Johnson WL, Giorgi IV. "High-risk" percutaneous transluminal coronary angioplasty. *Am J Cardiol.* 1988;61:336–376.
6. Borriello SL, Siegel SC, Fishman RF. Directional coronary atherectomy: a new treatment for coronary artery disease. *Heart Lung.* 1994;23:199–204.
7. Hudgins C, Sorenson G. Directional coronary atherectomy: a new treatment for coronary artery disease. *Crit Care Nurse.* 1994;2;61–66.
8. Topol EJ. Caveats about elective coronary stenting. *N Engl J Med.* 1994;331:539–541.
9. Noto TJ, Johnson LW, Krone R, et al. Cardiac catheterization 1990: a report of the Registry of the Society for Cardiac Angiography and Interventions. *Cathet Cardiovasc Diag.* 1991;24:75–83.
10. Hofman PA. Critical path method: an important tool for coordinating clinical care. *J Quality Improve.* 1993; 19:235–246.
11. Coffey RJ, Richards JS, Remmert CS, LeRoy SS, Schoville RR, Baldwin PJ. An introduction to critical paths. *Quality Manage Health Care.* 1992;1:45–54.
12. Zander K. Focusing on patient outcome: case management in the 90s. *Dim Crit Care Nurs.* 1992;3:127–129.
13. Zander K. Toward a fully integrated Caremap and case management system. *New Definition.* 1993;8:1–3.
14. Crummer MB, Carter V. Critical pathways—the pivotal tool. *J Cardiovasc Nurs.* 1993;7:30–37.
15. Redick EL, Stroud AR, Kurack TB. Expanding the use of critical pathways in critical care. *Dimens Crit Care Nurs.* 1994;13:316–321.
16. Huttner CA, Doran KA, Pritzker MC, Ahern CK. Clinical progression development by phases within an episode of illness: acute myocardial infarction. In: Spath PL, ed. *Clinical Paths: Tools for Outcomes Management.* Chicago, Ill: American Hospital Publishing;1994:231–242.
17. Gordon M. *Nursing Diagnosis: Process and Application.* New York, NY: McGraw-Hill;1987.
18. Martin KS, Scheet NJ. *The Omaha System: Application for Community Health Nursing.* Philadelphia, Pa: WB Saunders; 1992.
19. Ellers B. Innovation in patient-centered education. In: Gerteis M, Edgman-Levitan S, Daley J, Delbanco TL., eds. *Through the Patient's Eyes.* San Francisco, Calif: Jossey-Bass; 1993:96–118.
20. Gaw B. Motivation to change life-style following PTCA. *Dimens Crit Care Nurs.* 1992;2:68–74.
21. Tosone NC, Marcley DM, Thielen JB, Vyhlidal SK. Discharge teaching for the directional coronary atherectomy patient. *Dimen Crit Care Nurs.* 1994;13:208–217.
22. Murphy MC, Fishman J, Shaw RE. Education of patients undergoing coronary angioplasty: factors affecting learning during a structured educational program. *Heart Lung.* 1989;18:36–45.

Creating a Practice Partnership:
A Clinical Application of
Case Management

Colleen M. Lucas, Eric J. Dierks, and Nadine Parker

In the book *The Seven Habits of Highly Effective People,* Covey (1990) identifies important characteristics for thriving in one's personal and professional life. These habits are particularly crucial for the clinical nurse specialist to cultivate and practice. One of these habits, "seek first to understand . . . then to be understood" (p. 237) is well heeded as a guiding principle for consultations and other role functions. When followed, listening to understand communicates value and interest in the perspective of others. Accepting what is important to another person and the value placed on this importance builds the foundation for creating new practice relationships and strengthening existing ones. Furthermore, as a change agent, the clinical nurse specialist must truly understand the needs of the institution and provider in meeting the demands for health care reform before effective change can occur.

Current priorities call for matching the needs of institutions and payers for improved cost management with the needs of providers for improved patient outcomes. The clinical nurse specialist, who fully understands these needs, is in a pivotal position for effecting organizational change. As a consumer of research, expert clinician, consultant, and educator, the clinical nurse specialist is well prepared to steer the development of team partnerships for improved management of cost and clinical outcomes. One

method of addressing these improvements has been through the use of case management approaches. Case management provides a framework for developing practice agreements among team members. These agreements streamline communication among the many care providers and provide a consistent set of expectations for both team and patient. When the agreements are in writing and delineate the sequence of care with expected responses, they may also serve as a quality and cost management tool.

In the fall of 1993, the development of practice pattern agreements were begun for the head and neck surgery population undergoing free flap reconstruction. The surgeon performing the majority of the free flap surgeries initiated consultation from the surgical clinical nurse specialist to develop consistent standards of care for these patients. This casetype was targeted because of the complexity of the associated care, the many team members involved, the many handoffs of care across the continuum, and the potential for improved cost management. Some information on the surgical procedure is provided to gain appreciation for the risks and benefits of the surgery and the functional and emotional contribution made to the patient's quality of life.

BACKGROUND INFORMATION

The use of free tissue transfers ("free flaps") involving skin, muscle, and bone from distant

Adv Prac Nurs Q 1995; 1(2): 49–63

sites to reconstruct defects resulting from cancer surgery has increased tremendously during the past decade. The development of dependable techniques for the performance of microvascular anastomoses to donor vessels in the neck has made this the reconstructive modality of choice in the head and neck area. Microsurgical revascularization of these free flaps is successful in over 90% of cases. Segments of tongue, floor of the mouth, palate, or pharyngeal walls can be reliably reconstructed with the radial forearm flap. This thin, pliable skin flap from the inner surface of the wrist adapts itself well to the oral environment and enables the patient to recover good speech articulation and swallowing. Continuity defects of the mandible can be reconstructed with the fibula flap. This flap often includes a panel of skin from the lower leg that can replace the overlying gum tissue and can also carry some muscle and fat for restoration of cheek and jaw line contours. Less commonly, the removal of a malignant tumor from a head and neck site may require a large volume of soft tissue for reconstruction. The rectus abdominous muscle provides a moderate soft tissue volume, and the latissimus dorsi muscle provides a large amount of soft tissue that can be used in such instances. Resection of the cervical esophagus can now be reconstructed using a segment of jejunum, which allows excellent restoration of the swallowing conduit to the stomach. All of these flaps provide minimal morbidity in terms of loss of function at the donor site and serve to speed the healing of these difficult patients.

These advances in the quality of reconstruction have not come without a price. Previous, simpler reconstructive techniques could be performed by the same surgeon who performed the tumor ablation. The added complexity and specialized skills necessary for microvascular surgery have generally mandated that a second surgeon or even a second surgical team be used for the harvest of the free flap and the microvascular anastomosis. The added complexity and the tedious microsurgery have added from 2 to 5 hours to the duration of these already lengthy operations. The success of the entire reconstruc-

tion rests on the patency of an artery and a vein that may be one millimeter in diameter. The patency of the anastomosis requires careful, frequent monitoring, usually in an intensive care unit setting. All of these factors conspire to increase the cost of the care of a head and neck cancer patient significantly over the costs incurred by older, simpler reconstructive techniques.

Are the results worth the higher cost? Emotional function has been found to be significantly linked with extent and type of surgical procedure (Bjordal, Kaasa, & Mastekaasa, 1994). Vaughn, Bainton, and Martin (1992) compared oral cancer patients who had been reconstructed with free flaps with those treated by previous techniques and found a significant difference in the quality of life between these two groups. The benefits are indisputable; however, the spiraling costs may limit the availability of this technology in our present era of aggressive cost containment and managed care. Case management with continuum of care clinical paths offers a mechanism for cost containment while actually improving patient care through standardization of procedures, materials, and care coordination.

UNDERSTANDING THE CASETYPE

The first step in getting started in standardizing care was to fully understand the casetype trajectory, care requirements, and the sequence of care. The goal of this step was to profile the care and progress of the typical patient having this surgery.

Definition of the casetype

To gain further understanding of the casetype, standard or routine cases were reviewed via medical record, financial, and length of stay data. In preparation for accessing the data, the casetype needed to be defined consistent with data sort and query features. With the assistance of the medical records manager of data services, the casetype was defined as consisting of patients having reconstruction with a free flap graft following radical neck dissection surgery. With this definition, data could be sorted by procedure codes 40.41 or 40.42, identifying radical neck dissection as the primary or secondary procedure. It was determined that sorting patients by diagnosis-related group (DRG) instead of procedure code would be less helpful, since DRG assignment also reflects comorbidities, complications, diagnoses, and other procedures.

Gathering the initial data

Once defined, standard medical record reports were obtained to identify patients in the casetype and their related financial and clinical information. From fiscal year 1994 information, 12 patients were categorized as being in the casetype. Standard deviations for length of stay and charge data were calculated to determine the variability in the casetype and potential for guideline or practice standards development. From this step, two patients were identified as outliers, with a length of stay and charges greater than one standard deviation from the mean. In each case, medical problems unrelated to the free flap reconstruction resulted in a prolonged hospital stay. These two patients were dropped from further analysis, and a new standard deviation for length of stay (1.04 days) and charges ($7,042) was calculated for the remaining group.

Itemized charges by revenue center were then obtained to identify variations in practice and patient need. From these charges and previous medical record reports, standard or routine cases were identified for further study. These cases were selected based on the following criteria: percutaneous endoscopic gastrostomy tube (PEG) placed prior to admission, completion of preadmission process prior to surgery, absence of need to return to the operating room (OR) for a second surgery, and discharge to home. Surgeon team members confirmed selected cases and chart review of these cases was completed. Daily care and corresponding patient responses to the care were outlined for each patient. The information was then collated to identify pat-

terns of care and response. These patterns represented the profile of care or current practice standard. This standard was then ready to be translated into a clinical path format.

DRAFTING THE CLINICAL PATH

The accepted institutional format for the clinical path, sequences care from preadmission to hospital discharge. The format was adapted from a previous version in use at one of our system hospitals (Cardinal, Kraushar, & Wagie, 1994). Care is clustered into 11 aspects of care and six categories of patient response or outcome. The aspects of care include medical consults; diagnostics; assessments; procedures and treatments; medications; nutrition, fluids, and IV; therapies; activity; teaching; psychosocial and spiritual; and discharge planning. Categories of patient response or outcomes include physiologic, nutrition, self-care/safety/mobility, learning, psychosocial, and discharge. New to the format for this path was an intraoperative component, developed by the OR Clinical Coordinator for Head and Neck Surgery. Care was clustered into key aspects of care and sequenced in blocks of time. Most preoperative and postoperative time sequences are by the day; the intraoperative component divides time into the phases of the operative procedure.

NEGOTIATING PRACTICE AGREEMENTS

When the draft clinical path was completed, agreement on the represented practice patterns was sought. Agreement was needed because what had previously been implicit was now explicit and would serve as a quality standard. Furthermore, the validity of the now explicit standard needed verification. To reach agreement and fully understand the perspective of each team member, multidisciplinary reviews were held. The surgeons and team members from Preadmission Services, Speech Therapy, Cancer

Rehabilitation, Visiting Nurses, Nutrition Services, Pharmacy, surgery, and acute care nursing added to and further sequenced the outlined care.

Specific issues that were negotiated were the following:

1. *Timing of referrals.* The cancer rehabilitation social worker, speech therapist, and dietitian all wanted access to the patient prior to surgery, yet referrals were inconsistently made or communicated too late for team members to complete in their daily schedule. Pre-admission Services was unclear as to which patients required referral and sometimes did not know until the patient arrived in the clinic with orders in hand. *Solution:* Pre-printed physician orders were developed to address all three referral options. The surgeon selects needed referrals and communicates this to Pre-admission Services prior to the patient's scheduled visit.

2. *Timing and sequencing of diagnostics.* Laboratory tests were duplicated or omitted as a result of overlapping orders for nutrition management. Routine care of these patients includes enteral feedings via a PEG tube. Evaluation and adjustment of nutrition management requires sequenced laboratory tests, which have traditionally been completed in addition to laboratory tests required for managing the patient's surgical response. *Solution:* Laboratory tests were timed and sequenced to provide evaluation of both nutritional and other physiological parameters without overlap. Pre-printed physician orders were developed to outline this sequence from Pre-admission through recovery. The orders serve as a guideline for care and are modified based on individual patient condition.

3. *Frequency of monitoring and patient placement.* Flap viability is of primary concern after surgery, requiring hourly monitoring of the graft site for Doppler pulse and color changes. The frequency of monitoring adds to the already heavy nursing workload for these patients. Matching patient need with nursing staff skill and staffing level needed to be addressed. *Solu-*

tion: Standards for monitoring and airway management were incorporated into the clinical path to guide both frequency and amount of care required. Patients remain in the intensive care unit (ICU) the first two nights after surgery when acuity is higher and then are transferred to the general surgery nursing unit. The nurses on this unit are experienced in postsurgical care and airway management and have gained expertise in the management of this casetype. Doppler machines are left at the bedside to increase assessment efficiency. Again, the pre-printed orders structure the frequency and duration of assessment, which is hourly until the fifth postoperative day.

4. *Discharge planning.* The team agreed that discharge planning needs to start prior to admission, but the best way to incorporate this plan into the new structure required more discussion. Referrals prior to discharge would help, but home health nursing needed to be involved earlier in planning the discharge with the patient. Furthermore, teaching for self-care was not consistently initiated early enough nor were learning materials made available to the patient. *Solution:* Standards were incorporated into the path that further time and sequence care. Bolus tube feedings begin on the third postoperative day, with teaching about self-management of bolus feedings initiated by the fourth postoperative day. Available teaching materials are listed on the path and could be introduced earlier depending on patient learning readiness. Since approximately 75% to 80% of the patients require a tracheostomy and are not extubated until the fifth postoperative day, we have found initiating teaching on the fourth postoperative day coincides with learning readiness for most patients. To further support coordination of discharge planning with home care nursing, the need for a Visiting Nurse Association (VNA) referral is included in the pre-printed physician orders and the path. To address continuity of teaching, in-hospital nurses and home care nurses use the same teaching materials (see Figure A1 in the Appendix).

IMPLEMENTING THE PRACTICE STANDARDS

Once agreements had been reached on the clinical path components, the path was ready to be implemented. Pre-printed physician orders were used to support the timing and sequencing of care. In addition to the information previously referenced, the orders outline usual care from preadmission to post-ICU transfer. The orders consist of three parts: preadmission and preoperative; postoperative ICU; and transfer out of ICU orders (see Figures A2, A3, and A4).

The clinical path incorporates the physician orders as well as the practice patterns of the other team members. The path begins in the surgeon's office when the preadmission orders are initiated and faxed to the preadmission clinic. The pre-admission clinic nurse, schedules the clinic appointment with the patient, makes the referrals requested on the orders, and sets up a patient record. At the time of the clinic visit, the focus is on completing baseline diagnostics, assessments, and preoperative teaching. If previous referrals have been made, preoperative speech and nutritional evaluations are completed. Since many of these patients have a postoperative tracheostomy, preoperative evaluation is important for both baseline assessment and patient involvement.

The path continues through the preoperative short stay unit, the OR, ICU, and post-ICU transfer. Practice patterns include: antiembolic stockings applied in short stay, prior to the 8- to 10-hour surgery and discontinued when the patient is up and ambulating three times a day (postoperative day three); postoperative ventilator support and monitoring in the ICU; and weaning from the ventilator and initiation of PEG tube feedings postoperative day one. By the second postoperative day, the patient is transferred to the surgical unit and close hourly monitoring of the flap continues. Additionally, on transfer a VNA consult for discharge planning occurs, the patient is weaned from IV to per PEG pain medication, and IV fluids are decreased as tube feeding rate increases. By day four, bolus feedings are established and patient teaching is initiated. Patients are usually ready by the sixth postoperative day for discharge, and with the VNA, continue their recovery at home.

EVALUATING THE IMPACT OF THE CHANGE

At the end of 6 months, the clinical path and pre-printed orders had been used for 14 patients. Data analysis similar to the baseline analysis was conducted. Standard deviations for length of stay and charge data were calculated, identifying two patients exceeding the means by more than one standard deviation. These two patients were dropped from further analysis, and a new standard deviation for length of stay (1.7 days) and charges ($5,137) were calculated for the remaining group. Comparisons between the pre- and postclinical path groups were then made. With the preclinical path group, 80% of the patients required hospitalization for 8 days or longer. In the postclinical path group, only one patient (8%) was still hospitalized on the eighth postoperative day. Average length of stay dropped by 25% from pre- to postclinical path; charges and costs were reduced by 15% to 20%.

The clinical path should be modified to reflect the new anticipated length of stay of 5 to 6 days. The sequencing of care has subsequently been modified to better reflect patient differences. More specifically, physical therapy has been integrated in the path for patients after fibula flap, and the teaching of trachea care when discharge with a tracheostomy is anticipated.

At this point, the major thrust of clinical path development has been standardization of practices. To gain a better idea as to the impact of the path on the patient's recovery and to further improve the patient's response to care, variance tracking is being initiated. Key indicators of variance have been identified from chart review. These indicators are printed on a tracking tool format already in use for other casetypes at our institution (see Figures A5 and A6). The concurrent tracking of variances and later analysis by the interdisciplinary team has been found to be an effective means for identifying care improvement opportunities focused on the patient.

•   •   •

In the team partnership that has developed, the clinical path is the vehicle through which the interdisciplinary practice patterns are communicated. More important, the path represents and communicates the interdependence among the team members, and between the team and the patient in achieving expected outcomes. This integration of care at the patient level means patients experience a consistent approach among team members. Recovery occurs more quickly and patients display an increased confidence in their ability to manage their own care after discharge. Even though shortening the length of stay was not the initial goal, in the 6 months since initiation, length of stay has dropped and charges have been reduced. Variance tracking is now being implemented to understand trends in patient responses and provide the data needed for further modifying practice patterns.

REFERENCES

Bjordal, K., Kaasa, S. K., & Mastekaasa, A. (1994). Quality of life in patients treated for head and neck cancer: A follow-up study 7 to 11 years after radiotherapy. *International Journal of Radiation Oncology, Biology, Physics, 28*(4), 847–856.

Cardinal, J., Kraushar, V. K., & Wagie, T. (1994). Implementation of episodic case management in a managed care organization. In R. S. Howe (Ed.), *Case management for healthcare professionals.* Chicago, IL: Precept Press.

Covey, S.R. (1990). *The seven habits of highly effective people* (Fireside edition). New York, NY: Simon & Schuster.

Vaughn, E. D., Bainton, R., & Martin, I. C. (1992). Improvement in morbidity of mouth cancer using microvascular free flap reconstruction. *Journal of Cranio-Maxillo-Facial Surgery, 20*(3), 132–134.

Appendix

Legacy Portland Hospitals
Emanuel Hospital & Health Center
Good Samaritan Hospital & Medical Center
Legacy Infusion Services
Legacy Visiting Nurse Association

P A T I E N T   T E A C H I N G   S H E E T

TUBE FEEDING: SYRINGE METHOD

1. Maintain a position of 30˚ or more during the feeding.

2. Wash hands and gather supplies. Determine syringe type, catheter or Luer Lock tip.

3. Prepare liquid formula:

    a. Check expiration date on label or can.

    b. Shake the can or bottle well.

    c. Wipe the top of the container with a clean cloth before opening it.

    d. If you do not use all of the formula cover the opened can and store it in the refrigerator.

    e. Write the date and time on the opened container. **If the formula is not used in 24 hours, throw it away.**

4. Prepare powdered formula according to directions.

5. Check tube placement – See "How to Check Nasogastric/Gastric Tube for Proper Placement.

6. Check residuals – See "Checking for Residuals" under Enteral Instructions.

7. Remove the plunger from the syringe, rinse syringe with tap water then attach the syringe to the feeding tube.

8. While holding the syringe upright, pour the formula into the syringe. Allow it to run in slowly by gravity. Add more formula before the syringe empties to keep air from entering the stomach and causing bloating or gas.

9. By raising the syringe the formula will go in more quickly and by lowering it the formula will run in more slowly. The feeding should last 10–30 minutes.

10. After all the formula has been given, flush feeding tube with luke warm water or as directed by physician.

11. Remove the syringe and cap the feeding tube.

12. Wash the syringe in hot soapy water. Rinse thoroughly in warm water then allow to air dry. Store your equipment in a clean area.

Figure A1. Patient teaching sheet.

Legacy Portland Hospitals

PHYSICIAN'S ORDERS

Date & Time	ORDERS: ANOTHER BRAND OF GENERICALLY EQUIVALENT OR APPROVED THERAPEUTICALLY EQUIVALENT PRODUCT MAY BE ADMINISTERED UNLESS CHECKED	🕐

HEAD AND NECK with FREE FLAP

PRE-ADMISSION

1. Consent to be signed for:_____
2. Notify WWICU of planned admission.
3. Notify Cancer Rehab of planned admission.
4. Speech therapy consult for communication options.
5. Nutrition consult.
6. LABS: Pre-albumin; CBC; Acute chem profile; room air ABG. **Do not draw blood from arm to be used for graft donor.**
7. ECG if > 3 months or if abnormal; CXR if > 3 months or if abnormal
8. Instruct: NPO after midnight the night before surgery
9. Notify MD of any abnormal labs
10. PEG scheduled for_____.
11. **No blood draw or IV in donor arm.**
12. Other:

DAY OF ADMIT/PRE-OP

1. Activity as tolerated
2. NPO
3. Start IV with 18-20 guage cath with macro drip line with extension - no heparin lock. **Do not start IV in donor arm.**
4. **No blood draw or IV in donor arm.**
5. IV solution: Plasmalyte A 1000cc @ TKO
6. Ancef® 1.0 gm IV and Flagyl® 500mg IV, on call to OR.
   Alternative: Clindamycin phosphate (Cleocin®) 900 mg IV, on call to OR.
7. Type & cross ___ units ___PRBCs ___Autologous ___Designated donor
8. Other pre-op meds per Anesthesia.
9. Pneumatic sequential compression stockings.
10. Chlorhexidine gluconate (Peridex®), 20 ml oral rinse, hold 1 min. and expectorate. Repeat.
11. Notify MD if:_____

    _____

12. Other:

MD Signature_____

Order # (needs order number)   (3/95)

Figure A2. Physician's order for preadmission and day of admittance for head and neck with free flap.

Legacy Portland Hospitals

PHYSICIAN'S ORDERS

Date & Time	ORDERS: ANOTHER BRAND OF GENERICALLY EQUIVALENT OR APPROVED THERAPEUTICALLY EQUIVALENT PRODUCT MAY BE ADMINISTERED UNLESS CHECKED	🕐

POST-OPERATIVE HEAD AND NECK with FREE FLAP

1. Admit to ICU.
2. On arrival: Critical Care Panel 1, CXR
3. **LABS:** Hct @ _____ and then daily (call if <25)
   ABG for O_2 sats <93%;   Acute Chem Profile in a.m., daily.

4. Vital signs q 15" until stable, then per critical care routine
5. Doppler neck surface/flap and check color q 1 H. Call Resident **STAT** if color changes or pulse is lost.
6. Room temp 75-80° at all times
7. CVP readings q 6 H; continuous O_2 sats; I & O.
8. Call service if SBP >160, <90; DBP >100; T >38⁵; P >120, <60; R >30, <10; UO <50cc/H.
9. **Ventilator settings:** FiO₂ [_____], Vt [_____], Rate [_____], Mode VC or SIMV, PS [_____], PEEP [_____]. Adjust FiO₂ to keep sats >95%.
10. Respiratory therapy consult.
11. JPs to: ☐   100 cm H_2O wall suction   ☐   bulb suction
12. Routine trach care; **no trach ties or ties around neck.** Suction q 4 H and PRN.
13. Pneumatic pressure stockings.
14. Foley catheter. Notify service if UO <50cc/H
15. PEG to gravity until _____ , then clamp.
16. Keep tongue moist with saline if exposed.
17. **Medications:**
    a. Morphine sulfate 2-8 mg. IV, q 1 H, PRN.
       *If allergic to MS:*_____
    b. Midazolam (Versed®), 1-2 mg, IV q 1 H PRN agitation until _____. Hold for oversedation.
    c. Ancef® 1.0 gm IV and Flagyl®, q 8 H X 5 days.
       Alternative: Clindamycin phosphate (Cleocin®) 900 mg IV q 8 H x 5 days
    d. Cimetidine (Tagamet®), 300 mg, IV, q 6 H
    e. Droperidol (Inapsine®), .25 ml, IV, q 6 H, PRN N/V
    f. Chlorhexidine gluconate (Peridex®), 20 ml swish and espectorate BID (BID or via toothette, hold in mouth 1 minute)
    g. ASA 325 mg. rectal suppository daily. May give via PEG when tube feedings started.
    h. K+_____
    i. _____
    j. _____
18. **Activity:** Bedrest. HOB ↑ 30°. **Do not hyperextend neck or turn to extremes.**
19. NPO. Nutrition consult.
20. IV fluids: 1000 cc D 5 1/2 NS with 20 KCl @ _____cc/H. Follow with:_____

21. Keep donor arm/leg elevated.
22. Wound care BID: clean with 1/2 strength H_2O_2; antibiotic ointment. Begin post-op day 1.
23. Modified #5 Jackson metal trach tube with plug to bedside.

Resident/Fellow Signature_____ Beeper# _____

Order # (needs order number)   (3/95)

Figure A3. Physician's order for postoperative head and neck with free flap.

Legacy Portland Hospitals

PHYSICIAN'S ORDERS

Date & Time	ORDERS: ANOTHER BRAND OF GENERICALLY EQUIVALENT OR APPROVED THERAPEUTICALLY EQUIVALENT PRODUCT MAY BE ADMINISTERED UNLESS CHECKED	🕐

TRANSFER ORDERS POST-OPERATIVE HEAD AND NECK with FREE FLAP

1. Transfer to Unit 15.
2. VS routine, I&O, foley catheter. Suction at bedside.
3. Doppler neck surface/flap and check color q 1 H until post-op day 5, then routine with VS. Call resident STAT if color changes or pulse is lost.
4. Room temp 75-80°F at all times.
5. Call service if SBP >160, <90; DBP >100; T >38⁵; P >120, <60; R >30, <10; UO <50cc/H.
6. 40% O_2 per trach mask.
7. JPs to bulb suction.
8. Routine trach care, **no trach ties or ties around neck.** Bag and suction prn.
9. Pneumatic pressure stockings until patient ambulating.
10. **LABS:**   Post-Op Day 3: Hct, Acute Chem Profile
    Post-Op day 4: CBC, Pre-albumin
    Post-Op day 7: CBC, Acute Chem Profile, Pre-albumin

11. Clean PEG site daily. Refer to enteral feeding orders for formula and rate.
12. NPO, keep tongue moist with water or saline if exposed.
13. **Medications:**
    a. ☐ Lortab elixir _____ml. per FT q 3-4 H prn pain
       ☐ Potter's pain cocktail _____ml per FT q 3-4 H prn pain
    b. Morphine sulfate 2-6 mg. IV, q 2 H, PRN breakthrough pain
       If allergic to MS:
    c. Ancef® 1.0 gm IV and Flagyl 500 mg IV q 8 H. DC after last dose post-op day 4.
       If allergic to penicillin: Clindamycin phosphate (Cleocin®) 900 mg IV q 8 H. DC after last dose post-op day 4.
    d. Cimetidine (Tagamet®), 5 ml of 300 mg/5ml liquid per FT q 6 H
    e. Chlorhexidine gluconate labeled for home use (Peridex®), 20 ml swish, hold in mouth 1 minute and expectorate BID (or BID via toothette, hold in mouth 1 minute)
    f. ASA 325 mg. daily per PEG.
    g. K + per PEG tube _____
    h. _____
    i. _____
14. D 5 1/2 NS with 20 KCl @ ____ ml/H, or _____ @ ____ ml/H.
    ↓ IVF rate as tube feeding rate increases, to maintain total fluid intake of _____ml/H.
15. **Therapy:**
    ☐ Speech Therapy eval.
    ☐ Physical Therapy eval.
    ☐ Occupational Therapy eval.
16. **Activity:** HOB ↑ 30°. **Do not hyperextend neck or turn to extremes.** Up in chair @ least TID. Begin progressive ambulation in a.m.
17. Keep donor arm/leg elevated.
18. Wound care BID: clean with 1/2 strength H2O2; apply antibiotic ointment.
19. VNA follow-up for home care needs.

Resident/Fellow Signature_____ Beeper# _____

Order # (needs order number)   (3/95)

Figure A4. Physician's transfer orders for postoperative head and neck with free flap.

Legacy Portland Hospitals
Portland, Oregon
LEGACY Health System

VARIANCE TRACKING TOOL

A Quality Improvement tool for identifying significant variances
505-2005 (3/95)

Dx/Surg/Proc: **HEAD and NECK with FREE FLAP**   Target LOS: **6 days**

Write variances as they occur and place initials in the adjacent column. Comment on actions taken. Record actions taken in the medical record.

	Day: POST-OP Date:	Day: POD 1 Date:	Day: POD 2 Date:	Day: POD 3 Date:
	No significant variances.	No significant variances.	No significant variances.	No significant variances.
PATIENT/FAMILY	Unable to obtain doppler pulse in flap	Unable to obtain doppler pulse in flap	Unable to obtain doppler pulse in flap	Unable to obtain doppler pulse in flap
	VS outside of stated parameters	VS outside of stated parameters	VS outside of stated parameters	VS outside of stated parameters
	O₂ sats <92% with prescribed O₂	Unable to wean from vent	Unable to wean from vent	Requires >2 doses IV MS for breakthrough pain
SIGNIFICANT	VS/activity indicate pain not well controlled	VS/activity indicate pain not well controlled	VS/activity indicate pain not well controlled	Tube feeding residual q8H >50 ml
	Altered orientation, thought process	Altered orientation, thought process	Not transferred to surgical unit	Does not ambulate in hall TID with assist
	Does not tolerate up in chair	Does not tolerate up in chair	Does not tolerate up in chair	
VARIANCES				
CLINICIAN				
SYSTEM				

Remove tracking tool from medical record at discharge and place in designated UBQI file.   DC date: _____   LOS: _____

blue/varitool.15

Figure A5. Variance tracking tool for head and neck with free flap for postoperative days 1–3.

VARIANCE TRACKING TOOL
A Quality Improvement tool for identifying significant variances
505-2005 (3/95)

Legacy Portland Hospitals
Portland, Oregon

LEGACY
Health Systems

Dx/Surg/Proc: **HEAD and NECK with FREE FLAP**   Target LOS: **6 days**

Write variances as they occur and place initials in the adjacent column. Comment on actions taken. Record actions taken in the medical record.

blue/varitool.15

	Day: POD 4 Date:	Day: POD 5 Date:	Day: POD 6 Date:	Day: POD 7 Date:
	No significant variances.	No significant variances.	No significant variances.	No significant variances.
PATIENT/FAMILY ANY VARIANCES CLINICIANS SYSTEM	Unable to obtain doppler pulse in flap	Unable to obtain doppler pulse in flap	Neck wound edges not approximated/ drainage present	
	Vital signs outside of stated parameters	Vital signs outside of stated parameters	Does not administer tube feedings independently	
	Requires >2 doses IV MS for breakthrough pain	Does not tolerate plugging of trach during sleep; shows sign/symptoms of respiratory distress	Does not identify awareness of support groups and options for obtaining needed support after discharge	
	Does not tolerate plugging of trach during sleep; shows sign/symptoms of respiratory distress	Does not ambulate independently with assist device (if fibula graft)	Does not verbalize plan for self-care after discharge	
	Does not ambulate/bear weight on operative leg	Does not administer tube feedings with assistance		
	Does not report understanding of tube feeding teaching sheets	Unable to state follow-up plan for care after discharge		

Remove tracking tool from medical record at discharge and place in designated UBQI file.

DC date:_____   LOS:_____

Figure A6. Variance tracking tool for head and neck with free flap for postoperative days 4–7.

Index

A

Accountability, Center for Case Management (CCMA), 104–105
Activity-based costing
  aggregate activities, 156
  case types, analysis of, 154–155
  cost drivers, for cost flow analysis, 156, 160, 162, 163
  cross-functional steering committee, 154
  DRG categories, 155, 166
  graphic example of, 161
  health care delivery profile, 155–156
  need for, 153–154
  numerical example of, 162–167
  training in, 160
  variance analysis report, 160, 162, 164
Acute care
  tools for, 30
  triggers for geriatric care, 119
Age
  acute care triggers, 119
  and case management services, 43
  and length of stay, 79
  and pricing, 175
AIDS. *See* HIV disease management
Alliant Health System, 131
Allied Services Act, 4
Alternative health care, home care, 186
Ambulatory care, tools for, 30
Arizona Health Sciences Center, managed care example, 16–18
Autonomy, definition of, 70

B

Back injuries. *See* Spinal cord injury; Spinal protocol
Beneficence, as ethical principle, 70
Benefit investigation, 169
Benefit substitution, 186
Brain injury. *See* Mild traumatic brain injury; Neurobehavioral case management
Broker model of case management, 3, 5

C

Candler County Hospital, nurse case management, 75–80
Capitation, meaning of, 181
Captive group, of group model HMO, 181
Cardiac procedures. *See* Interventional cardiology
Cardinal Hill Rehabilitation Hospital, program-management model, 213–218
Caregiver/clinician variance, 128–129
Care management, elements of, 86
CareMaps, quality improvement, 108
Case finding, 23
Case identification, 32–38, 43–44
  and age of patient, 43
  decision flowchart, 35
  demographic/social criteria, 32
  follow-up goals, 36
  goals for patient/family, 36
  high-risk group identification, 34
  questionnaire, 33

screening, meaning of, 43
utilization-based criteria, 32
Case management
conceptual framework, 5
definitions of, 28, 39, 233
goals of, 18, 28, 39–40, 51
historical view, 4, 18
process, stages in, 51
productivity factors, 32
Case management models, 4–5, 29
broker model, 3, 5
dominator model, 23
for Friendly Hills Healthcare Network, 29–38
for Health Plan of Nevada, 57–69
for Johns Hopkins Hospital, 53–56
partnership model, 23
systems of care model, 121–127
Case management program
case identification, 43–44
data availability, 42
financial benefits, 43, 45
guiding principles, 53–54
levels of intensity, 63
organizational assessment for, 40–43
outcome measures, 44–45
provider relationships, 40–41
staffing, 41–42
team in, 25, 54–55
timeline in development of, 61
training, 41–42
weakpoints in, 45–46
Case Management Society of America
(CMSA), 44
ethical principles, 70–72
practice standards, 104
Case management team
benefits of, 63–64
case review by, 25
functions, 55
meetings, 55, 64, 67
philosophy, statement of, 61
triad team, 54–55
Case manager
evaluation of, 103
functions of, 55, 168–169
practice standards, 104

skills required for, 56
traditional role of, 103–104
training, 56
Casetype, information about, 297–298
Causal modeling, 193–201
benefits of, 194, 197
and causality, 194
classic text on, 194
confirmatory factor analysis, 200
construct validity, 196
convergent validity, 196
discriminant validity, 196
exploratory model, 194–195
functions of, 193–194
goodness of fit, 200–201
Internet site for, 196
latent variables, 195, 200
matrix algebra, 196
measurement model, 196–197
model development, 194
modification indices, 201
results of, 199–200
SIMPLIS language, 196, 197–199
structural equation, 196, 197
syntax, 197–198
testing model, 197
Center for Case Management Accountability
(CCMA), 104–105
Clinical Information Network database, 227
Clinical nurse specialists (CNSs), 15–26
community case management, 20–26
expanded role of, 19–20
role functions, 19
work environment of, 15–16
Clinical pathways
elements of, 286, 298
for interventional cardiology, 286–295
postprocedure evaluation, 300–301
Clinical trax guidelines, 45
Community case management, 20–26
case example, 24
case finding, 23
case review, 25
dominator model, 23
levels of care, 22
limitations of, 82

partnership in, 20, 23
partnership model, 23
risk determination, 24–25
roles and communication in, 21
wellness perspective, 25
Community variance, 129
Competency indicators, quality improvement, 107
Complex case management
client problems, 66
elements of, 65
frequency/type of contact, 65–66
referral sources, 67
types of interventions, 66
Comprehensive case management
complexity of, 203–204
conceptual theory in, 204
factors affecting case managers, study, 204–211
and Medicaid reimbursement, 204
needs for, 210–211
opinion of case managers about, 209
problems/solutions related to, 207–209
Computerized case management
benefits of, 149
department-specific criteria, 148
diagnosis criteria, 147–148
interdepartmental process flow, 148
and referral criteria, 144, 146
skilled nursing facility criteria, 148
software development, 145–146
system requirements, 143–144
triage function, 146–147
Computers, variance data collection, 130–131
Concurrent review, 50
Consolidation, meaning of, 48–49
Construct validity, causal modeling, 196
Continuous quality improvement (CQI), 78, 107
case management plans, use of, 78
and variance management, 133
Continuum of care, 22, 29–31, 180, 182
Convergent validity, causal modeling, 196
Coordination of care, 67
Costs
benefit investigation, 169
benefits of case management, 43, 45

hard cost savings, 168–169
and integrated health management, 116
savings, examples of, 168
savings and managed care, 48, 50
soft cost savings, 169
and utilization management, 49, 50
See also Activity-based costing; Pricing
Critical pathways
development of, 77, 79
family/patient involvement, 132–133
functions of, 233
steering committee, role of, 134
Custodial setting, case management, 65

D

Databases, for pricing, 177
Deductive thinking, 214–215
Diagnosis-related groups (DRGs), 16, 19, 33
and activity-based costing, 155, 166
critical pathways developed from, 77, 79
Dilution, negative aspects of, 45–46
Direct contact model, of HMOs, 181
Discharge planning, 50
Discriminant validity, causal modeling, 196
Disease management programs, 171–172
compared with case management, 171–172
features of, 172
types of diseases, 171
Divergent thinking, 215
Dominator model, community case management, 23

E

Emergency department (ED)
case management in, 51
prospective review, 49–50
Empowerment of patient
meaning of, 99
and social support, 100
and telephonic case management, 98–100
Ethical principles, 70–72
beneficence, 70
justice, 71–72
nonmaleficence, 70

patient autonomy, 70
veracity, 72

F

Fee-for-service, meaning of, 181
First Databank company, 177
Fletcher Allen Health Care, 128, 131, 132
    variance management, 133–140
Friendly Hills Healthcare Network, case
    management model, 29–38

G

Geriatric Care Coordination Program, 118
Goodness of fit, causal modeling, 200–201
Group model, of HMO, 181

H

Harris Methodist Health System, integrated
    health management, 83–89
Health, definition of, 254
Health care delivery, continuum for, 22, 29–31,
    180, 182
Health Care Management Guidelines, 177
Health care system
    environmental changes related to, 15–16
        vertical integration of, 16, 17
Health Insurance Association of America
    (HIAA), 177
Health maintenance organizations (HMOs),
    181
    direct contact model, 181
    group model, 181
    independent physician association (IPA), 181
    network model, 181
    staff model, 181
Health Plan of Nevada, health management
    program, 57–69
Health promotion
    definition of, 254
    and telephonic case management, 98
Healthy Birth Act, 4
Henry Street Settlement House, 4
High-risk group
    complex case management, 65
    identification of, 34
    meaning of, 183

HIV disease management
    acute care, 267–268
    advanced state, 265
    antiretroviral therapies, 266
    beginning of care, 266
    care plan, 264–265
    continuum of care, 263, 264
    education/counseling, 268
    home care, 268–269
    hospice, 268–269
    linkage management, 269–270
    opportunistic infections, 266–267
    patient referral, 264
    staging tool, 270, 271–272
Home care, 184–192
    alternative health care, example of, 186
    continuum of services, 186
    cost–benefit analysis, 186
    elements of, 59–60
    funding/reimbursement for, 189–192
    HIV patients, 268–269
    managed care goal for, 185–186
    Medicare model, 184, 186
    surgical recovery, 188–189
    tools for, 31
    visiting physician program, 187–188
Hospice
    elements of care, 187
    funding/reimbursement for, 190
    HIV patients, 269
    tools for, 31
Hospital/system variance, 129
Hull House, 4

I

Independent group, of group model HMO, 181
Independent physician association (IPA),
    nature of, 181
Inductive thinking, 215
Inpatient cost, pricing of, 175
Integrated care
    definition of, 115–116
    model of, 183–184
Integrated health management
    cardiovascular health, example plan, 90–94
    care management, 86
    case management, 86–87
    components of, 83

cost factors, 116
goal of, 83
levels of, 84
management structure, 88
models of, 118
patient responsibilities, 119
physician/hospital partnership, 88–89
population needs assessment, 84–85
prevention, 116
primary care, 117–118
risk identification, 116–117
risk stratification, 118–119
strategic health plan, 85–86
wellness/prevention, 86
Integrated partnerships, elements of, 49
Interventional cardiology
cardiac health care notebook, 292–293
clinical pathway for, 286–295
community care manager, role of, 294–295
increase in use of procedures, 285
nurse care manager, role of, 293–294
Omaha System Problem Classification
Scheme (OSPCS), 287–291
patient education, 292
types of procedures, 284

J

Johns Hopkins Hospital, 131
case management initiative, 53–56
Justice, as ethical principle, 71–72

L

Latent variables
causal modeling, 195, 200
endogenous type, 195
exogenous type, 195
Layering, negative aspects of, 45
Length of stay, analysis of, 79–80
Long-term care
need for, 31
tools for, 31

M

Managed care
Arizona Health Sciences Center example,
16–18

capitation, 181
and case management, 18, 20
case management, 50–52
consolidation, meaning of, 48–49
cost management by, 48, 50
definition of, 16–17
fee-for-service, 181
growth/efficiency concept, 48
growth of, 47–48
health maintenance organizations (HMOs),
181
and hospital changes, 48
integrated partnerships, 49
preferred provider organizations (PPOs), 181
utilization management, 49–50
Managed care organizations (MCOs), 48
Manuals, policies/procedures, 44
Medical supplies, pricing of, 176
Medicare Nursing Practice and Patient Care
Improvement Act, 4
Medicare Risk program, 18
Medicare Standard Analytical Files, 177
Metropolitan Life Insurance Company, 4
Mild traumatic brain injury
cognitive assessment, 240–242
definition of, 238–239
evaluation protocol, purpose of, 239
follow-up referral, 244
high-risk factors assessment, 242
medical assessment, 238, 239–240
patient education, 238, 242–243
Postconcussion Symptom Inventory, 243
posttrauma symptoms, 237–238
written instructions for patients, 240
Modification indices, causal modeling, 201

N

Narrowing, negative aspects of, 46
Network model, of HMO, 181
Neurobehavioral case management
elements of, 248
rehabilitation program, issues related to, 249
return to work, plan for, 250–253
New England model, nurse case management,
75–76
Nonacute care, pricing of, 175–176
Nonmaleficence, as ethical principle, 70
Nurse, clinical nurse specialists (CNSs), 15–26

Nurse case manager
  activities of, 9
  in broker model, 3, 5
  for Candler County Hospital, 75–80
  educational background, 10
  functions of, 55, 78–79
  learning background of, 9–10
  New England model, 75–76
  physician support, 77
  roles of, 11, 51
  survey of, 5–11
  telephonic case management, 97–101
  variance data collection, 132
Nursing
  domains of nursing practice, 97
  and program-management model, 217–218

O

Omaha System Problem Classification Scheme (OSPCS), 287–291
Omnibus Budget Reconciliation Act, 4
On-site case management, 64, 68
Outcome measures, 44–45, 51–52
  areas for, 45
  importance of, 44–45
Out-of-area case management, 64
Outpatient cost, pricing of, 175

P

PacifiCare, computerized case management, 142–149
Partnership model
  community case management, 23
  integrated partnerships, 49
Path analysis, 193
Patient education
  HIV patients, 268
  interventional cardiology, 292
  mild traumatic brain injury, 238, 242–243
  patient teaching sheet (tube feeding), 302
  spinal cord injury patient, 255
Patient/family variance, 128, 129
Patient responsibilities, integrated health management, 119
Personal Health and Social History (PHSH), 58

Pharmacy
  case management, 189
  drug pricing, 176
Physician cost
  home care physicians, 190
  pricing of, 175
Physician's orders, example of, 303–305
Population, needs assessment, 84–85
Population-based case management, integrated health management, 83–89
Practice agreements
  and clinical path, 300
  content of, 299
  development of, 298–299
Preferred provider organizations (PPOs), nature of, 181
Preterm birth
  prevention guidelines, 100–101
  telephonic case management, 96–101
Prevailing Health Care Charges System (PHCS), 177
Prevention, 29–30
  activities, 30
  barriers to, 116
  integrated health management, 116
  primary prevention, 101
  secondary prevention, 101
  tertiary prevention, 171
  tools for, 30
Pricing
  age–sex factors calculation, 175
  alternative normative data, 177
  area factors calculation, 175
  baseline rate calculation, 173
  cost components calculation, 174–175
  cost rate calculation, 176
  databases used, 177
  data for capitation rates, 175–176
  data subsetted diagnosis, 173–174
  difficulties related to, 173
  and encounter data, 175–176
  home care, 189–192
  membership data analysis, 174
  PMPM cancer example, 178–179
  risk/stop loss issues, 179
  total program cost, 176
  See also Costs

Primary care, 117–118
  definition of, 117
  level in continuum of care model, 22
Primary care physician, role of, 170–171
Primary prevention, goal of, 101, 116, 171
Problem-based learning
  benefits of, 274
  case example, 279–280
  clinical reasoning process, 277–278
  compared with classroom learning, 281–282
  learning outcomes, 280–281
  limitations of, 283
  practice setting, 275
  practicum learning model, 275–277
  student objectives, 274–275
Program of All-Inclusive Care of the Elderly (PACE), 116
Program for Healthcare Innovations, 220–222
Program-management model, 213–218
  discipline-management model, 214
  issues related to, 215–216
  and medication errors, 217
  organizational chart, 214
  and organizational flexibility, 214–215
  patient outcomes, 216
  size of nursing staff and patient falls, 216–218
  substitute for nursing director, 217–218
Prospective review, 49–50

Q

Quality council, 124–125
Quality improvement
  CareMaps, 108
  competency indicators, 107
  continuous quality improvement, 107
  implementation of, 112, 114
  maintenance indicators, 106–107
  quality projects, 109–110
  rate-based indicators, 107–108
  research, use of, 110
  sentinel events, 110, 112
  structural indicators, 107
  and variance tracking, 108–109, 133
Quality improvement teams, 222–223
Quality Management Services department, 219–229
  clinical evaluation unit, 225–226
  cost/stay reduction efforts, 222
  mission of, 219
  outcomes from, 227–229
  physician feedback, 220, 227
  Program for Healthcare Innovations, 220–222
  quality improvement teams, 222–223
  utilization review initiatives, 220
Quality planning team, functions of, 122
Quarternary level, in continuum of care model, 22

R

Rate-based indicators, quality improvement, 107–108
Regression analysis, 193
Rehabilitative care, elements of, 60
Resource-based relative value scale (RBRVS), 177
Retrospective chart review, variance data collection, 130
Retrospective review, 50
  benefits of, 50
Risk determination, 24–25, 116–117
  elements of, 24–25, 117
  issues/questions related to, 117
  Personal Health and Social History (PHSH), 58
  risk stratification, levels of, 118–119
Risk issue, pricing, 179
Robert Packer Hospital, trauma case management, 233–236
Robert Wood Johnson Hospital, 131
Role theory, 5

S

Secondary care level, in continuum of care model, 22
Secondary prevention, goal of, 101, 116, 171
Sentinel events, quality improvement, 110, 112
SIMPLIS language, causal modeling, 196, 197–199
Social health maintenance organization (SHMO), 116

Social support, and empowerment of patient, 100
Social worker, functions of, 55
Socioeconomic status, and length of stay, 79–80
Specialty case management, 31–38
    activities, 32
    case identification, 32–38
    goals of, 31–32
Spinal cord injury
    information source on, 256
    levels of intervention, 256
    patient education, topics for, 255
    physical fitness activities, 255–256
Spinal protocol
    case manager, role of, 260
    effects of implementation of, 260–262
    medication, 258
    physical therapy protocol, 260
    physician procedures, 259
    spinal protocol steps, 259
Staffing, case management program, 41–42
Staff model, of HMO, 181
Statistical techniques
    causal modeling, 193–201
    path analysis, 193
    regression analysis, 193
Stop loss
    aggregate, 179
    and pricing, 179
Structural indicators, quality improvement, 107
Subacute care, 64–65
    services for, 60
Substituted benefits, 190
Surgery, home recovery, 188–189
Surveys, of nurse case manager, 5–11
Symbolic interactionism, 5
System of care model, 121–127
    assessment of health care effectiveness, 124
    care management, 124
    clinical aims, 124, 125
    continuum of care, 122, 123
    patient management, 123–124
    quality council, 124–125
    quality planning team, 122
    value chain model, 125–126

T

Teams
    case management team, 63–64
    quality improvement teams, 222–223
    Quality Management Services department, 223–224
    Systems Improvement teams, 224–225, 226
    See also Case management team
Telephonic case management
    and health promotion, 98
    nurse functions in, 97–98
    and patient compliance, 96
    and patient empowerment, 98–100
    preterm birth, 96–101
    settings for, 96
Tertiary care
    in continuum of care model, 22
    examples of, 31
    patient goals, 36
    tools for, 31
Tertiary prevention, goal of, 116, 171
Training
    in activity-based costing, 160
    case management program, 41–42
    case manager, 56
Trauma case management, 233–236
    critical pathways, 233–234
    patient management difficulties, 233
    postdischarge, 234
Triage, computerized, 146–147

U

University of Iowa Hospitals and Clinics, quality improvement, 106–114
University of Massachusetts Medical Center, Quality Management Services department, 219–229
Utilization management
    concurrent review, 50
    and costs, 49, 50
    by nurse, 54, 55
    prospective review, 49–50
    retrospective review, 50
    and variance tracking, 136
Utilization review nurse, 20

V

Value chain model, 125–126
  benefits of, 125
  value chain for clinical aim, 126
Variances
  in activity-based costing, 160, 162, 164
  and case management, 132–133
  categories of, 128–129
  classification schemes, 128–130
  computerized pathway approach, 130–131
  and continuous quality improvement (CQI),
    133
  definition of, 128
  documentation of, 130, 134, 136
  Fletcher Allen Health Care example, 133–140
  management of, 136–140
  and quality improvement, 108–109
  and utilization management, 136
  variance analysis, 131–132
  variance data, collection of, 130–131, 136
  variance tracking tool, 306–307
Veracity, as ethical principle, 72
Vertical integration, health care management,
    16, 17
Volunteers
  for care of seniors, 58–59
  positions held, 59

W

Wellness
  definition of, 254
  health-related activities, 25
Wellness level, in continuum of care model, 22
Work, brain-injured return to, 250–253